Strategies for Student Success on the

NEXT GENERATION NCLEX® (NGN)
TEST ITEMS

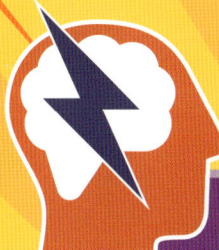

2ND EDITION

Strategies for Student Success on the

NEXT GENERATION NCLEX® (NGN) TEST ITEMS

Linda Anne Silvestri PhD, RN, FAAN, ANEF
Nursing Instructor
University of Nevada, Las Vegas
Las Vegas, Nevada;
President, Nursing Reviews, Inc., and Professional Nursing Seminars, Inc.
Owner, Silvestri's NurseForward, LLC
Henderson, Nevada;
Next Generation NCLEX® (NGN) Consultant, Thought Leader, and Subject Matter Expert
Elsevier Inc.

Angela Elizabeth Silvestri PhD, APRN, FNP-BC, CNE
Associate Professor and Associate Dean for Entry and Prelicensure Education
University of Nevada, Las Vegas
Las Vegas, Nevada;
President, Nurse Prep, LLC
Owner, Silvestri's NurseForward, LLC
Henderson, Nevada;
Next Generation NCLEX® (NGN) Consultant and Subject Matter Expert
Elsevier Inc.

Donna D. Ignatavicius MS, RN, CNE, CNEcl, ANEF, FAADN
Speaker and Curriculum Consultant for Academic Nursing Programs
Founder, Boot Camp for Nurse Educators
President, DI Associates, Inc.
Littleton, Colorado;
Next Generation NCLEX® (NGN) Consultant, Thought Leader, and Subject Matter Expert
Elsevier Inc.

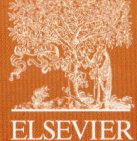

Elsevier
3251 Riverport Lane
St. Louis, Missouri 63043

STRATEGIES FOR STUDENT SUCCESS ON
THE NEXT GENERATION NCLEX® (NGN) TEST ITEMS, SECOND EDITION   ISBN: 978-0-443-24602-9

Copyright © 2026 by Elsevier Inc. All rights are reserved, including those for text and data mining, AI training, and similar technologies.

For accessibility purposes, images in electronic versions of this book are accompanied by alt-text descriptions provided by Elsevier. For more information, see https://www.elsevier.com/about/accessibility.

Publisher's note: Elsevier takes a neutral position with respect to territorial disputes or jurisdictional claims in its published content, including in maps and institutional affiliations.

No part of this publication may be reproduced or transmitted in any form or by any means, electronic or mechanical, including photocopying, recording, or any information storage and retrieval system, without permission in writing from the publisher. Details on how to seek permission, further information about the Publisher's permissions policies and our arrangements with organizations such as the Copyright Clearance Center and the Copyright Licensing Agency, can be found at our website: www.elsevier.com/permissions.

This book and the individual contributions contained in it are protected under copyright by the Publisher (other than as may be noted herein).

Notice

Practitioners and researchers must always rely on their own experience and knowledge in evaluating and using any information, methods, compounds or experiments described herein. Because of rapid advances in the medical sciences, in particular, independent verification of diagnoses and drug dosages should be made. To the fullest extent of the law, no responsibility is assumed by Elsevier, authors, editors or contributors for any injury and/or damage to persons or property as a matter of products liability, negligence or otherwise, or from any use or operation of any methods, products, instructions, or ideas contained in the material herein.

Previous edition copyrighted 2023.

Associate Content Strategist: Grace Onderlinde
Content Development Manager: Danielle Frazier
Senior Content Development Specialist: Rae Robertson
Publishing Services Manager: Catherine Jackson
Senior Project Manager: Jodi Willard
Design Direction: Amy Buxton

Typeset by GW Tech

Printed in India

Last digit is the print number: 9 8 7 6 5 4 3 2 1

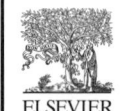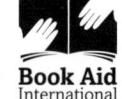

In loving memory of my parents and Angela's grandparents, Arnold Lawrence and Frances Mary, who opened my door of opportunity to this amazing profession of nursing. My memories of their love, support, and words of encouragement will remain in my heart forever!

And, to my husband, Larry, for being my rock of support through all of my life's journeys. And finally, to all nursing students, you have chosen to be a part of an incredible profession, and the rewards will be never-ending as you touch the lives of so many on your journey.

Linda Anne Silvestri

To my husband, Brent, who has supported my work since the day we met. I will always remember how he anticipated what I would need to be successful in this journey.

To nursing students, you have chosen a wonderful profession that will give back to you what you are putting in now. You can do this!

Angela Elizabeth Silvestri

To my husband, Charles, who continues to encourage me in all of my professional endeavors; and to my entire family, who has supported my work as an author and consultant for many decades.

To nursing students, who have chosen the caring profession that can change the lives of so many; and to nurse educators, whose passion and role modeling continues to shape the future of the nursing profession.

Donna D. Ignatavicius

About the Authors

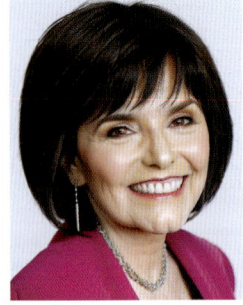

Linda Anne Silvestri, PhD, RN, FAAN, ANEF

Linda is a well-known nurse educator, entrepreneur, and philanthropist whose professional aspirations focus on assisting nursing students to become successful. She has been teaching nursing students at all levels of nursing education for many years. Dr. Silvestri is currently a nursing instructor at the University of Nevada, Las Vegas (UNLV). She earned her PhD in Nursing from UNLV and conducted research on self-efficacy and the predictors of NCLEX® success. Her research findings are published in the *Journal of Nursing Education and Practice*. Dr. Silvestri has received several awards and honors. In 2019 she was inducted as a Fellow into the very prestigious American Academy of Nursing and in 2023 was inducted as a Fellow into the very esteemed Academy of Nursing Education for her national and international contributions to nursing education. In 2012 she received the UNLV School of Nursing Alumna of the Year Award. In 2010 she received the School of Nursing Certificate of Recognition for the Outstanding PhD Student. Dr. Silvestri is a member of several national nursing organizations, some of which include the Honor Society of Nursing, Sigma Theta Tau International, the National League for Nursing, the American Nurses Association, and the American Academy of Nursing. Dr. Silvestri is a successful Elsevier author of numerous best-selling NCLEX® preparation resources on national and international levels. She also served as an Elsevier Consultant and Subject Matter Expert for the Next Generation NCLEX® (NGN) and has presented numerous webinars to both faculty and students on NCLEX® preparation and success. Dr. Silvestri is the President and Owner of Nursing Reviews, Inc. and Professional Nursing Seminars, Inc. Both companies are dedicated to helping nursing graduates achieve their goals of becoming licensed nurses. Partnered with Angela Silvestri, Linda is the co-owner of Silvestri's NurseForward LLC, a company committed to globally assisting students and graduates with testing success and preparing for professional nursing practice.

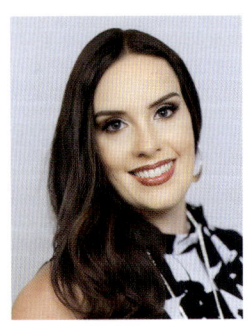

Angela Elizabeth Silvestri, PhD, APRN, FNP-BC, CNE

Angela Silvestri is a well-known nurse educator, researcher, and author. She has been teaching and working in university administrative roles for the past 10 years at all levels of nursing education. She has experience teaching across the program and in both classroom and clinical settings and working with graduate students on their culminating projects and research dissertations. She is currently serving in a leadership role as the Associate Dean for Entry and Prelicensure Education at the University of Nevada, Las Vegas (UNLV). Angela earned a bachelor's in Nursing and a bachelor's in Sociology from Salve Regina University in Newport, Rhode Island, and a master's and PhD in nursing education from UNLV. She also has a post-master's graduate certificate in advanced practice and is a board-certified family nurse practitioner. She is a Scholar in Sigma Theta Tau's New Academic Leadership Academy and the American Association of Colleges of Nursing Elevating Leaders in Academic Nursing. Angela is passionate about college student success. She works as a family nurse practitioner with faculty, staff, and students on managing primary and episodic health care needs at UNLV's Student Wellness Center and Faculty and Staff Treatment Center. Dr. Silvestri is a successful Elsevier author of numerous best-selling NCLEX® preparation resources on national and international levels. She also served as an Elsevier Subject Matter Expert for the Next Generation NCLEX® (NGN). This passion also comes through in her work at the School of Nursing teaching leadership and licensure exam preparation as well as in publishing research and best-selling licensure exam review resources on national and international levels.

Partnered with Linda Silvestri, Angela is the co-owner of Silvestri's NurseForward LLC, a company committed to globally assisting students and graduates with testing success and preparing for professional nursing practice.

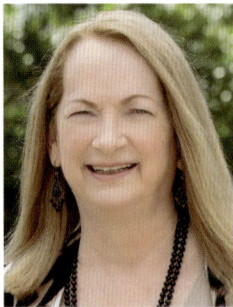

Donna D. Ignatavicius, MS, RN, CNE, CNEcl, ANEF, FAADN

Nationally recognized as an expert in nursing education and medical-surgical nursing, Donna, better known as "Iggy," has a wealth of experience in education, clinical nursing, and administration. Through her company, DI Associates, Inc., Iggy speaks at national and state conferences, such as the Boot Camp for Nurse Educators®, and provides consultation on such topics as curriculum transformation and NGN preparation. In addition, she is the primary author of a number of articles, chapters, and books including the 11th edition of her leading textbook, *Medical-Surgical Nursing: Concepts for Clinical Judgment and Collaborative Care*, which was published in 2024. In 2007 Iggy was inducted as a Fellow into the very prestigious Academy of Nursing Education for her national contributions to nursing education. In 2021 she was also inducted as a Fellow into the Academy of Associate Degree Nursing for her national influence and contributions to programs preparing students for nursing practice. Iggy obtained her initial Certified Nurse Educator® credential in 2016 (recertified in 2021) and her Certified Academic Clinical Educator® credential in 2020.

Reviewers

Eileen H. Gray, DNP, RN, CPNP
Nursing Instructor
University of Nevada, Las Vegas
Las Vegas, Nevada;
Consultant
Nursing Reviews, Inc.
Henderson, Nevada

Tami Little, DNP, RN, CNE
Adjunct Instructor of Nursing
Pittsburgh Technical College
Oakdale, Pennsylvania

David Petersen, MSN-Ed, RN
Assistant Professor of Academics
Chamberlain University
Phoenix, Arizona

Karen Petersen, MSN-L, RN
Assistant Professor of Nursing
Chamberlain University
Phoenix, Arizona

Acknowledgments

We want to acknowledge the many people from Elsevier who were such a significant part of our journey as we prepared this revised resource for nursing students. First and foremost, we extend our deepest appreciation to Heather Bays-Petrovic, former Content Strategist, for accepting our proposal for the second edition and promoting our vision for this project and for supporting us every step of the way from start to finish. Thank you, Heather! We also extend our sincere gratitude to Rae Robertson, Senior Content Development Specialist, for her guidance, patience, and support throughout the preparation of the manuscript; Jodi Willard, Senior Project Manager, for her outstanding efforts to ensure consistency throughout the manuscript and for maintaining organization of all our manuscript; Amy Buxton, Senior Book Designer; and Catherine Jackson, Publishing Services Manager. We thank all of you for your willingness and flexibility to design this resource ensuring that our ideas and vision were executed and for your consistent attention to the many details in our manuscript. We also want to thank Bruce Seibert and Bala Cherukumili for their patience and assistance in implementing our requests in developing the electronic platform that accompanied the first edition, and Santhoshkumar Govindaraju, Senior Producer, for his assistance in the second edition. A very grateful and appreciative "thank you" from us to all of you. We could not have achieved our aspirations for this resource without you! Finally, we want to thank the reviewers for this edition—your feedback ensured our provision of the highest level of quality test items that mirror the realities of professional practice. Thank you!

Preface

Welcome to the second edition of *Strategies for Student Success on the Next Generation NCLEX® (NGN) Test Items!*

This revised text is focused on providing you with the latest information about the Next Generation NCLEX® (NGN) along with practice questions that will prepare you to successfully answer the newest test item types on today's NCLEX®. This book highlights general NGN Tips for student success and unique test-taking strategies that you'll only find in this resource! Chapter 1 introduces the clinical judgment (CJ) cognitive skills on which the NGN test items are based. Chapter 2 presents examples of the current NGN test item types. Chapters 3 to 8 describe the CJ cognitive skills and present enhanced test-taking strategies on how to answer practice items that measure each skill. Chapter 9 demonstrates how Stand-Alone items and Unfolding Case Studies are presented on the NGN, and Chapter 10 provides an NGN Practice Test to apply what you learned throughout the book. The answers, rationales, enhanced test-taking strategies, content areas, and CJ cognitive skill(s) for each practice question throughout all chapters are presented at the end of the book. In addition, the priority concepts are identified. The specific focus of each chapter is summarized below.

Organization of the Book

- Chapter 1, *Introduction to the Clinical Judgment Process,* describes how clinical judgment builds on the nursing process and introduces you to the six essential cognitive skills of the NCSBN Clinical Judgment Measurement Model (NCJMM). These cognitive skills are the basis for the NGN test item types.
- Chapter 2, *Introduction to the NGN and the NGN Test Item Types,* explains the purpose and design of the NGN and presents the newest test item types. An example of each item type is presented, and the correct responses are provided with rationales.
- Chapter 3, *Strategies for Answering NGN Questions: Recognize Cues,* describes the CJ cognitive skill *Recognize Cues,* which requires you to identify relevant clinical findings and decide which findings are of *immediate* concern and *most* important based on the clinical scenario. This chapter also identifies test items and enhanced test-taking strategies that you can use when answering items that measure this skill. Examples of these test items allow you the opportunity to practice applying these strategies within the chapter and in the practice test at the end of the chapter.
- Chapter 4, *Strategies for Answering NGN Questions: Analyze Cues,* describes the CJ cognitive skill *Analyze Cues,* which requires you to connect or link relevant cues to the clinical scenario, interpret these cues, and establish their significance. This chapter also identifies test items and enhanced test-taking strategies that you can use when answering items that measure this skill. Examples of these test items allow you the opportunity to practice applying these strategies within the chapter and in the practice test at the end of the chapter.
- Chapter 5, *Strategies for Answering NGN Questions: Prioritize Hypotheses,* describes the CJ cognitive skill *Prioritize Hypotheses,* which requires you to establish and rank client needs or hypotheses in order of priority. This chapter also identifies test items and enhanced test-taking strategies that you can use when answering items that measure this skill. Examples of these test items allow you the opportunity to practice applying these strategies within the chapter and in the practice test at the end of the chapter.
- Chapter 6, *Strategies for Answering NGN Questions: Generate Solutions,* describes the CJ cognitive skill *Generate Solutions,* which requires you to use knowledge of evidence-based solutions about treatments and interventions that would address identified client needs and modify them to meet priorities of care. This chapter also identifies test items and enhanced test-taking strategies that you can use when answering items that measure this skill. Examples of these test items allow you the opportunity to practice applying these strategies within the chapter and in the practice test at the end of the chapter.
- Chapter 7, *Strategies for Answering NGN Questions: Take Actions,* describes the CJ cognitive skill *Take Actions,* which requires that you perform appropriate and necessary interventions based on the client's situation and generated solutions. This chapter also identifies test items and enhanced test-taking strategies that you can use when answering items that measure this skill. Examples of these test items allow you the opportunity to practice applying these strategies within the chapter and in the practice test at the end of the chapter.
- Chapter 8, *Strategies for Answering NGN Questions: Evaluate Outcomes,* describes the CJ cognitive skill *Evaluate Outcomes,* which requires that you examine outcomes and measure client progress toward meeting those outcomes. This chapter also identifies test items and enhanced test-taking strategies that you can use when answering items that measure this skill. Examples of these test items allow you the opportunity to practice applying these strategies within the chapter and in the practice test at the end of the chapter.
- Chapter 9, *Stand-Alone Items and Unfolding Case Studies: The Role of Contextual Factors in Making Clinical Judgments,* describes the differences between Stand-Alone items and Unfolding Case Studies. Samples of Stand-Alone items (including Bow-tie and Trend items) are illustrated as well as Unfolding Case Studies. The chapter also identifies the contextual factors that influence the

ability of the nurse to make appropriate clinical judgments when caring for a client. Additionally, enhanced test-taking strategies that you can use when answering questions accompanying each type of case study are included.

- Chapter 10, *NGN Practice Test: Putting It All Together*, provides you with the opportunity to practice all of the types of test items on the NGN, starting with Unfolding Case Studies and ending with Stand-Alone Bow-tie and Trend items.

Special Features of the Book

- *NGN tips within each chapter*. These unique tips provide the student with key points to remember, such as the NGN item type or cognitive skill (CS) features.
- *In-chapter sample questions* are presented in Chapters 3 to 9 to provide examples of the NGN test item types that best measure the CJ cognitive skill(s) presented in the chapter. Each question within the chapter specifies the priority concepts and content area being tested. The answer, rationale, enhanced test-taking strategy, and references are also presented to help students learn the thinking process needed to select the correct test item response.
- *End-of-chapter practice* questions are presented at the end of Chapters 3 to 8 to provide the opportunity for students to apply what they learned in each chapter and experience answering selected test items that measure each of the NCSBN's CJ cognitive skills. Chapter 9 presents Stand-Alone items (both Bow-tie and Trend items) and Unfolding Case Studies and identifies the contextual factors (environmental and individual factors) that influence the ability of the nurse to make appropriate clinical judgments when caring for a client.
- *A comprehensive practice test* is presented in Chapter 10 to allow students to apply what they learned in Chapters 1 to 9. Students have the opportunity to answer multiple Unfolding Case Studies and Stand-Alone items representing all clinical specialty areas. The priority concepts, content area, answer, rationale, enhanced test-taking strategy, and reference for each test item are provided at the end of the book.

- *Enhanced test-taking strategies for the NGN*. This unique feature walks students through the thinking process needed to navigate complex NGN cases. Each strategy explains how to apply the cognitive skill when considering the information presented in the clinical scenario. Each question is accompanied by enhanced test-taking strategies that are presented both narratively and in table format to guide the student through a logical thinking process and to suit multiple learning styles. This thinking process with test-taking strategies will also help students be successful on nursing course exams.
- *Thinking Space*. The Thinking Spaces located in the margins of the book are places for personal note taking. The student can use these spaces to write down new and important information they want to remember. To become most familiar with the cognitive skills and to build CJ skills, using the Thinking Space to make important linkages between clinical scenario information and the cognitive skill will reinforce the aspects of the NCJMM model as the student is studying and preparing for the NGN.

Special Features Found on Evolve

The book includes 24 single-case sample questions and 36 single-case practice questions (each with 1 NGN item), 6 Stand-Alone items (3 Bow-tie and 3 Trend items), and 4 Unfolding Case Studies (each with 6 NGN items). This equals a total of 90 NGN items in the book. The Evolve site accompanying this resource provides the student with all of the sample and practice test questions in the book plus additional practice questions. There are 84 single cases (each with 1 NGN item), 26 Stand-Alone items (Bow-tie and Trend items), and 36 Unfolding Case Studies (each with 6 NGN items). Altogether, there are a total of 326 NGN items on Evolve.

The Evolve site lists various category selections. You can select by type of question—either single case, Stand-Alone items (Bow-tie or Trend items) or an Unfolding Case Study. You can also select by the specific cognitive skill, content area, or priority concept. The table below illustrates the various categories for selection.

Types	Cognitive Skills	Content Areas	Priority Concepts
Single case	Recognize Cues	Foundations of Nursing	Clotting
Stand-Alone item	Analyze Cues	Obstetric-Newborn Nursing	Cognition
Unfolding Case Study	Prioritize Hypotheses	Medical-Surgical Nursing	Elimination
	Generate Solutions	Mental Health Nursing	Fluid and Electrolyte Balance
	Take Actions	Pediatric Nursing	Gas Exchange
	Evaluate Outcomes	Pharmacology	Glucose Regulation
			Immunity
			Infection
			Inflammation
			Mobility
			Mood and Affect
			Perfusion
			Reproduction
			Sensory Perception
			Stress and Coping
			Tissue Integrity

How to Use This Book

For Students

As implied in the title, this book was written to help you be successful when answering the test item types that are part of the Next Generation NCLEX® (NGN). The first two book chapters present a review of the CJ process and the NGN item types. The test item types are based on the six cognitive (thinking) skills needed for safe, appropriate clinical judgment and readiness for nursing practice. Be sure that you are very familiar with this information before beginning to practice answering the test questions later in the book.

Chapters 3 to 8 describe each CJ cognitive skill and provide general NGN Tips on how to answer test items that measure each skill. Sample NGN test items are then presented with the Rationale and enhanced Test-Taking Strategy for the correct and incorrect responses, followed by six end-of-chapter practice questions for you to answer. The practice questions in each chapter represent all content specialties. The rationale and enhanced test-taking strategy that you can use for each question to determine the correct answers are described in detail, with tables to help organize the information in each question. In addition, each test item is labeled by priority nursing concepts and content specialty. References are also provided to help you review the content associated with each test item if needed.

When working through Chapters 3 to 8, start with Chapters 3 and 4 early in your program so you can learn how to determine the most important client findings in a clinical scenario and what they mean (*Recognize Cues* and *Analyze Cues*). When you feel you have mastered these cognitive skills, work through Chapter 5, which will help you learn to prioritize client needs and the care required to meet them. Chapters 6 and 7 are focused on helping you learn to plan and implement nursing actions to meet the client's needs. Finally, Chapter 8 will assist you in determining whether the client's condition has improved after care has been implemented.

After working through Chapters 3 to 8 and when you feel ready to put all of the cognitive skills together, Chapter 9 provides examples for NGN Unfolding Case Studies and Stand-Alone items and points out the contextual (environmental and individual) factors considered in the care of the client. Chapter 10 presents a comprehensive practice test that simulates what you can expect on the NGN. The rationale and enhanced test-taking strategy for each practice test item in these chapters are described in detail. Additional single-case items, Stand-Alone items, and Unfolding Case Studies are available on the Evolve site. Each accompanying practice test item includes a rationale, an enhanced test-taking strategy, the content specialty, priority nursing concepts, and reference(s).

For Faculty

This book is designed for you to use as it is organized, beginning with helping students learn what clinical judgment is and gain an understanding of each of the essential CJ cognitive skills as described in Chapter 1. Students in their first nursing course should learn how to use these skills to make safe, appropriate clinical judgments to ensure client safety. If students are already making clinical judgments using these skills, Chapter 1 could be used for review. Then, students should become familiar with the NGN test design and item types as presented in Chapter 2. Finally, by the end of the first semester (or other term), students should learn how to *Recognize Cues* and *Analyze Cues* (Chapters 3 and 4). These cognitive skills focus on assessing the client, discerning how to determine which client findings are most important, and deciding what those findings mean. End-of-chapter practice questions can be used online or during class, simulation pre- or post-briefing, or clinical post-conference. The test items can be assigned to students as individuals or in groups to answer. Regardless of where or how practice test items are used, such as in the classroom, online, lab sessions, or clinical setting, be sure to review the answers, rationales, and strategies for arriving at the correct response(s) to identify and improve students' thinking process as needed.

As students progress through the program, they should focus on how to prioritize care to determine what nursing actions they would plan and implement. Part of this thinking process includes an assessment to decide if the actions were effective and the client's condition has improved. Therefore students would next focus on Chapters 5 to 8. Again, you can assign the practice items to students as individuals or in groups and review the items to help students improve their thinking skills as needed.

Chapters 9 and 10 put together all of the cognitive skill steps and NGN test item types—both Stand-Alone items and Unfolding Case Studies. These chapters can be used whenever students are applying the individual CJ cognitive skills and considering contextual (environmental and individual) factors to successfully answer the test items in preparation for the NGN. Assign these practice Unfolding Case Studies and Stand-Alone items as individual student practice to determine any skill areas where improvement is needed. Students needing improvement can then review any of the six earlier chapters (Chapters 3 to 8) to hone their thinking skills.

Faculty Tool Kit

The Faculty Tool Kit was created to guide faculty in using this book with their students at any stage in the program to prepare them for the NGN.

The Tool Kit:
- Furnishes a guide for how to use this book, *Strategies for Student Success on the Next Generation NCLEX® (NGN) Test Items,* to prepare students for the NGN
- Provides chapter-to-chapter strategic points to emphasize to students and ways to prepare students for answering NGN test items
- Provides suggestions for using the Evolve site accompanying this book

- Presents step-by-step guides for writing Stand-Alone items and Unfolding Case Studies
- Presents step-by-step guides for writing NGN items
- Specifies NCSBN resources that focus on the NGN for students and faculty
- Provides Elsevier resources and references for preparing students for the NGN

Additional Resources for Students

- Ignatavicius, D. D. (2025). *Developing Clinical Judgment for Professional Practice and NGN Readiness* (2nd ed.). St. Louis: Elsevier.

    This recently revised and expanded workbook helps students preparing to become RNs learn how to develop NCSBN's six CJ cognitive skills through practice in answering the newest NGN test item types, including Unfolding Case Studies and Stand-Alone items. Clinical scenarios are presented from more basic care to complex, multisystem care of clients in multiple specialty areas that can be used across the curriculum.

- Ignatavicius, D. D., & Little, T. K. (2026). *Developing Clinical Judgment for Practical/Vocational Nursing Practice and NGN Readiness* (2nd ed.). St. Louis: Elsevier.

    This workbook helps students preparing to become LPNs or LVNs learn how to develop the NCSBN's six CJ cognitive skills through practice in answering the newest NGN test item types, including Unfolding Case Studies and Stand-Alone items. Clinical scenarios in multiple specialty areas are included, with a primary emphasis on the care of older adults in a variety of health care settings, and can be used throughout the entire curriculum.

- Ignatavicius, D. D. & Andersen, S. (2025). *Alfaro's Clinical Judgment in Nursing: A How-to Practice Approach* (8th ed.). St. Louis: Elsevier.

    This totally revised resource helps students learn how to develop each of the six CJ cognitive skills they will need to be ready for today's nursing practice. Thinking exercises in each chapter allow students to practice what they learn, and multiple NGN practice test items are available in the last chapter of the book with additional practice on the Evolve site.

- Silvestri, L. A., & Silvestri, A. E. (2023). *Saunders Comprehensive Review for the NCLEX-RN® Examination* (9th ed.). St. Louis: Elsevier.

    This is an excellent resource to use both while you are in nursing school and in preparation for the NCLEX® examination. This book contains 20 units with 70 chapters, and each chapter is designed to identify specific components of nursing content. Each chapter includes clinical judgment boxes that illustrate application of the cognitive skills to a clinical scenario. The book and accompanying software contain more than 5200 practice questions and include NGN items and alternate item format questions. The software also contains a 75-question preassessment test that generates an individualized study calendar. A postassessment test is included as well as case studies and accompanying NGN item type practice questions.

- Silvestri, L. A., & Silvestri, A. E. (2024). *Saunders Q&A Review for the NCLEX-RN® Examination* (9th ed.). St. Louis: Elsevier.

    This book and accompanying Evolve site provide you with more than 6000 practice questions based on the NCLEX-RN® test plan. Each practice question includes a priority nursing tip that provides you with a piece of important information to remember that will help you answer questions on nursing exams and on the NCLEX® examination. The chapters in this book are uniquely designed and are based on the NCLEX-RN® examination test plan framework, including Client Needs and Integrated Processes. The software also contains a 75-question preassessment test that generates an individualized study calendar. A postassessment test is included as well. Alternate item format questions and case study and NGN item type practice questions are included. Case studies and NGN items include Bow-tie and Trend items, single-episode case studies, and Unfolding Case Studies. With practice questions focused on the Client Needs, Integrated Processes, and Clinical Judgment/Cognitive Skills, you can assess your level of competence.

- Silvestri, L. A., & Silvestri, A. E. (2024). *HESI/Saunders Online Review for the NCLEX-RN® Examination* (4th ed.). St. Louis: Elsevier.

    The online NCLEX-RN® review course provides a systematic and individualized approach and addresses all areas of the test plan identified by the National Council of State Boards of Nursing, Inc. This self-paced online review contains 10 interactive, multimedia-rich modules featuring animations and videos, practice questions, end-of-lesson case studies, and much more! A diagnostic pretest generates a study calendar to guide your review. NCLEX®-style questions—including NGN items and every type of alternate item format question—are provided, concluding with a comprehensive examination that will sharpen your test-taking skills. In addition, case studies and accompanying NGN practice questions are included. Unique videos that simulate a live review course focus on difficult subjects such as dysrhythmias and make them easier to understand.

- Silvestri, L. A., & Silvestri, A. E. (2026). *Saunders 2026-2027 Clinical Judgment and Test-Taking Strategies* (9th ed.). St. Louis: Elsevier.

    This book is designed for both RN and PN nursing students and provides a foundation for understanding and unpacking the complexities of NCLEX® exam questions, including alternate item formats and NGN items. *Saunders 2026–2027 Clinical Judgment and Test-Taking Strategies* takes a detailed look at all of the test-taking strategies you will need to know in order to pass any nursing examination, including the NCLEX® examination. Special nursing content tips are integrated along with other tips, such as clinical preparation tips and life-planning tips. There are 1200 practice questions included, so you can apply the testing strategies. Case studies and NGN items and practice test questions are also included on the Evolve site accompanying this resource.

- Silvestri, L. A., & Silvestri, A. E. (2024). *Saunders Comprehensive Review for the NCLEX-PN® Examination* (9th ed.). St. Louis: Elsevier.

    This is an excellent resource to use both while you are in nursing school and in preparation for the NCLEX® examination. This book contains 20 units with 70 chapters, and each chapter is designed to identify specific components of nursing content. Each chapter includes clinical judgment boxes that illustrate application of the cognitive skills to a clinical scenario. The book and accompanying Evolve site contain more than 4500 practice questions and include NGN items and alternate item format questions. The software also contains a 75-question preassessment test that generates an individualized study calendar. A postassessment test is also included as well as case studies and accompanying NGN item type practice questions.

- Silvestri, L. A., & Silvestri, A. E. (2023). *Saunders Q&A Review for the NCLEX-PN® Examination* (6th ed.). St. Louis: Elsevier.

    This book and accompanying Evolve site provide you with more than 5900 practice questions based on the NCLEX-PN® test plan. Each practice question includes a priority nursing tip that provides you with a piece of important information to remember that will help you answer questions on nursing exams and on the NCLEX® examination. The chapters in this book are uniquely designed and are based on the NCLEX-PN® examination test plan framework, including Client Needs and Integrated Processes. The software also contains a 75-question preassessment test that generates an individualized study calendar. A postassessment test is included as well. Alternate item format questions and case study and NGN item type practice questions are included. Case studies and NGN items include Bow-tie and Trend items, single-episode case studies, and Unfolding Case Studies. With practice questions focused on the Client Needs, Integrated Processes, and Clinical Judgment/Cognitive Skills, you can assess your level of competence.

- Silvestri, L. A., & Silvestri, A. E. (2023). *HESI/Saunders Online Review for the NCLEX-PN® Examination* (3rd ed.). St. Louis: Elsevier.

    The online NCLEX-PN® review course provides a systematic and individualized approach and addresses all areas of the test plan identified by the National Council of State Boards of Nursing. This self-paced online review contains 10 interactive, multimedia-rich modules featuring animations and videos, practice questions, end-of-lesson case studies, and much more! A diagnostic pretest generates a study calendar to guide your review. NCLEX®-style questions—including NGN items and every type of alternate item format question—are provided, concluding with a comprehensive examination that will sharpen your test-taking skills. In addition, case studies and accompanying NGN practice questions are included. Unique videos that simulate a live review course focus on difficult subjects such as dysrhythmias and make them easier to understand.

Contents

CHAPTER 1
Introduction to the Clinical Judgment Process, 1
What Is the Purpose of Today's NCLEX® and How Is It Designed?, 1
Why Was There a Need for NCLEX® Change?, 2
What is the NCSBN'S Definition and Model of Clinical Judgment?, 2
What Are the Six NCSBN Clinical Judgment Cognitive Skills?, 4
How Are the Six Clinical Judgment Skills Measured on Today's NCLEX®?, 8
How Can You Prepare for Today's NCLEX®?, 9

CHAPTER 2
Introduction to the NGN and the NGN Test Item Types, 10
Test Item Types Used for Unfolding Case Studies, 10
Test Item Types Used for Stand-Alone Test Items, 23

CHAPTER 3
Strategies for Answering NGN Questions: Recognize Cues, 26
What Are Cues?, 26
How Are Client Findings (Cues) Presented in an NGN Clinical Scenario?, 26
Which Client Findings Are Relevant?, 27
Which Relevant Client Findings Require Immediate Follow-Up?, 28
What Types of Clinical Scenarios May Be Included on the NGN?, 28
Which NGN Item Types Optimally Measure *Recognize Cues*?, 28
Practice Questions, 37

CHAPTER 4
Strategies for Answering NGN Questions: Analyze Cues, 40
How Do You Analyze Cues?, 40
How Does Analyzing Cues Help You Guide Client Care?, 40
How Do You Analyze Cues in an NGN Clinical Scenario?, 41
What Will You Think About to Analyze Cues in This Clinical Scenario?, 43
Which Client Findings Are Most Important When Analyzing Cues?, 44
When Might You Need to Analyze Cues in a Clinical Situation?, 44
Which NGN Item Types Optimally Measure *Analyze Cues*?, 44
Practice Questions, 55

CHAPTER 5
Strategies for Answering NGN Questions: Prioritize Hypotheses, 60
What Do Hypotheses Mean?, 60
What Does Prioritizing Mean?, 60
What to Consider When Prioritizing Hypotheses, 60
External Factors and Prioritizing Hypotheses, 61
How Do You Know That You Need to Prioritize?, 63
What Strategies Can You Use to Prioritize Hypotheses?, 64
How Do You Prioritize Hypotheses in an NGN Clinical Situation?, 65
What Will You Think About to Prioritize Hypotheses in This Clinical Scenario?, 66
Which NGN Item Types Optimally Measure *Prioritize Hypotheses*?, 66
Practice Questions, 74

CHAPTER 6
Strategies for Answering NGN Questions: Generate Solutions, 79
What to Consider When Generating Solutions, 79
The Plan of Care and Generating Solutions, 79
How Do You Know That You Need to Generate Solutions?, 79
How Do You Generate Solutions in an NGN Clinical Situation?, 80
What Will You Think About to Generate Solutions in This Clinical Scenario?, 81
Which NGN Item Types Optimally Measure *Generate Solutions*?, 81
Practice Questions, 89

CHAPTER 7
Strategies for Answering NGN Questions: Take Actions, 93
How Do You Know What Actions to Take?, 93
How Will Nursing Actions Be Tested?, 94
Which NGN Item Types Optimally Measure *Take Actions*?, 94
Practice Questions, 101

CHAPTER 8
Strategies for Answering NGN Questions: Evaluate Outcomes, 105
How Do You Evaluate Outcomes?, 105
How Will *Evaluate Outcomes* Be Tested?, 105
NGN Question Stems Addressing *Evaluate Outcomes*, 106
Which NGN Item Types Optimally Measure *Evaluate Outcomes*?, 106
Practice Questions, 114

CHAPTER 9
Stand-Alone Items and Unfolding Case Studies: The Role of Contextual Factors in Making Clinical Judgments, 120

What Are Stand-Alone Items?, 121
What Are Unfolding Case Studies?, 133
How Are Stand-Alone Items and Unfolding Case Studies Different?, 133

CHAPTER 10
NGN Practice Test: Putting It All Together, 143

Unfolding Case Studies, 143
Stand-Alone Items, 170

Answers to Practice Questions, 177

References and Bibliography, 319

CHAPTER 1

Introduction to the Clinical Judgment Process

>THINKING SPACE

This chapter will help you understand the latest change in the NCLEX® and the clinical judgment process that serves as the basis for the newest test item types, often referred to as the Next Generation NCLEX® (NGN). After a brief review of the NCLEX® design, the cognitive (thinking) skills needed to make safe, evidence-based clinical judgments are introduced. General NGN Tips are provided to help you relate each cognitive skill with the current NCLEX®.

The NCLEX® has included the newest NGN item types since April 2023, and they are described in detail in Chapter 2 of this book. Specific Test-Taking Strategies that will help you correctly answer these new items are provided throughout other chapters of this book and accompany all sample and practice questions in the book and on the Evolve site. Be sure to review this chapter *before* reading the rest of this book or practicing NGN questions!

What Is the Purpose of Today's NCLEX® and How Is It Designed?

As you know, prelicensure nursing education programs like the one you're currently in prepare students for eligibility to take either the NCLEX-RN® or the NCLEX-PN® after graduation. Nursing national licensure examinations are developed and updated under the direction of the National Council of State Boards of Nursing (NCSBN). This organization also oversees the administration of the NCLEX® in the United States, Canada, and other countries.

The primary purpose of the NCSBN is to *protect the public* by providing competency assessments, such as the NCLEX®, that are sound and secure. The NCLEX® is comprehensive and reflects current nursing practice. To ensure examination currency, the NCSBN collects and analyzes nursing practice data every 3 years from thousands of graduates to determine what knowledge and activities are required in their role as new nurses. This information is used to develop the content of the NCLEX® and is organized in a new licensure test plan every 3 years (https://www.ncsbn.org/testplans.htm). The test plan is organized by four major Client Needs Categories, some of which have subcategories. In addition, six Integrated Processes are defined and included throughout the NCLEX® Test Plan as listed in Box 1.1.

The NCLEX® measures the new graduate's minimum competence in safety to ensure public protection through a variety of test items. Most of the test items on this exam are either Multiple Choice or Multiple Response, also known as Select All That Apply (SATA) questions. For each of these item types, client information is presented in one to two sentences followed by a question about the nurse's role in client care. Examples of these traditional test item types are presented in Box 1.2.

As you'll notice in these traditional test items, each question focuses on what the nurse would do or say in response to specific client data. Only the client information that is the most important, relevant, or, in some cases, of immediate concern to the nurse is presented. The answer is then selected from a list of choices provided. The

⚡ THINKING SPACE

BOX 1.1	NCLEX-RN® Test Plan Organizing Concepts
Integrated Processes	**Client Needs Categories/Subcategories**
Nursing Process[a]	Safe and Effective Care Environment
Teaching and Learning	• Management of Care[b]
Communication and Documentation	• Safety and Infection Control
Caring	Health Promotion and Maintenance
Culture and Spirituality	Psychosocial Integrity
Clinical Judgment	Physiological Integrity
	• Basic Care and Comfort
	• Pharmacological and Parenteral Therapies[c]
	• Reduction of Risk Potential
	• Physiological Adaptation

[a]This Integrated Process on the NCLEX-PN® Test Plan is the Problem-Solving Process.
[b]This Client Needs subcategory on the NCLEX-PN® Test Plan is Coordinated Care.
[c]This Client Needs subcategory on the NCLEX-PN® Test Plan is Pharmacological Therapies.

narrow focus of these test items often does not represent the scope of actual nursing practice and does not allow measurement of clinical judgment. Rather, these types of items reflect whether the candidate can distinguish between right and wrong. At this point in your education, you likely are very familiar with these item types on your course exams.

Why Was There a Need for NCLEX® Change?

Although national NCLEX® first-time pass rates for both RN and PN graduates have increased for the past several years, health care employers continue to report increasing errors in client care and lack of appropriate clinical judgment skills among new nursing graduates. A literature review conducted by the NCSBN found that 50% of all nurses have been involved in at least one client error. Sixty percent of those errors were the result of poor clinical judgment (NCSBN, 2018). In response to these data, the NCSBN began to question if the NCLEX® was measuring "the best thing" to protect the public.

An analysis of activities performed by practicing RNs and RN role experts confirmed the importance of sound clinical judgment skills for many tasks and activities performed by entry-level nurses. This analysis also highlighted that nurses today make more complex decisions to provide safe care for clients with higher acuity and advanced age (NCSBN, 2018).

The NCSBN literature review also found that the nurse's primary practice activity is the ability to problem solve and critically think—thinking processes needed for making appropriate clinical judgments. *Problem solving* is the process of developing and evaluating nursing solutions or approaches to client conditions. *Critical thinking* can be described as a process requiring the use of logic and clinical reasoning to identify the strengths and weaknesses of nursing solutions or approaches to client problems. The NCSBN built on these process descriptions to create a definition and model of clinical judgment to be used as a basis for developing new NCLEX® test item types.

What Is the NCSBN'S Definition and Model of Clinical Judgment?

As a result of the literature review, nursing practice analyses, and input from a variety of nurse clinicians and educators, the NCSBN developed this definition of clinical judgment:

> *Clinical judgment is defined as the observed outcome of critical thinking and decision making. It is an iterative process with multiple skills that uses nursing knowledge*

CHAPTER 1 Introduction to the Clinical Judgment Process   3

> **BOX 1.2   Examples of Traditional Multiple Choice and Multiple Response NCLEX® Test Items**
>
> **Example 1: Multiple Choice Item**
> The nurse is planning care for a client admitted to the hospital with a diagnosis of acute pancreatitis and controlled hypertension. What is the nurse's **priority** for the client's care at this time?
>
> ☐ Administer an antiemetic medication.
> ☐ Manage the client's acute pain.
> ☐ Monitor the client's blood pressure.
> ☐ Administer supplemental oxygen.
>
> Answer:
> The nurse is planning care for a client admitted to the hospital with a diagnosis of acute pancreatitis and controlled hypertension. What is the nurse's **priority** for the client's care at this time?
>
> ☐ Administer an antiemetic medication.
> ☒ Manage the client's acute pain.
> ☐ Monitor the client's blood pressure.
> ☐ Administer supplemental oxygen.
>
> **Example 2: Multiple Response (Select All That Apply) Item**
> The nurse is assessing an adolescent who was taken to the ED for threatening to commit suicide. Which of the following questions would be the **most appropriate** for the nurse to ask the client at this time? **Select all that apply.**
>
> ☐ "What made you want to kill yourself?"
> ☐ "Do you have a plan for killing yourself?"
> ☐ "Do you plan to kill yourself with anyone else?"
> ☐ "Is this the first time you've threatened to kill yourself?"
> ☐ "Did you write a suicide note to explain why you are doing this?"
>
> Answer:
> The nurse is assessing an adolescent who was taken to the ED for threatening to commit suicide. Which of the following questions would be the **most appropriate** for the nurse to ask the client at this time? **Select all that apply.**
>
> ☐ "What made you want to kill yourself?"
> ☒ "Do you have a plan for killing yourself?"
> ☒ "Do you plan to kill yourself with anyone else?"
> ☐ "Is this the first time you've threatened to kill yourself?"
> ☐ "Did you write a suicide note to explain why you are doing this?"

THINKING SPACE

to observe and assess presenting situations, identify a prioritized client concern and generate the best possible evidence-based solutions in order to deliver safe client care (NCSBN, 2023).

So, what does this definition mean for you as a nursing student and future professional nurse? Think about these key points in the definition to make effective clinical judgments:

- Recognize that clinical judgment is the result or *outcome of thinking* to make decisions about client care when potential or actual health conditions occur. The same process of thinking to make clinical decisions occurs repeatedly as you manage client conditions *(iterative process)*.
- Acquire and recall *nursing knowledge* to make appropriate clinical judgments. (However, having knowledge does not guarantee that an accurate or appropriate clinical judgment will be made.)

THINKING SPACE

> **BOX 1.3 Examples of Environmental and Individual Factors That Influence Clinical Judgment**
>
> | Examples of Environmental Factors | Examples of Individual Factors |
> |---|---|
> | Environment | Knowledge |
> | Medical records | Skills |
> | Time pressure | Specialty |
> | Task complexity | Prior experience |
> | Resources | Level of experience |
> | Cultural considerations | Candidate characteristics |
> | Client observation | |
> | Consequences and risks | |

- Learn how to *prioritize* a client's need for care based on the data presented in a clinical situation.
- Be familiar with the *best current evidence* regarding a presented client situation so you can plan possible solutions or approaches for care to keep the client *safe*.

You will want to acquire these skills and a strong knowledge base during your nursing program to be ready for a dynamic, complex health care system and the current NCLEX®.

After the NCSBN developed its definition of clinical judgment, the organization created a model of clinical judgment called the NCSBN Clinical Judgment Measurement Model (NCJMM). As the name implies, this model was created to measure the nursing graduate's ability to make clinical judgments. Although it is not important for you to be familiar with the entire model, it is essential that you master the clinical judgment process. The NCJMM identifies six cognitive skills that are needed to make safe appropriate clinical judgments and serve as the basis for the new NGN test item types. These skills are listed in Layer 3 of the NCJMM and are introduced in the next section of this chapter.

The NCJMM also identifies factors that influence the ability of nurses to make appropriate clinical judgments. Examples of these Environmental and Individual factors, as specified in Layer 4 of the NCJMM, are listed in Box 1.3. Environmental factors are those that influence the nurse's clinical decision making in the health care setting. Individual factors are those related to the nursing graduate candidate taking the NCLEX®.

What Are the Six NCSBN Clinical Judgment Cognitive Skills?

The current NCLEX® includes new test item types that measure the six cognitive skills of clinical judgment. Chapters 3 through 8 in this book describe these skills in more detail and present examples of the newest NGN test items designed to measure the ability to use each skill. The cognitive skills essential for clinical judgment are listed in Box 1.4 with key questions that explain the focus of each skill.

Recognize Cues

For clients in any health care setting, the nurse collects health data from a number of sources. *Cues* are client findings or assessment data that provide information for nurses

> **BOX 1.4 Clinical Judgment Cognitive Skills With Key Questions**
>
> **Recognize Cues:** What matters most (and now)?
> **Analyze Cues:** What could it mean?
> **Prioritize Hypotheses:** Where do I start?
> **Generate Solutions:** What can I do?
> **Take Actions:** What will I do?
> **Evaluate Outcomes:** Did it help?

as a basis for making safe appropriate clinical judgments and can be divided into the following four major types. Chapter 3 describes these sources of cues in more detail.

- Environmental cues (e.g., presence of family member)
- Client observation cues (e.g., signs and symptoms)
- Medical record cues (e.g., lab values or vital signs)
- Time pressure cues (e.g., rapid clinical decline)

In actual clinical practice, the nurse reviews all client findings to determine which data are most important, relevant, and require immediate follow-up. To help you *Recognize Cues,* ask yourself which client data are most important in the clinical presentation. Carefully review the client's presenting data, such as vital signs and medical diagnosis, to determine their relevance in various contexts. For example, a heart rate of 140 would require immediate follow-up for a middle-aged adult, but is within the typical range for a newborn.

In some cases, the client has a history of one or more acute and/or chronic health conditions. For example, an older adult with a long history of COPD may have a PaO_2 of 65 mm Hg. This arterial oxygen level seems abnormal because it is below the usual range of 80 to 100 mm Hg. However, for *this* client, the low arterial oxygen level is likely not important or of immediate concern because it is expected. Many clients with advanced COPD have chronically low arterial oxygen, but they compensate by using breathing techniques combined with low-flow supplemental oxygen.

Analyze Cues

After relevant cues have been identified in a client scenario, the nurse organizes and links them to the client's clinical presentation. Ask yourself: "What do the relevant or most important client findings mean or indicate at this time?" For example, consider a middle-aged client who had a small bowel resection 2 days ago and begins having increasing abdominal pain, distention, vomiting, and absent bowel sounds. These data, when grouped together, are consistent with a possible postoperative paralytic ileus. To connect these assessment findings with an ileus, you need knowledge of pathophysiology, especially signs and symptoms.

In some clinical presentations, the client may have *multiple* relevant cues that are associated with several different conditions. Box 1.5 illustrates an NGN-style test item that measures the ability to analyze cues for an older adult hospitalized for a urinary tract infection and sepsis. In this Thinking Activity, you would need to review each client finding to determine if it is consistent with one or more of the specified conditions. In this example, one finding may be consistent with two or three client conditions, such as generalized weakness and acute confusion. However, dyspnea on exertion is associated with only one of the listed conditions—anemia. The correct responses to the Thinking Activity are found in Box 1.6.

In other clinical presentations, the client may not be experiencing an actual health condition, but is *at risk* for one or more potential conditions. For example, the client who recently had a spontaneous vaginal delivery is at risk for postpartum hemorrhage within the first 24 hours, particularly if the uterus becomes boggy (a client observation cue).

▶THINKING SPACE

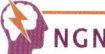

NGN TIP

Remember: To *Recognize Cues,* carefully review the client's assessment data like developmental age and history to help determine if findings are relevant and require immediate follow-up.

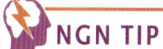

NGN TIP

Remember: To *Analyze Cues,* you are not required to make a medical diagnosis but rather will be expected to connect or link client findings with selected client conditions or health problems, either actual or potential.

BOX 1.5	Example of a Thinking Activity That Requires the Ability to *Analyze Cues*		
Client Findings	**Dehydration**	**Hypernatremia**	**Anemia**
Generalized weakness			
Acute confusion			
Dry mouth			
Increased heart rate			
Dyspnea on exertion			

BOX 1.6 Answers to Example of a Thinking Activity That Requires the Ability to *Analyze Cues*

Client Findings	Dehydration	Hypernatremia	Anemia
Generalized weakness	X	X	X
Acute confusion	X	X	X
Dry mouth	X	X	
Increased heart rate	X	X	X
Dyspnea on exertion			X

In some client clinical presentations then, part of the thinking process to *Analyze Cues* is to identify if cues are linked to or consistent with potential conditions.

Prioritize Hypotheses

After organizing, grouping, and linking relevant client findings with actual or potential client conditions, the next cognitive skill requires you to narrow down what the data mean and prioritize the client's needs for care. Although you may have learned about priority decision-making models such as the ABCs or Maslow's Hierarchy of Needs, these models are often not very useful in helping you make clinical judgments in more complex clinical situations.

To *Prioritize Hypotheses,* review and evaluate each of the client's needs in the clinical presentation. Then rank them to decide what is *most likely* the priority health condition or need. Evaluate factors in the clinical situation such as urgency, risk, difficulty, and time sensitivity for the client. For example, consider this clinical situation:

> A 42-year-old postpartum client who just gave birth to a third child in 4 years reports severe "afterbirth pains" of 9 on a 0 to 10 pain intensity scale. The client also reports having problems with getting the baby to latch for breast-feeding/chest-feeding. The nurse assesses that the client has a boggy uterus and is saturating a peri-pad every 20 to 30 minutes.

In this example, the client has three conditions that you would evaluate and rank in this order:
1. Excessive postpartum bleeding due to boggy uterus
2. Severe abdominal pain due to uterine contractions
3. Difficulty with breast-feeding/chest-feeding due to inability of baby to latch

The priority for the client at this time is to manage excessive postpartum bleeding because the client could become hypovolemic and develop shock, which is potentially life-threatening. In this situation, managing the client's bleeding is more *urgent* than managing severe pain or breast-feeding/chest-feeding difficulty.

Generate Solutions

After identifying the client's priority need or condition in a given clinical presentation, you want to think about all possible actions that can be used to resolve or manage the condition. To assist in selecting the possible actions or approach to care you might include, first determine what outcomes are desired or expected for the client. For example, consider this scenario:

> The birth parent of an 11-year-old brings the child to the ED for a right forearm injury experienced as a result of a scooter accident. The nurse observes that the child is crying and guarding the right arm, which is swollen, deformed, and bruised. The child is left-handed. During the head-to-toe assessment, the nurse notes old bruising on the left side of the child's chest and scarring on both upper thighs. Both knees have large abrasions with small stones and dirt embedded in them. The child denies having had

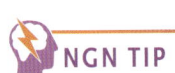

NGN TIP

Remember: The urgency of a clinical situation, the likelihood of a medical complication, and the risk to the client are the most important factors that will help you *Prioritize Hypotheses.* The complexity and difficulty of the clinical presentation and any time constraint for managing the client are also important in some situations.

any previous accidents or injuries. An x-ray confirms a right nondisplaced metaphyseal ulnar fracture.

In this example, the child has an acute injury and signs of previous injuries, possibly from abuse. The desired outcomes would include that the child:
- States that pain is no more than a 2–3 on a 0 to 10 pain intensity scale
- Does not experience neurovascular compromise in the right arm
- Has decreased swelling of the right arm
- Will experience healing of bilateral knee abrasions without infection
- Is safe at home (no neglect or abuse) with the birth parent or other family/significant other

The next skill in this thinking process is to generate multiple potential nursing actions that could achieve the desired outcomes for the priority client need(s). Also identify which actions would be avoided or are not indicated. To develop a list of actions for this pediatric client, you need knowledge of child development, fracture treatment, child abuse, and pain management.

Potential nursing actions may focus on additional assessments, such as collecting additional information about the client. For instance, the nurse would likely want to interview the birth parent to obtain information about the old bruising and scarring observed on the child's chest and thighs. Other potential actions that could help achieve the desired outcomes in this clinical situation include:
- States that pain is no more than a 2–3 on a 0 to 10 pain intensity scale
  - Administer nonopioid pain medication; avoid opioids if possible.
  - Provide distraction for the child, such as an iPad or gaming device.
  - Reassure the child that analgesics will be available as needed after discharge.
- Does not experience neurovascular compromise in the right arm
  - Assist in applying a right synthetic forearm cast.
  - Monitor the child's right arm neurovascular status after cast application.
- Has decreased swelling of the right arm
  - Apply an ice pack to the arm outside the cast, and teach the child about the need to use ice for the next 24 hours.
  - Teach the child to keep the arm elevated as much as possible.
- Will experience healing of bilateral knee abrasions without infection
  - Cleanse both knees to remove debris and dirt.
  - Apply triple antibiotic ointment on open areas, and cover with clean gauze.
  - Apply topical lidocaine to knees to decrease pain.
- Is safe at home (no neglect or abuse) with the birth parent or other family/significant other
  - Communicate concern about the child's safety to the primary health care provider.
  - Consult with the social worker about the child's potential safety risk, family situation, and possible change in placement.
  - Report potential child abuse to Child Protective Services (CPS).

After the list of potential actions has been identified for each desired outcome, determine which actions should be implemented to meet the priority needs of the client in the *Take Actions* process.

Take Actions

Deciding which actions to implement is the focus of this clinical judgment skill. After generating a list of possible actions, determine the most appropriate action or combination of actions to resolve or manage the client's priority health conditions. Also determine how each action will be implemented. Examples of methods to accomplish or implement nursing actions include what to communicate, document, perform, administer, teach, or request from a primary health care provider or other member of the health care team.

For example, in the pediatric clinical presentation described in the previous section on *Generate Solutions,* you might request a consultation with the social worker to interview the birth parent about the child's injuries and home situation. Social workers are

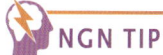
THINKING SPACE

NGN TIP

Remember: To *Generate Solutions* to meet a client's priority needs, determine the client's desired or expected outcomes first.

experts in interviewing and addressing family situations, and they can determine if the child's injuries are potentially consistent with abuse.

When deciding on how to implement nursing actions, avoid memorized textbook methods or procedures. Instead, consider the elements of the clinical situation to determine which approach to use. For example, teaching the birth parent about the care of the child after discharge would be appropriate for most situations. However, in the pediatric clinical example, you might *not* want to teach the birth parent about home care after discharge from the ED until it is determined whether the child will go home with the birth parent. If abuse is suspected, the child would be removed from the current family situation.

> **NGN TIP**
>
> **Remember:** When deciding to *Take Actions,* avoid memorized textbook methods and procedures; instead, customize your action to meet the needs of the client in the clinical presentation.

Evaluate Outcomes

The last clinical judgment thinking skill is to determine if the interventions implemented for the client resolved or effectively managed the health condition(s). The best way to make that determination is to compare what the desired or expected outcomes are with current client findings or observed outcomes. Ask yourself, "Which assessment findings/signs and symptoms indicate that the client's condition has improved?" "Which findings indicate that the client's condition has not improved or worsened?"

For example, consider this clinical situation:

A 78-year-old client has been hospitalized for 6 days for exacerbation of chronic heart failure. On admission, the client was placed on supplemental oxygen and IV furosemide for peripheral edema and impending pulmonary edema. The physician adjusted the client's cardiac medications and restricted salt intake (no added table salt). The nurse preparing for the client's discharge performs a head-to-toe assessment to determine the effectiveness of heart failure management. The nurse documents the following client findings:

- *Lungs clear with no adventitious breath sounds*
- *No shortness of breath when walking short distances*
- *Lost 5 lb (2.3 kg) during hospital stay*
- *Bilateral ankle and foot edema decreased from 3+ to 1+*
- *States planning to continue using table salt at home*

In this example, all of the client findings at the time of discharge demonstrate that the actions used to manage heart failure were effective because the client is improving. However, the client plans to continue using table salt at home, which could contribute to another exacerbation of heart failure. The nurse may need to reinforce teaching about the relationship of sodium to fluid retention.

> **NGN TIP**
>
> **Remember:** To *Evaluate Outcomes,* compare desired or expected client outcomes with current observed outcomes.

How Are the Six Clinical Judgment Skills Measured on Today's NCLEX®?

The current NCLEX® is composed of traditional test item types and NGN test item types. The total number of test items ranges between 85 and 150 total questions. The six NCJMM cognitive skills introduced in this chapter are measured through use of a variety of test items that are embedded into two types of case studies—the Unfolding Case Study and the Stand-Alone item. Both types of cases present a clinical scenario and include part of a medical record similar to the record shown in Fig. 1.1. Additional medical record tabs may be included as the client presentation requires.

The *Unfolding Case Study* presents the client over time through several phases of care. It is often referred to as the NGN Case Study. The time between phases can be minutes, hours, or even days. The client may initially be evaluated in an ED, acute care hospital, clinic, school, or urgent care center. As the clinical presentation changes, or "unfolds," test items require that the candidate use the information in the current phase of the client's care to answer each question. All nursing candidates have three NGN Unfolding Case Studies with six questions each. Each of the six questions represents one of the clinical judgment cognitive skills discussed earlier.

The nurse is caring for an 87-year-old client in the Urgent Care Center.

| History and Physical | Nurses' Notes | Orders | Laboratory Results |

2010: Brought to Urgent Care by family with report of extreme fatigue, shortness of breath, and worsening cough over the past 2 days. Client alert & oriented × 1 (person only). Family states client's mind is usually very sharp. Bilateral lower lobe crackles. Diffuse chest pain, especially when moving. S_1 and S_2 heart sounds present; no murmurs or gallops. Abdomen soft and round; BS present in all 4 quadrants. Able to move all extremities. Cap refill <3 sec bilaterally. VS: T 100.2°F (37.9°C); HR 104 and irregular; RR 24; BP 122/78; SpO_2 89% on RA.

FIG. 1.1 An example of medical record tabs that present client information.

The *Stand-Alone item*, sometimes referred to as the Stand-Alone clinical judgment item, presents a client at one point in time and includes one of the NGN test item types. Each item measures one or more of the six clinical judgment cognitive skills. Nursing candidates have varying numbers of Stand-Alone items, depending on the candidate's ability in taking the exam.

How Can You Prepare for Today's NCLEX®?

One of the best ways to prepare for today's NCLEX®, especially the NGN items, is to practice multiple test questions in the Unfolding Case Study and Stand-Alone item formats. NGN practice questions are located at the end of Chapters 3 through 8 of this book. Chapter 9 illustrates Stand-Alone and Unfolding Case Studies with appropriate NGN test items. Chapter 10 is a comprehensive NGN Practice Test that includes questions in all specialty areas. Answers, rationales, test-taking strategies, specialty content areas, priority concepts, clinical judgment cognitive skill(s), and references are available for all sample and practice questions in this book.

In addition to the questions in this book, multiple Stand-Alone items and Unfolding Case Studies with accompanying questions are available for your practice on the Elsevier Evolve site. Categories for selection of questions on Evolve include Content Area, Priority Concepts, and Clinical Judgment Cognitive Skill.

In addition to using this book, other resources such as the *Developing Clinical Judgment* workbooks written by one of this book's authors (D.D.I.) provide thinking exercises to help you master the six cognitive skills to make appropriate clinical judgments. If you need help with basic NCLEX® test-taking strategies and want beginning practice with NGN test items, two of this book's authors (L.A.S. and A.E.S.) created a book entitled *Clinical Judgment and Test-Taking Strategies.* All of these books are included in the NGN Resource list at the end of this book.

Now that you have been introduced to the six cognitive skills needed to make appropriate clinical judgments, you are ready to learn about the specific NGN test item types. The next chapter describes and illustrates examples of these test items.

CHAPTER 2

Introduction to the NGN and the NGN Test Item Types

⚡ THINKING SPACE

The six clinical judgment cognitive (thinking) skills introduced in Chapter 1 are measured on the current NCLEX® (also called the Next-Generation NCLEX® [NGN]) through test item formats that are embedded into two types of clinical scenarios—the Unfolding Case Study and the Stand-Alone item. Both scenarios present common, realistic clinical situations that new graduates will likely encounter. As mentioned in Chapter 1, client data for each test item are presented as part of a medical record under selected tabs such as:

- Orders
- Nurses' Notes
- Progress Notes
- Laboratory Results
- Diagnostic Results
- Vital Signs
- History and Physical
- Nursing Flow Sheet

This chapter describes the item types that are part of the Unfolding Case Studies and the two Stand-Alone items. An example of each item type is presented, and correct responses are provided with brief rationales. Multiple examples of all item types, each with a detailed Rationale, Test-Taking Strategy, Content Area, Priority Concepts, Cognitive Skill(s), and Reference, are presented in later chapters of this book.

Most NGN items are scored using partial credit rather than being completely correct or incorrect. This means that for most NGN items, you will receive credit for any correct responses but will not receive credit for incorrect responses.

> **NGN TIP**
>
> **Remember:** Client data presented in the NGN test item formats are part of a medical record. Be sure to read all information presented about the client.

> **NGN TIP**
>
> **Remember:** Expect each unfolding case on the NGN to present client data that change over time (minutes, hours, days) and six NGN test items, each measuring one of the six clinical judgment cognitive skills.

⚡ Test Item Types Used for Unfolding Case Studies

The Unfolding Case Study, also known as the NGN Case Study, begins with a client presentation and the initial data describing the clinical situation. The client either is experiencing or is at risk for an urgent or emergent health condition resulting from clinical deterioration or a medical complication. As the clinical scenario unfolds or evolves, the client's condition changes over time through several phases of care. Six NGN test items are included as part of each Unfolding Case Study.

Twelve test item types are integrated into the Unfolding Case Studies as part of the current NCLEX®. Table 2.1 organizes these item types by major category. The item types that may be included in Unfolding Case Studies are described in the following sections.

Matrix/Grid Test Items

The two types of Matrix/Grid test items include the Matrix Multiple Choice and Matrix Multiple Response. Both types are structured in a tabular format with at least four rows and three columns.

TABLE 2.1 NGN Test Item Types Used for Unfolding Case Studies

NGN Test Item Category	NGN Test Item Type in Each Category
Matrix/Grid	Matrix Multiple Choice Matrix Multiple Response
Multiple Response	Multiple Response Select All That Apply Multiple Response Select N Multiple Response Grouping
Drop-Down	Drop-Down Cloze Drop-Down Rationale Drop-Down In Table
Drag-and-Drop	Drag-and-Drop Cloze Drag-and-Drop Rationale
Highlight	Highlight-In-Text Highlight-In-Table

THINKING SPACE

Matrix Multiple Choice Test Item

For a Matrix Multiple Choice test item, you would select *only one response for each row,* as shown in the example in Sample Question 2.1. This example item measures the clinical judgment cognitive skill of *Evaluate Outcomes.*

Sample Question 2.1 — Example of a Matrix Multiple Choice Test Item

The nurse is caring for a 70-year-old client in the acute orthopedic unit.

Nurses' Notes

0745: Client preparing for discharge today after having a cemented right total knee arthroplasty (TKA) and is preparing to go home with a daughter. Reviewed discharge instructions with client and provided written copy to both client and daughter.

For each client statement, select whether the statement indicates understanding or no understanding of the health teaching provided.

Client Statement	Understanding	No Understanding
"I'll call my surgeon if my incision gets red or has drainage."	☒	☐
"I can stop taking my blood thinner when I get home."	☐	☒
"I'll have physical therapy for about a week."	☐	☒
"I'm allowed to bear weight as tolerated on my right leg."	☒	☐
"I can probably drive in a few months."	☒	☐

Rationale: As indicated in the test item, the client's statements that are not correct and show that the client does not understand the health teaching include: "I can stop taking my blood thinner when I get home," and "I'll have physical therapy for about a week." Clients who have total joint arthroplasty (especially knee and hip) are at a high risk for venous thromboembolism—DVT or PE. To help prevent these problems, the client is prescribed an oral anticoagulant, which is typically continued for 10 days to several weeks after surgery and should be taken after the client is discharged from the acute care unit. The client would call the surgeon if the incision becomes red and/or has drainage because these symptoms indicate possible infection.

After surgery, most clients have 3 to 6 weeks of physical therapy depending on the type of prothesis and the client's overall health and tolerance. The surgical joint is often stiff, painful, and swollen, which limits the client's range of motion; however, weight bearing to tolerance helps promote ambulation and increase muscle strength. Physical therapy plus exercises that clients practice every day help improve joint function and independence. The client will be allowed to drive when muscle strength and joint mobility improve. Driving is difficult until the surgical knee is able to flex more than 90 degrees. This goal may not be achieved for 6 to 8 weeks or more after surgery.

Matrix Multiple Response Test Item

By contrast, the Matrix Multiple Response test item asks you to select one or more responses for each row of the presented table. Sample Question 2.2 shows an example of this type of item to measure the clinical judgment cognitive skill of *Analyze Cues*.

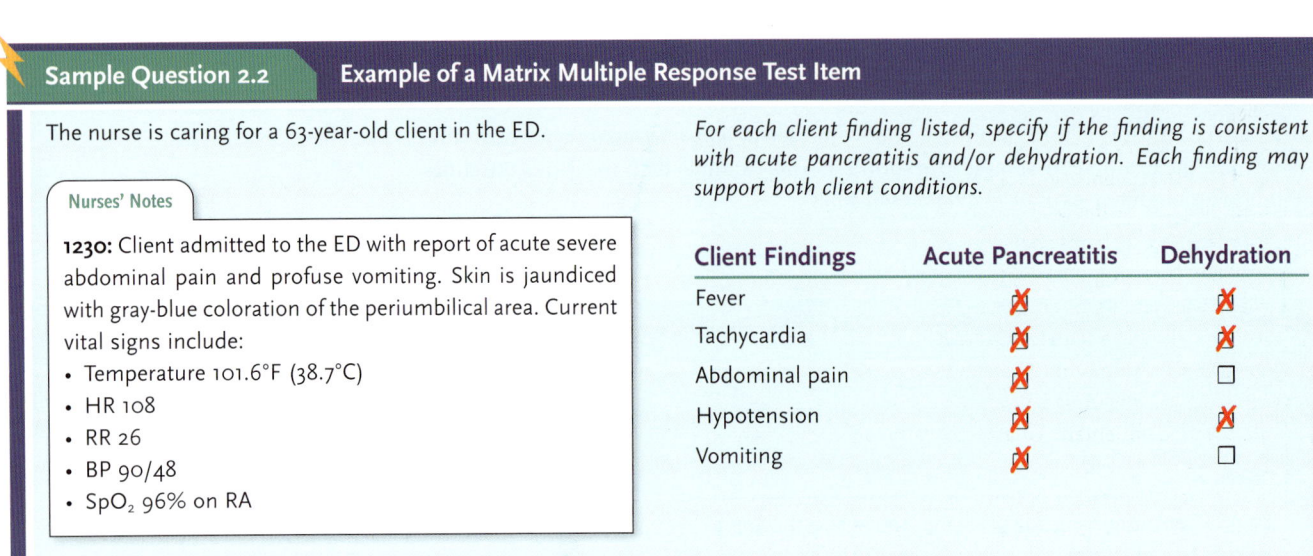

Sample Question 2.2 — Example of a Matrix Multiple Response Test Item

The nurse is caring for a 63-year-old client in the ED.

Nurses' Notes

1230: Client admitted to the ED with report of acute severe abdominal pain and profuse vomiting. Skin is jaundiced with gray-blue coloration of the periumbilical area. Current vital signs include:
- Temperature 101.6°F (38.7°C)
- HR 108
- RR 26
- BP 90/48
- SpO$_2$ 96% on RA

For each client finding listed, specify if the finding is consistent with acute pancreatitis and/or dehydration. Each finding may support both client conditions.

Client Findings	Acute Pancreatitis	Dehydration
Fever	X	X
Tachycardia	X	X
Abdominal pain	X	☐
Hypotension	X	X
Vomiting	X	☐

Rationale: The client has classic signs and symptoms of acute pancreatitis, including an acute onset of severe abdominal pain, nausea and vomiting, and gray-blue coloration of the abdomen, especially around the umbilical area. Vomiting can cause dehydration but is not a symptom of dehydration. The client's vital signs reveal fever, tachycardia, and hypotension, which are common in clients with pancreatitis. These vital sign changes are also common in clients who are dehydrated.

Multiple Response Test Items

Multiple Response test items have been a large part of the NCLEX® for many years. Traditional items present a short clinical scenario with five or six options. The correct response(s) could be one, some, or all options (see Box 1.2 in Chapter 1 for an example). Since the implementation of the NGN, there are three variations of the traditional Multiple Response test item:
- Multiple Response Select All That Apply
- Multiple Response Select N
- Multiple Response Grouping

Multiple Response Select All That Apply Test Item

The format for the Multiple Response Select All That Apply test item that is part of the Unfolding Case Studies is similar to the traditional NCLEX® format. However, the item has at least 5 choices and no more than 10 choices. The correct response could be one, some, or all options (see Sample Question 2.3). This example measures the clinical judgment cognitive skill of *Analyze Cues*.

Sample Question 2.3 — **Example of a Multiple Response Select All That Apply Test Item**

The nurse is caring for an 81-year-old client in an acute care medical unit.

Nurses' Notes

1430: Admitted to acute care unit from an assisted-living facility with a low-grade fever and acute confusion. The client's family tells the admitting nurse that the client had a stroke 2 years ago that resulted in left hemiparesis and urinary incontinence; the client has been in the assisted-living facility for the past 5 months. Client has a long history of type 2 diabetes mellitus (DM), which has been well controlled. During the visit today, the family noted that the client was lethargic, confused, and unable to ambulate with a walker like usual. POC testing in the ED indicated the presence of multiple bacteria in the client's urine and FSBG of 581 mg/dL (32.3 mmol/L). Currently the client is alert and disoriented. Unable to carry on conversation. Skin warm and dry; mucous membranes dry. Breath sounds clear throughout lung fields with no adventitious sounds. S_1 and S_2 present and irregular. Able to move all extremities. Cap refill >3 sec. Peripheral pulses present. VS: T 100.8°F (38.2°C); HR 102; RR 22; BP 88/46; SpO$_2$ 91% on RA.

Which of the following conditions does the client **most likely** have at this time? **Select all that apply.**

- ☒ Urosepsis
- ☒ Delirium
- ☒ Dehydration
- ☐ Diabetic ketoacidosis
- ☐ Transient ischemic attack
- ☒ Hyperglycemic hyperosmolar syndrome

Rationale: This test item asks you to *Analyze Cues* based on relevant client findings that require immediate follow-up. The findings indicate that the client could have a urinary tract infection (UTI) as evidenced by multiple bacteria in the urine. Fever, acute confusion, and a low BP suggest that the client is dehydrated. Acute confusion is also known as *delirium,* a common assessment finding in older clients who have dehydration. Because the client has type 2 diabetes, the client also is likely experiencing a diabetic complication called *hyperglycemic hyperosmolar syndrome.* The client's elevated blood glucose and dehydration are consistent with a hyperglycemic hyperosmolar state.

THINKING SPACE

Multiple Response Select N Test Item

The Multiple Response Select N test item is similar to the Multiple Response Select All That Apply item, except that the number of required correct responses is specified in the question. This test item also has at least five options but no more than 10 options from which to choose. Sample Question 2.4 shows an example of this type of item to measure the clinical judgment cognitive skill of *Recognize Cues* for an adult client who has new onset of signs and symptoms.

Sample Question 2.4 — Example of a Multiple Response Select N Test Item

The nurse is caring for a 52-year-old female client in the ED.

Nurses' Notes

2205: Admitted to ED with report of acute onset dyspnea and back pain that started about an hour ago. The client's medical history includes type 2 diabetes mellitus (DM), obesity, hypertension, hypercholesteremia, and asthma. Client is alert and oriented × 4. Skin warm and dry. Occasional inspiratory wheezes heard throughout lung fields. S_1 and S_2 present and irregular. Able to move all extremities. Cap refill <3 sec. Peripheral pulses present. VS: T 98.8°F (37.1°C); HR 78; RR 26; BP 148/90; SpO_2 92% on RA.

*Select the **5** client findings that require **immediate** follow-up.*

- ☒ Dyspnea
- ☒ Back pain
- ☐ Temperature
- ☐ History of obesity
- ☐ History of diabetes
- ☒ Tachypnea
- ☐ Occasional inspiratory wheezes
- ☒ Elevated BP
- ☒ SpO_2

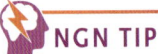

NGN TIP

Remember: When reviewing client findings to *Recognize Cues*, first determine what is most relevant for that particular client in the clinical situation. Organize these findings to determine which data are consistent with specific client conditions to *Analyze Cues*.

⚡ THINKING SPACE

Rationale: The client's new assessment findings include dyspnea and back pain, which could indicate a potentially life-threatening myocardial infarction (MI) that could be life-threatening. Female clients with an MI often present with findings that differ from those in males, including having back or jaw pain. The client's RR and BP are both elevated and need immediate follow-up, but the temperature is normal. The peripheral oxygen saturation level is below the expected level of 95% for a middle-aged client. This finding combined with dyspnea could be life-threatening because the heart may not be adequately perfusing due to lack of oxygen. Occasional wheezes are expected in a client with a history of asthma. The medical history may help explain or predict the current client condition, but it is not relevant at this time for planning nursing care.

Other examples of stems for Multiple Response Select N test items with the associated cognitive skills being measured include:

- Select the **2** priority health conditions that the client is experiencing. *Prioritize Hypotheses*
- Select the **4** actions that the nurse would take at this time for the client. *Take Actions*
- Select the **5** findings that indicate the client is improving. *Evaluate Outcomes*

Multiple Response Grouping Test Item

The Multiple Response Grouping test item is similar to the Multiple Response Select All That Apply item except that the options are presented in categories or by group in a table with a minimum of two columns and three rows. Each category, often a body system, has two to four options per row and requires selection of at least one response option. Sample Question 2.5 shows an example of this type of item to measure the clinical judgment cognitive skill of *Take Actions*.

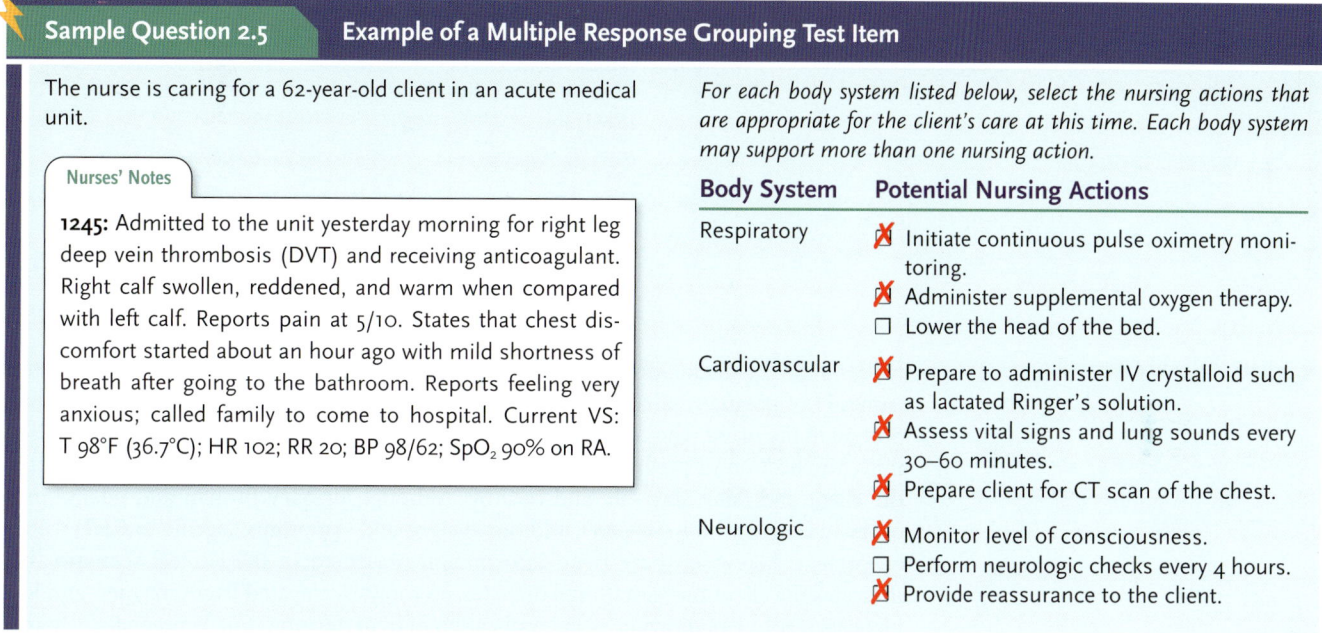

Rationale: The client has shortness of breath and a low SpO$_2$ for which the nurse would raise the head of the client's bed (not lower it) and immediately start oxygen therapy. The client's blood pressure is low, causing the heart rate to increase. An IV crystalloid-like lactated Ringer's solution would help increase blood volume and the client's blood pressure. If the BP continues to decrease, a vasopressor such as dobutamine may be ordered. VS and lung sounds are monitored frequently (every 30 to 60 minutes), and the client needs to be prepared for a chest CT scan or CT angiogram to confirm a possible pulmonary embolus (PE). Although the nurse does not need to perform a neurologic assessment every 4 hours, the client's LOC should be monitored due to a decreasing blood pressure and possible hemoptysis (cough with blood-streaked sputum) that can occur in some clients who have a PE.

> **NGN TIP**
>
> **Remember:** When selecting which nursing actions are appropriate for a client in a specific clinical scenario, consider the independent and collaborative interventions to manage the priority client condition.

Drop-Down Test Items

For any Drop-Down test item, you will need to click on the word [Select] to access the options for a fill-in-the-blank item to complete the sentence(s). For the NGN, there are three variations of the Drop-Down test item:
- Drop-Down Cloze
- Drop-Down Rationale
- Drop-Down in Table

⚡THINKING SPACE

Drop-Down Cloze Test Item

The Drop-Down Cloze and Drop-Down Rationale test items are very similar. Both variations present a sentence with blanks that you will need to fill in with options provided for each blank. The Drop-Down Cloze item has a minimum of one sentence and a maximum of three sentences with one or more drop-down menus per sentence. Sample Question 2.6 shows an example of this type of item to measure the clinical judgment cognitive skills of *Analyze Cues* and *Prioritize Hypotheses* for a pregnant client.

Sample Question 2.6 — Example of Drop-Down Cloze Test Item

The nurse is caring for a 28-year-old client in the OB clinic.

Nurses' Notes

1550: 32-week pregnant client in for monthly OB visit. Reports having several mild to moderate headaches during the past week. Gained 10 lb (4.5 kg) since last visit 4 weeks ago. States baby is very active, especially at night; FHR 146. VS: T 99°F (37.2°C); HR 92 and regular; RR 20; BP 150/92; SpO_2 94% on RA. Urine protein 1+. 2+ pitting edema in both feet and ankles.

Complete the following sentences by selecting from the lists of options provided.

The nurse reviews the assessment findings and recognizes that the client *most likely* has **preeclampsia**. The *priority* for this client's care is to **ensure maternal and fetal safety**.

Options for 1	Options for 2
Chronic kidney disease (CKD)	Admit the client to the hospital
Gestational diabetes	Ensure maternal and fetal safety
Preeclampsia	Restrict the client's fluid intake
HELLP syndrome	Place the client on a special diet

THINKING SPACE

Rationale: The client most likely has preeclampsia because the client is in the third trimester of pregnancy, has an elevated BP, has dependent pitting edema, and is spilling protein in the urine. The client has also had several headaches, which could be related to this complication of pregnancy. The most important desired outcome is to ensure that the client and baby stay safe and healthy. Although urinary protein and edema may occur in clients who have CKD, additional signs and symptoms specific to CKD would be present. Likewise, there is no information presented in the clinical scenario that indicates the client has gestational diabetes. Hemolysis, elevated liver enzymes, and low platelets (HELLP) syndrome is a complication of hypertension during pregnancy. In this condition, HELLP develops before the 37th week of pregnancy but can occur shortly after the baby is delivered. There are no assessment findings that support the client has a HELLP problem.

Drop-Down Rationale Test Item

The Drop-Down Rationale test item also uses a cloze (fill-in-the-blank) format in a cause-and-effect sentence. Using the clinical scenario and client data from the Drop-Down Cloze item in Sample Question 2.6, Sample Question 2.7 shows an example of this type of item to measure the clinical judgment cognitive skill of *Analyze Cues*.

Sample Question 2.7 — Example of a Drop-Down Rationale Test Item

The nurse is caring for a 28-year-old client in the OB clinic.

Nurses' Notes

1550: 32-week pregnant client in for monthly OB visit. Reports having several mild to moderate headaches during the past week. Gained 10 lb (4.5 kg) since last visit 4 weeks ago. States baby is very active, especially at night; FHR 146. VS: T 99°F (37.2°C); HR 92 and regular; RR 20; BP 150/92; SpO_2 94% on RA. Urine protein 1+. 2+ pitting edema in both feet and ankles.

Complete the following sentence by selecting from the lists of options provided.

The nurse reviews the assessment data and determines that the client *most likely* has **preeclampsia** as evidenced by **hypertension and proteinuria**.

Options for 1	Options for 2
CKD	Pitting edema and weight gain
Gestational diabetes	Hypertension and proteinuria
Preeclampsia	Fever and headaches
HELLP syndrome	Fetal heart rate and SpO_2

Rationale: The client most likely has preeclampsia because the client is spilling protein in the urine and has an elevated BP. Having severe headaches would also be significant, but the headaches are mild to moderate, which is not significant for a pregnant client unless the client is developing additional visual changes. Having pitting edema does not necessarily indicate that the client is preeclamptic, but it can occur in clients with this complication. The fetal heart rate is within normal limits, and the client does not have a fever or tachycardia. Although the SpO_2 is slightly below 95%, the client or fetus does not have any known respiratory distress, and this finding is not a criterion for preeclampsia. Although urinary protein and edema may occur in clients who have CKD, additional signs and symptoms specific to CKD would be present. Likewise, there is no information presented in the clinical scenario that indicates the client has gestational diabetes. Hemolysis, elevated liver enzymes, and low platelets (HELLP) syndrome is a complication of hypertension during pregnancy. In this condition, HELLP develops before the 37th week of pregnancy but can occur shortly after the baby is delivered. There are no assessment findings that support the client has a HELLP problem.

Drop-Down in Table Item

The Drop-Down in Table test item provides categories of options from which you would need to select. These options are often grouped by body system. Sample Question 2.8 shows an example of this type of item to measure the clinical judgment cognitive skill of *Generate Solutions*.

▶ THINKING SPACE

Sample Question 2.8 — Example of a Drop-Down in Table Test Item

The nurse is caring for an 18-year-old client in the Urgent Care Center.

Nurses' Notes

1740: Family accompanying client who has a long history of eating disorder, major depressive disorder, asthma, and severe anxiety. Started college this semester and living on campus with roommate. Reports having frequent episodes of palpitations, weakness, and intermittent abdominal pain currently described as 3/10. Denies chest pain. Fainted yesterday while having drinks with friends; fell and hit the back of the head. Has had increased issues with memory and attention over the past 24 hours; reports headache as dull and persistent since the fall; pain at 4/10. Alert and oriented × 4. PERRLA. Skin and hair very dry; wears a wig due to alopecia. Old right thigh dressing for cuts made 3 days ago; states that cuts are seeping and burning. Old cutting scars on left thigh and both upper arms. Lungs clear throughout; no adventitious or abnormal breath sounds. S_1 and S_2 present and irregular. Abdomen slightly distended; exaggerated bony prominences. Able to move all extremities; muscle wasting present. Peripheral pulses present; pedal pulses 1+ bilaterally. Cap refill <3 sec. Current weight 98 lb (44.5 kg); height 5 ft. 7 in. (1.7 m); BMI 15.3. VS: T 99°F (37.2°C); HR 102; RR 22; BP 86/44; SpO_2 95% on RA.

The nurse is planning care for the client. Complete the following table by selecting one potential nursing action for each body system from the lists of options provided.

Body System	Potential Nursing Actions
Cardiovascular	Draw labs for electrolytes
Neurologic	Request a head CT scan
Integumentary	Assess right thigh wounds

Options for 1	Options for 2	Options for 3
Draw labs for electrolytes	Perform hourly neuro checks	Assess right thigh wounds
Start continuous cardiac monitoring	Request a head CT scan	Initiate antibiotic therapy
Prepare client for cardiac ablation procedure	Administer analgesic for headache	Apply new right thigh dressing

Rationale: The client has a history of an eating disorder and a very low BMI, indicating an inadequate intake of vital nutrients. The client's tachycardia, weakness, and palpitations suggest the client may have fluid and/or electrolyte imbalances that would be confirmed by stat labs. Because the client denies chest pain and there is no indication that the client had a baseline ECG, continuous cardiac monitoring is not indicated at this time but may be needed later. There is no indication that the client needs a cardiac ablation. While the client's neurologic status needs to be monitored, an hourly assessment is not needed because the client is alert and oriented × 4, has PERRLA, and can move all extremities. Because the client hit the back of the head and has one known episode of syncope, a head CT scan is needed to determine if the client has a traumatic brain injury (TBI), a potentially life-threatening condition. An analgesic should not be given until the TBI is ruled out. The client's recent cuts should be assessed for healing and possible infection. Although a new dressing may need to be applied, this action is not more important than the wound assessment. If the client has an infection, then treatment would be indicated.

Drag-and-Drop Test Items

Drag-and-Drop test items are similar to traditional NCLEX® Drag-and-Drop/Ordered Response items in that you will need to click on several options and move them to complete one or more sentences. At least two types of NGN test items use this format: the Drag-and-Drop Cloze item and the Drag-and-Drop Rationale item.

Drag-and-Drop Cloze Test Item

The Drag-and-Drop Cloze test item is very similar to the Drop-Down Cloze item. Instead of clicking on the blanks to obtain a drop-down selection of options, you will need to click on the correct responses to move them into the blanks to complete one or more sentences. Sample Question 2.9 shows an example of this type of item to measure the clinical judgment cognitive skill of *Analyze Cues*.

Sample Question 2.9 — Example of a Drag-and-Drop Cloze Test Item

The nurse is caring for a 17-year-old client in the ED.

Nurses' Notes | **Laboratory Results**

2330: Client brought to ED by friends stating client drank more than 8 beers and multiple "shots" at a party earlier this evening. Client started shaking and having difficulty breathing. Currently very drowsy but able to arouse. Oriented to self and place. Unable to follow conversation at times. Breath sounds clear in all lung fields; no adventitious or abnormal breath sounds; S_1 and S_2 present and regular. Abdomen soft and round; bowel sounds present × 4. Moves all extremities slowly. Peripheral reflexes diminished. Skin cyanotic and clammy. VS: T 97.2°F (36.2°C); HR 52 and irregular; RR 10 and irregular; BP 82/45; SpO_2 87% on RA.

0015: Stat lab results reviewed; physician aware.

Nurses' Notes | **Laboratory Results**

Laboratory Test and Reference Range	0015
Blood alcohol level (BAL) 0.31 g/dL (310 mg/dL) (0.0 g/dL)	0.31 g/dL (310 mg/dL)
Blood glucose (74–106 mg/dL [4.1–5.9 mmol/L])	50 mg/dL (2.8 mmol/L)
Sodium (136–145 mEq/L [136–145 mmol/L])	129 mEq/L (129 mmol/L)
Potassium (3.5–5.0 mEq/L [3.5–5.0 mmol/L])	3.3 mEq/L (3.3 mmol/L)

Complete the following sentence by selecting from the list of word choices below.

The nurse recognizes that the client is **most likely** experiencing <u>alcohol intoxication</u>.

Word Choices

Alcohol use relapse
Wernicke-Korsakoff syndrome
Substance withdrawal syndrome
Alcohol intoxication

Rationale: The client's findings are consistent with rapid alcohol intoxication, sometimes called *alcohol poisoning*. A client who has a BAL of over 0.08 g/dL is usually identified as having alcohol intoxication; this client's BAL is 0.31 g/dL. At this high level of blood alcohol, the client would be expected to experience nausea and vomiting, memory blackouts, and decreased vital sign values. The client is not experiencing findings associated with withdrawal, such as delirium tremens (DTs), nausea, and headache. It is not known whether the client has a history of alcohol or other substance use. Clients who have Wernicke-Korsakoff syndrome are often comatose or severely confused. This client is drowsy but arousable at this time.

THINKING SPACE

Drag-and-Drop Rationale Item

The Drag-and-Drop Rationale test item is very similar to the Drop-Down Rationale item in that this item also uses a cloze format in a cause-and-effect sentence. Instead of clicking on the blank to obtain a drop-down selection of options, you will need to click on the correct responses in the list of word choices to move them to the blanks to complete the sentence. The sentence may have two blanks (dyad) or three blanks (triad) to complete. Sample Question 2.10 shows an example of this type of item to measure the clinical judgment cognitive skill of *Prioritize Hypotheses*.

Sample Question 2.10 — **Example of a Drag-and-Drop Rationale Test Item**

The nurse is caring for an 18-year-old client in the Urgent Care Center.

Nurses' Notes

1740: Family accompanying client who has a long history of eating disorder, major depressive disorder, asthma, and severe anxiety. Started college this semester and living on campus with roommate. Reports having frequent episodes of palpitations, weakness, and intermittent abdominal pain currently described as 3/10. Denies chest pain. Fainted yesterday while having drinks with friends; fell and hit the back of the head. Has had increased issues with memory and attention over the past week; reports headache as dull and persistent since the fall at 4/10. Alert and oriented × 4. PERRLA. Skin and hair very dry; wears a wig due to alopecia. Old right thigh dressing for cuts made 3 days ago; states that cuts are seeping and burning. Old cutting scars on left thigh and both upper arms. Lungs clear throughout; no adventitious or abnormal breath sounds. S1 and S2 present and irregular. Abdomen slightly distended; exaggerated bony prominences. Able to move all extremities; muscle wasting present. Peripheral pulses present; pedal pulses 1+ bilaterally. Cap refill <3 sec. Current weight 98 lb (44.5 kg); height 5 ft 7 in. (1.7 m); BMI 15.3. VS: T 99°F (37.2°C); HR 102; RR 22; BP 86/44; SpO$_2$ 95% on RA.

Complete the following sentence by selecting from the list of word choices below.

The **priority** need at this time is to manage the client's <u>traumatic brain injury</u> that resulted from <u>falling</u>.

Word Choices

Suicidal ideation
Wound infection
Traumatic brain injury
Cutting
Falling

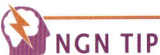

NGN TIP

Remember: When answering either a Drag-Down Rationale or Drag-and-Drop Rationale test item that measures *Analyze Cues* or *Prioritize Hypotheses*, be sure that the client condition that you select is supported by the client findings presented in the clinical scenario in a cause-and-effect relationship.

Rationale: The client has several actual and potential health conditions that need to be further evaluated and managed. However, the client's fall caused a headache that is rated at a 4/10 on a 0 to 10 pain intensity scale as well as memory/attention issues. As a result of the fall, the client likely has a traumatic brain injury, which is a potentially life-threatening condition. The client stated that the right thigh wound is draining, but it is not known whether or not the wound is infected. The client's skin cutting is not life-threatening, therefore it is not the priority for care. The client does not have a fever, therefore it is unlikely that the client has a systemic infection. There is no indication that the client is experiencing suicidal ideation.

Highlight Test Items

Highlight test items require you to identify information in the clinical scenario to answer the question by highlighting the correct responses with the computer mouse or, in a print product, with a marker. This type of item is used most often to measure the clinical judgment cognitive skill of either *Recognize Cues* or *Evaluate Outcomes*. The two variations of this test item are the Highlight-in-Text and Highlight-in-Table items.

Highlight-in-Text Test Item

As discussed earlier for the NGN test items, clinical scenarios are presented as part of a client's medical record under tabs such as Nurses' Notes or Health History. This information provides client assessment data, referred to as *client findings*. Highlight test items ask you to identify the client findings that require immediate follow up *or* to identify findings that indicate effectiveness of nursing care. Sample Question 2.11 shows an example of this type of item to measure the clinical judgment cognitive skill of *Recognize Cues*.

Sample Question 2.11 — **Example of a Highlight-in-Text Test Item**

The nurse is caring for a 31-year-old client in the ED.

*Highlight the findings that require **immediate** follow-up.*

Nurses' Notes

0040: Client with a history of type 1 diabetes mellitus (DM) admitted with ==nausea and vomiting, diaphoresis, and headache==. Has been working out on home gym equipment, but worked out longer than usual with extra-heavy weights late tonight. Started ==feeling "light-headed"== about an hour ago and checked FSBG, which was 62 mg/dL (3.4 mmol/L). Drank a glass of fruit juice, but FSBG decreased to 46 mg/dL (2.8 mmol/L). Began feeling nauseated and vomited several times, which prompted a call to 911. Wondering if constipation for the past week is contributing to these problems. Had COVID-19 4 weeks ago and has been very fatigued since that time. Lungs clear throughout, and bowel sounds present × 4. Stat blood work shows current blood glucose is ==50 mg/dL (2.8 mmol/L)==. VS: T 98.4°F (36.9°C); HR 89; ==RR 28==; ==BP 146/88==. IV fluids started; given one dose of ondansetron at 0120.

Rationale: The client has DM type 1, indicating that the client is taking insulin for glucose control. The client began having symptoms that indicate the client's blood glucose was too low, including nausea and vomiting, diaphoresis, light-headedness, and headache. The client tested the FSBG to confirm the hypoglycemia. These findings prompted the ED nurse to perform a stat lab draw to confirm the low blood glucose level, which was 50 mg/dL (2.8 mmol/L). Vital signs are within normal limits except for BP and respirations, which are elevated. Any of these relevant client findings could become life-threatening and need immediate follow-up. The client's concern about constipation is not important at this time and could be addressed later. The remaining assessment data are within normal limits and expected.

THINKING SPACE

Highlight-in-Table Test Item

The second variation of the Highlight test item is the Highlight-in-Table test item. For this item type, you may be asked to highlight the client findings affecting selected body systems that require immediate follow up. Or, you may be asked to highlight the laboratory results that require immediate follow up. Sample Question 2.12 shows an example of this type of item to measure the clinical judgment cognitive skill of *Recognize Cues*.

Sample Question 2.12 — Example of a Highlight-in-Table Test Item

The nurse is caring for a 28-year-old client in the trauma unit.

Highlight the findings that require **immediate** follow-up.

Nursing Flow Sheet

Time	0815
Vital Signs	T 98.1°F (36.7°C); HR 96; RR 14, BP 178/72; SpO$_2$ 98% on mechanical ventilation
Neurologic	PERRLA; unable to follow commands; intubated and sedated with propofol and fentanyl
Cardiac	S$_1$ and S$_2$ present; normal sinus rhythm; cap refill <3 sec; ==bounding pulses present in all extremities==; 1+ nonpitting edema in both feet
Pulmonary	==Fine crackles in both lung bases== #7.5 ETT secured at 20 cm; Ventilator Settings: Assist Control, Rate 14, Fio$_2$ 50%, PEEP 9 cm H$_2$O
Gastrointestinal	Bowel sounds active × 4
Genitourinary	Indwelling urinary catheter
Integumentary	Skin warm and dry; ecchymosis and massive bruising on face, chest, and back from previous physical assault Central venous access device (CVAD) in right jugular vein
I&O	Intake since 0400: • IV fluids 500 mL Output since 0400: • ==Urine: 50 mL== • Characteristics: ==cloudy, no odor, cola-colored== • Bowel: none

THINKING SPACE

Rationale: The client has high blood pressure with oliguria (scant urine) less than 30 mL/h and evidence of fluid volume excess, including bounding pulses, crackles in both lung bases, and pitting edema. These client findings are potentially life-threatening and may affect electrolyte levels, therefore they require immediate follow-up by the nurse. Cola-colored urine could indicate hematuria from possible internal bleeding resulting from the physical assault. All other client findings are within normal parameters except for the heart rate, which is 100 and meets the definition of tachycardia. However, the client's pain level from the assault could have increased the heart rate and would be monitored; the heart rate is not at a life-threatening level at this time.

Test Item Types Used for Stand-Alone Test Items

As described in Chapter 1, Stand-Alone test items present a client situation with assessment data similar to that in the first phase of an Unfolding Case Study. However, the client's condition does not change or evolve over time unless data are presented in a trend format. The two types of Stand-Alone items on the current NCLEX® are the Bow-tie test item and the Trend test item. Both items can measure more than one or more clinical judgment cognitive skills.

Bow-tie Test Item

The Bow-tie test item provides a clinical scenario that includes client data at one point in time. The correct responses to the item are placed into three parts of a "figure" that looks like a bow-tie or butterfly using drag-and-drop technology. A Bow-tie test item measures all six clinical judgment cognitive skills (see Sample Question 2.13).

> **NGN TIP**
>
> **Remember:** To answer a Bow-tie item, first identify relevant data and organize the data to determine the client's condition. Then review the choices under Potential Conditions, and select the one that best matches your analysis. After selecting or dragging the client condition into the middle section of the Bow-tie figure, decide on the Nursing Actions that would be appropriate to manage the client condition and the Parameters that a nurse would need to monitor to determine if those actions were effective.

Sample Question 2.13 — Example of a Bow-tie Test Item

The nurse is caring for a 25-year-old client in the postpartum unit.

Nurses' Notes

0810: Surgical Day. G1P1 had full-term cesarean section 4 hours ago. Alert and oriented × 4. Breath sounds clear throughout lung fields; no adventitious sounds. S_1 and S_2 present and regular. Abdomen tender with firm fundus at umbilicus; bowel sounds present but faint × 4. Reports surgical pain at 4/10. Small amount of lochia on pad. Taking fluids without nausea or vomiting. Abdominal dressing dry and intact. Urinary catheter draining large amount of clear, light-yellow urine. SCDs in place. VS: T 98.6°F (37°C); HR 77; RR 16; BP 110/60; SpO_2 97% on RA. History of obesity and gestational diabetes mellitus (DM). Current FSBG 123 mg/dL (6.8 mmol/L).

1025: Client reports feeling short of breath with chest discomfort. Feels like heart is beating "extra fast." Crying and does not want to talk with lactation specialist or have baby now. VS: T 99.2°F (37.3°C); HR 114; RR 24; BP 132/88; SpO_2 92% on RA. Client assisted into upright position, and Rapid Response initiated.

Complete the diagram by identifying from the choices below to specify what potential condition the client is likely experiencing, **2** nursing actions that are appropriate to take, and **2** parameters the nurse would monitor to assess the client's progress.

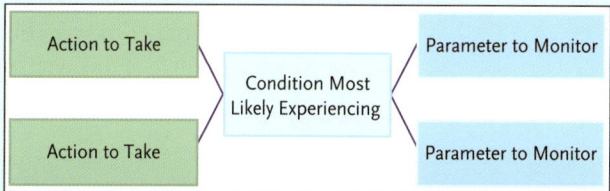

Actions to Take	Potential Conditions	Parameters to Monitor
Perform an electrocardiogram (ECG)	Stable angina	Urinary output
Prepare client for pulmonary imaging studies	Pulmonary embolism	Pain level
Monitor vital signs every 4 hours	Postpartum hemorrhage	SpO_2
Initiate supplemental oxygen therapy	Diabetic ketoacidosis (DKA)	Blood glucose
Administer fast-acting insulin		Vital signs

Answer

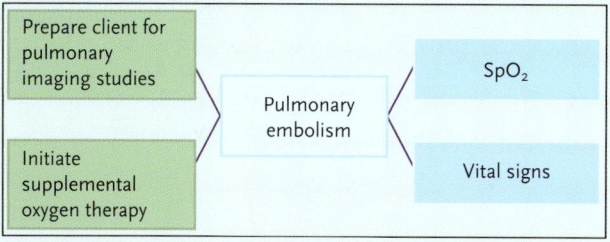

Rationale: Clients who give birth, especially via cesarean section, are at higher risk for venous thromboembolism (VTE) (deep vein thrombosis and pulmonary embolism [PE]) when compared with those who did not recently give birth. PE typically manifests with sudden-onset chest pain and dyspnea. Although the client has a slightly elevated blood glucose level, there is no indication of DKA. Therefore IV insulin is not necessary at this time. The client's chest pain and dyspnea when resting might indicate unstable angina, but most clients with *stable angina* do not have dyspnea or shortness of breath. Therefore an ECG is not indicated at this time. Once the diagnosis of PE is confirmed by imaging studies, such as pulmonary angiography and V/Q scan, the nurse would anticipate administering an anticoagulant to prevent the clot(s) from becoming larger, and oxygen to manage the client's dyspnea. Vital signs should be monitored more often than every 4 hours, usually every 30 to 60 minutes. To ensure that the treatment is effective, the nurse would monitor the client's SpO$_2$ levels via pulse oximetry as well as vital signs. Pain level would not be the most important parameter to monitor because it is more subjective than vital signs. Monitoring urinary output or blood glucose is not helpful to determine the progress of a PE.

Trend Test Item

Similar to the Bow-tie item, the Trend test item begins with a client situation that includes assessment data. These findings, however, include multiple data points over time in the clinical scenario, such as vital signs, I&O, lab values, and Nurses' Notes entries. The test question for this type of item may be any of the 12 item types used for the Unfolding Case Studies as described earlier in this chapter. The trend test item can measure one or more of the six clinical judgment cognitive skills. Sample Question 2.14 shows an example of this type of item.

Sample Question 2.14 — Example of a Trend Test Item

The nurse is caring for a 14-year-old client admitted to the 23-hour Observation Unit.

Vital Signs | **Nurses' Notes**

Vital Signs	1900	0100	0700 (current)
Temperature	100° F/37.8°C	100.8° F/38.2°C	101.6° F/38.7°C
HR	82	90	94
RR	16	18	16
BP	112/74	96/58	100/64

Vital Signs | **Nurses' Notes**

1900: Admitted with moderate abdominal pain (6/10) that started early this morning. Reports nausea with no appetite since yesterday, and vomited twice this morning. Bowel sounds present × 4; abdomen soft and slightly distended. Awaiting results of abdominal x-ray and ultrasound. IV of 5%D/0.45%NS infusing via left forearm catheter at 100 mL/h. Maintaining NPO. Given IV antiemetic.

0100: Imaging studies show excessive intestinal gas and enlarged appendix with inflammation. Resident on call notified. Increased IV rate to 125 mL/h. Lab called for stat results of CMP. Potassium and sodium slightly decreased; other labs WNL. Bowel sounds present × 4; abdomen more distended than at 1900. States pain is increasing to 8/10. Placed in a sitting position. No additional vomiting episodes.

0700: Surgical resident in to examine client. IV continuing to infuse at 125 mL/h. Remains NPO. Temperature increased. States nausea is improving.

The nurse consults with the surgical resident about the client's plan of care. Which of the following orders would the nurse anticipate? Select all that apply.

- ☐ Obtain informed consent.
- ☒ Prepare client for surgery.
- ☐ Place a nasogastric tube and clamp.
- ☐ Type and crossmatch for 2 units of packed RBCs.
- ☒ Administer IV antibiotic 1 hour prior to surgery.
- ☒ Change IV to lactated Ringer's solution at 125 mL/h.

Rationale: According to imaging studies, the client has appendicitis and requires an appendectomy to remove the inflamed appendix before it could possibly rupture and cause peritonitis. The surgeon or surgical resident (not the nurse) is responsible for explaining the surgical procedure and potential complications, including death, and obtaining informed consent from the parents in this case. The nurse prepares the client for surgery by reinforcing health teaching and completing the preoperative checklist. The IV solution likely needs to be changed to lactated Ringer's solution because this isotonic solution is used to maintain or increase blood volume for clients who have or are at risk for low BP. An IV antibiotic may be given either an hour before surgery or at the surgical opening in the OR. Because the client has not had additional vomiting and will likely have laparoscopic surgery, the nasogastric tube is not necessary. There is no information indicating that the client will need a transfusion of 2 units of packed RBCs.

NGN TIP

Remember: Before answering a Trend test item, review all information presented and determine the significance of changes in assessment data across time. The test question for this type of item may be any of the 12 types used for the Unfolding Case Studies.

CHAPTER 3

Strategies for Answering NGN Questions: Recognize Cues

Recognize Cues is a CJ cognitive skill needed for nurses to make safe, appropriate clinical judgments. When clinical deterioration or a major change in a client's condition is not recognized, death or permanent disability from a complication of illness or lack of care can result. This event is referred to as "failure to rescue." Clients most at risk for clinical deterioration or major condition change include:
- Clients who had recent surgeries
- Clients who are emergently admitted to acute care
- Clients with acute or preexisting health conditions
- Clients recovering from critical conditions

Preventing negative outcomes when a client clinically worsens is crucial and requires that nurses have keen observation and thinking skills. Therefore being able to *Recognize Cues* is an essential skill to ensure client safety and quality of care and is measured both on the NGN and by your instructors on course exams.

What Are Cues?

As discussed in Chapter 1, *cues* are client findings or assessment data that provide information for nurses as a basis for making clinical judgments. Table 3.1 lists common sources and examples of client findings that may be presented as part of an NGN clinical scenario.

How Are Client Findings (Cues) Presented in an NGN Clinical Scenario?

Unfolding Case Studies on the NGN begin with a clinical scenario that could be presented in several ways. To make the scenario as realistic as possible, client findings are displayed as part of a medical record similar to the accompanying figure.

History and Physical

Admitting Problem: LUQ abdominal pain with rectal bleeding

History of Present Illness: Last week this 72-year-old widow residing in an independent living senior center began noticing bright red blood on tissue after having a BM. Since then, the client has had bright red blood in the toilet every time the client defecates. Yesterday the client also started having LUQ abdominal pain, which worsens during the night. Admitted through the ED.

Current Medications:
- Acetaminophen 650 mg orally every 4–6 hours PRN for joint pain
- Metoprolol XL 100 mg orally every morning for hypertension
- Calcium carbonate 1000 mg chewable tabs twice each day for osteopenia
- Clopidogrel 75 mg orally every day for atrial fibrillation

TABLE 3.1 Common Sources and Examples of Client Assessment Findings

Sources of Client Findings	Examples of Client Findings
History data provided by client or family	History of past and present illness, family history, medications, surgeries, allergies
Physical assessment findings	VS, breath sounds, heart sounds, pain level
Behavioral findings	Alcohol use, tobacco use, illicit drug use, mental health status
Laboratory test results	Basic metabolic panel (BMP), complete blood count (CBC)
Imaging test results	X-rays, MRI, CT scan impressions

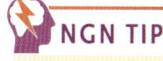

NGN TIP

Remember: Relevant client findings make a significant difference in achieving optimum outcomes for the client and help determine the nurse's priority for client care.

NGN test items that measure the ability to *Recognize Cues* require you to distinguish between which presented client findings are *relevant* (cues that are directly related to client outcomes or priority of care) and *not relevant* (cues that are *not* directly related to client outcomes or priority of care).

Which Client Findings Are Relevant?

When determining which client findings are relevant, you'll need to *first* consider if they are within the normal or usual parameters you learned from your nursing textbooks. Then recall that clients are individuals whose baseline findings can vary depending on many diverse factors, including age, race, ethnicity, and culture. For instance, consider the client findings in the following clinical scenario.

The nurse is caring for a 91-year-old client in the ED.

THINKING SPACE

> **Nurses' Notes**
>
> **1540:** Client brought by EMS to the ED after falling at home. The client's family explains to the nurse that the client has "always been stubborn by insisting on doing everything independently." While the family went out to buy groceries, the client climbed onto a stepstool to reach something in a cabinet over the refrigerator. Client apparently lost balance and was found on the kitchen floor. Alert and oriented × 2 (person and place); reports pain at 10/10. Whimpering and holding right hip. Right leg and foot externally rotated; right leg shorter than left leg. Cap refill >3 sec in both feet. VS: T 96.8°F (36°C); HR 90 and regular; RR 22; BP 142/88; SpO$_2$ 92% on RA.

In this clinical scenario, the findings that are *not* within the usual or normal range for most adults include:

- Temperature = 96.8°F (36°C)
- Respirations = 22
- BP = 142/88
- SpO$_2$ = 92% (on RA)
- Alert and oriented × 2 (person and place)
- States that pain is 10/10
- Whimpering and holding right hip
- Right leg and foot externally rotated
- Right leg shorter than left leg
- Capillary refill >3 sec in both feet

Although each of these findings is not within the usual or normal range for most adults and *could be* relevant, a body temperature of 96.8°F (36°C) is *expected* for older adults as a normal physiologic change associated with aging. So, for *this* client, a low body temperature is *not relevant* in this clinical situation. Another expected finding for any healthy adult is being alert and oriented × 4 (person, place, time, and situation). However, this client is oriented to only person and place. After a fall with injury for an older adult, it would be *expected* that the client might be disoriented, especially considering the amount of pain

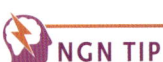

THINKING SPACE

being experienced. Therefore the deficit in two parameters for orientation (time and situation) is likely *not* relevant or of immediate concern to the nurse at this time.

Another example of an abnormal but expected finding for this client is the BP of 142/88, which is above the recommended normal range for adults. This elevation in BP could be relevant. However, this client is an older adult who is in severe pain owing to trauma from a fall, so the BP elevation is likely *not relevant*. As you may recall, when clients are in severe pain, they experience a sympathetic nervous system response. As a result, BP and HR increase. If the client's pain is effectively managed, the BP may return to a normal level or to the client's baseline.

The client's RR is slightly elevated (22), and the SpO_2 is slightly low at 92%. However, the client is in severe pain, so these data are probably not relevant in this clinical situation. An individual's oxygen saturation level tends to decrease with advanced age, so 92% may be expected and likely not relevant for this client who is apparently not in respiratory distress. Because older adults usually have arteriosclerosis as a physiologic change of aging, it would also be expected that the client would have decreased distal perfusion and a capillary refill of greater than 3 seconds.

The most *relevant abnormal* data are related to the client's trauma resulting from the fall. These data include:

- States that pain is 10/10
- Whimpering and holding the right hip
- Right leg and foot externally rotated
- Right leg shorter than left leg

The CJ cognitive skill of *Recognize Cues* requires you to not only select relevant client findings, but also involves deciding which relevant findings are of *immediate* concern and *most* important to the nurse based on the clinical situation. This step determines how well you can identify client findings that must be followed up and managed immediately to prevent potential or actual life-threatening complications.

Which Relevant Client Findings Require Immediate Follow-Up?

In some clinical scenarios, client findings may be relevant, but not of *immediate* concern or important at this time. For example, the nurse assessing a child who sustains multiple traumatic injuries after a motor vehicle accident would need to follow up immediately on possible internal organ damage and hemorrhage. The child's history of well-controlled DM type 1 would be relevant for later in the client's plan of care, but it would *not* require immediate follow-up.

What Types of Clinical Scenarios May Be Included on the NGN?

As mentioned in Chapter 2, most NCLEX-RN® and NCLEX-PN® test items are traditional multiple choice and multiple response and present a short clinical scenario with only the essential information needed to answer the item. However, as also described in Chapter 2, the clinical scenarios for newer NGN test items are lengthier than scenarios for the traditional NCLEX® items and usually require multiple answers rather than just one. Most importantly, NGN items present realistic and comprehensive clinical scenarios that nurses are likely to encounter as new graduates. Box 3.1 provides examples of common clinical conditions requiring the ability to *Recognize Cues*.

Which NGN Item Types Optimally Measure *Recognize Cues*?

Many NGN test item types may be used to measure the CJ cognitive skill of *Recognize Cues*. The best item types for measuring this skill are listed in Table 3.2.

Examples of these item types that best measure *Recognize Cues* are presented in this chapter.

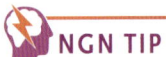

NGN TIP

Remember: When recognizing cues, do not interpret or analyze what is causing the client's findings or what nursing care may be required as a result.

NGN TIP

Remember: Use these strategies for NGN items that measure *Recognize Cues*:

1. Decide if each assessment finding is normal/usual or abnormal for the presented client.
2. If the client finding is abnormal, determine if it is expected in the clinical scenario; if the client finding is *expected*, it is likely *not relevant*. If the client finding is abnormal and *not expected*, it is likely *relevant* in the clinical scenario.
3. Decide which relevant client findings are most important and require immediate follow-up for the client in the clinical scenario.
4. For each client finding, ask yourself: Is this finding life-threatening or potentially life-threatening? If so, the finding is likely relevant and requires immediate follow-up.

BOX 3.1 Examples of Common Clinical Conditions Requiring the Ability to Recognize Cues

- Dysrhythmias
- Myocardial infarction (MI)
- Acute heart failure
- Respiratory compromise
- Pneumonia
- Gastrointestinal bleeding
- Intestinal obstruction/perforation
- Bleeding, hypotension, hypovolemia, shock
- Stroke
- VTE (DVT and PE)
- Infection, sepsis, septic shock
- Arterial occlusion
- Acute kidney injury (AKI)
- Compartment syndrome
- Abdominal trauma
- Chest trauma
- Fluid and electrolyte imbalances
- Mental health crisis/suicidal ideation
- Eating disorders
- Complications of pregnancy

TABLE 3.2 Test Items That Optimally Measure *Recognize Cues*

NGN Test Item Category	NGN Test Item Type in Each Category
Matrix/Grid	Matrix Multiple Choice
Multiple Response	Multiple Response Select All That Apply Multiple Response Select N Multiple Response Grouping
Drop-Down	Drop-Down Cloze Drop-Down Rationale Drop-Down In Table
Drag-and-Drop	Drag-and-Drop Cloze Drag-and-Drop Rationale
Highlight	Highlight-In-Text Highlight-In-Table

THINKING SPACE

Highlight Test Items to Measure *Recognize Cues*

Highlight test items provide a clinical scenario in text or table format with multiple client findings. When this item type is used to measure *Recognize Cues,* the test taker is required to highlight the relevant findings that require immediate follow-up by the nurse. The two variations of the Highlight test item are the Highlight-in-Text and Highlight-in-Table test items. Sample Question 3.1 illustrates a Highlight-in-Text item for an adolescent clinical scenario. The rationale and test-taking strategy to help you derive the correct responses in Sample Question 3.1 are also provided.

Sample Question 3.1 — **Highlight-in-Text:** *Recognize Cues*

The nurse is caring for a 16-year-old client in the acute behavioral health unit.

*Highlight the findings that require **immediate** follow-up.*

Nurses' Notes

1100: Alert and oriented x 4. <mark>Cut self last night (as the client has done previously)</mark> and doesn't understand the reason for inpatient admission. <mark>Client has been very depressed and was "planning to take parent's Xanax to help ease the emotional pain."</mark> Recognizes that family loves the client and is very supportive. Client's partner broke off a long-term relationship recently because the client is "too fat." As a result, <mark>client increased binge eating and purging to lose weight.</mark> Height 68 in. (173 cm); weight 108 lb (49 kg). BMI 16.4. Left upper thigh dressing in place with old bloody drainage. VS: T 98°F (36.7°C); HR 88; RR 18; BP 122/74.

▸ **THINKING SPACE**

Rationale: The client is a teenager who participates in cutting and was planning to use the family's antianxiety medication to manage emotional pain. The nurse would want to immediately follow up on the client's self-mutilation behaviors and whether the client is suicidal or has suicidal tendencies now to ensure safety. The client perceives self as too fat, although the client's BMI is 16.4, below the desired level, and *expected* for clients with eating disorders. As a result, the client binge eats and then purges, which is a major concern for the nurse owing to potentially life-threatening risks for inadequate nutrition and fluid and electrolyte imbalances. The nurse would want to collect more data about how long these eating behaviors have occurred and what previous body weights have been. The thigh dressing with old blood is expected because the client has been cutting. This finding is also not concerning at this time because there is no active or new bleeding. VS are within normal range.

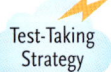

Test-Taking Strategy: Remember to first identify normal/usual or abnormal and expected (not relevant), and abnormal and not expected (relevant) client findings to determine which findings require immediate follow-up by the nurse. The client's findings can be categorized as shown in the table.

Client Findings	Abnormal and Not Expected (Relevant) and Requiring Immediate Follow-up	Normal/Usual or Abnormal but Expected (Not Relevant) and Not Requiring Immediate Follow-up
Alert and oriented × 4	☐	☒
Cut self	☒	☐
Depressed and "planning to take parent's Xanax"	☒	☐
Parents loving and supportive	☐	☒
Loss of long-term relationship	☐	☒
Thinks partner ended relationship because client is too fat	☐	☒
Increased binging and purging	☒	☐
Underweight for height	☐	☒
Thigh dressing with old bloody drainage (from cutting)	☐	☒
VS: T 98°F (36.7°C); HR 88; RR 18; BP 122/74	☐	☒

Recall that although adolescents often have a poor self-image and self-esteem if they are rejected by their peers, it is *not* normal/usual or expected for them to self-mutilate, binge and purge, and take psychoactive drugs to manage their stress. For this clinical scenario, then, all of the relevant client findings require immediate follow-up by the nurse, with most being unhealthy coping behaviors that can cause self-harm and potentially life-threatening conditions.

Content Area: Mental Health Nursing
Priority Concepts: Mood and Affect; Tissue Integrity
Reference(s): Halter, 2022, pp. 247–254, 342–344, 483–484

Drop-Down Test Items to Measure *Recognize Cues*

Drop-Down test items can be used to measure multiple cognitive skills needed to make clinical judgments, including *Recognize Cues*. Variations for Drop-Down items include the Drop-Down Cloze and Drop-Down Rationale items. For both variations, you need to select the correct response from a list of options provided for each empty blank in one to three sentences. Sample Question 3.2 presents a test item using the Drop-Down Cloze item to assess whether you are able to identify the relevant client findings that are of immediate concern to the nurse. The rationale and test-taking strategy to help you derive the correct responses in Sample Question 3.2 are also provided.

Sample Question 3.2 — Drop-Down Cloze: *Recognize Cues*

The nurse is caring for a 58-year-old client in the surgeon's office.

Nurses' Notes

0915: Follow-up postoperative visit today following right total knee arthroplasty 3 weeks ago. Alert and oriented × 4. Breath sounds clear throughout lung fields; denies dyspnea or chest pain. Using walker, but has not started outpatient PT due to lack of transportation. Has difficulty using stairs, but apartment is on first floor with ramp into building. Right knee incision open about 1/2 inch. (1.2 cm); draining thick yellowish purulent exudate. Erythema around incision extending approximately 1 inch. (2.5 cm). Client states that the incision "popped open" last week, which the client covered with gauze; knee pain ranges from 5–6/10. VS: T 100.6°F (38.1°C); HR 100; RR 20; BP 132/86; SpO$_2$ 95% on RA.

Complete the following sentence by selecting from the lists of options provided.

The client findings that require **immediate** follow-up are <u>yellowish purulent incisional drainage</u>, <u>T 100.6°F (38.1°C)</u>, and <u>erythema around incision</u>.

Options for 1	Options for 2	Options for 3
RR 20	T 100.6°F (38.1°C)	SpO$_2$ 95%
BP 132/86	HR 100	Difficulty using stairs
Yellowish purulent incisional drainage	5–6/10 knee pain	Erythema around incision

---

THINKING SPACE

Rationale: The client's incision is not healing as expected because it is open about ½ inch (1.2 cm) and draining yellowish purulent exudate. The incision should be closed and dry. An open wound could become or be infected, which could be life-threatening if the infection does not remain localized. Therefore these findings need immediate follow-up by the health care team. In addition, erythema extends beyond the incision, and the client has a low-grade fever. These findings require immediate follow-up because the client could be experiencing a systemic condition rather than a localized one that is confined to the incision. Although the client's heart rate is 100, it does not meet the definition of tachycardia which is a heart rate greater than 100. The client's BP is slightly elevated but not at a life-threatening or potentially life-threatening level. The elevation could be caused by anxiety, fever, or pain. Knee pain is also not life-threatening and does not require immediate follow-up. Although the client has not yet started PT, the client is able to ambulate with a walker and is able to get out of the apartment as needed using the ramp instead of the steps. The respiratory rate and peripheral oxygen saturation level (SpO$_2$) are within normal parameters.

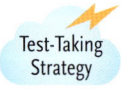

Test-Taking Strategy: Remember to first identify normal/usual or abnormal and expected (not relevant), and abnormal and not expected (relevant) client findings to determine which findings require immediate follow-up by the nurse. The client's findings can be categorized as shown in the table.

Client Findings	Abnormal and Not Expected (Relevant) and Requiring Immediate Follow-Up	Normal/Usual or Abnormal but Expected (Not Relevant) and Not Requiring Immediate Follow-Up
RR 20	☐	☒
BP 132/86	☐	☒
Yellowish purulent incisional drainage	☒	☐
T 100.6°F (38.1°C)	☒	☐
HR 100	☐	☒
5–6/10 knee pain	☐	☒
SpO$_2$ 95%	☐	☒
Difficulty using stairs	☐	☒
Erythema around incision	☒	☐

Next, review the findings that are abnormal and not expected for this particular client. These client findings are the significant cues in this clinical scenario and provide the correct responses to this test item measuring *Recognize Cues*.

Content Area: Foundations of Care
Priority Concepts: Tissue Integrity; Infection
Reference(s): Potter et al., pp. 460–461

Multiple Response Test Items to Measure *Recognize Cues*

Three variations of the Multiple Response test item can be used to measure any of the six CJ cognitive skills: Multiple Response Select All That Apply, Multiple Response Select N, and Multiple Response Grouping. When this type of item is used to measure *Recognize Cues,* a clinical scenario describing a client with multiple client findings is presented. Then these findings are listed in the test item, where you will be asked to select the relevant choices that require immediate follow up in the scenario. Sample Question 3.3 illustrates a Multiple Response Select N item. With this type of item, you are asked to select a specific number of choices. The rationale and test-taking strategy to help you derive the correct responses in Sample Question 3.3 are also provided.

Sample Question 3.3 — Multiple Response Select N: *Recognize Cues*

The nurse is caring for a 75-year-old client in the ED.

Nurses' Notes

2030: Brought to ED by community volunteer after finding long-time unhoused client lying in alley behind a dumpster. Client drowsy, moaning, and unable to answer questions or follow commands. Unable to assess client's orientation. Volunteer shares that client is a veteran; has history of substance use disorder (primarily heavy alcohol use) and hypertension, but does not regularly take prescribed antihypertensive drugs. Client known to ED; no history of diabetes mellitus. PERRLA, slightly sluggish. Breath smells of alcohol. Crackles heard in bilateral lung bases; chest barrel-shaped. S_1 and S_2 present; no abnormal cardiac sounds. Abdomen soft and round; BS present × 4. Peripheral pulses 2+ except in right foot. No right pedal pulse via Doppler ultrasound. Right leg extremely pale, mottled, and cooler than left leg. VS: T 97.6°F (36.4°C); HR 60 and regular; RR 14; BP 194/98; SpO_2 94% on RA.

*Select the **3** findings that require **immediate** follow-up.*

- ☐ Drowsiness
- ☐ Alcohol use
- ☐ Crackles in lung bases
- ☒ BP 194/98
- ☐ HR 60 and regular
- ☐ SpO_2 94% on RA
- ☒ Absent right pedal pulse
- ☒ Pale, cool, mottled right leg
- ☐ Unable to follow commands

THINKING SPACE

Rationale: The client is drowsy and unable to follow commands or answer questions. This level of consciousness is expected due to heavy alcohol use and would not require immediate follow-up. However, the nurse would monitor for changes in neurologic status for possible worsening of the client's condition. Crackles in the client's lung bases would also not require immediate follow-up because this adventitious breath sound is often heard in clients who have a barrel-shaped chest as a result of possible COPD. The client's SpO_2 is slightly below the expected range of 95% or higher. However, the client is older and is not experiencing respiratory distress. Older adults often have an SpO_2 between 90% and 94% without any respiratory compromise. The client's pulse is within the normal range (60–100) and regular, therefore the nurse would not need to follow up on this finding but would continue to monitor the client's vital signs. However, the client's blood pressure is very high, which could cause a stroke or other acute hypertensive complication. The nurse would immediately follow up on the client's elevated blood pressure because it could be potentially life-threatening. The findings related to the client's right leg are very concerning because the leg is pale, cool, and mottled with an absent pedal pulse. These findings require immediate follow-up because they indicate inadequate peripheral perfusion, which could lead to damage to or loss of the client's leg.

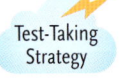

Test-Taking Strategy: Remember to first identify normal/usual or abnormal and expected (not relevant), and abnormal and not expected (relevant) client findings to determine which findings require immediate follow-up by the nurse. The client's findings can be categorized as shown in the table.

CHAPTER 3 Strategies for Answering NGN Questions: Recognize Cues

Client Findings	Abnormal and Not Expected (Relevant) and Requiring Immediate Follow-Up	Normal/Usual or Abnormal but Expected (Not Relevant) and Not Requiring Immediate Follow-Up
Drowsiness	☐	☒
Alcohol use	☐	☒
Crackles in lung bases	☐	☒
BP 194/98	☒	☐
HR 60 and regular	☐	☒
SpO$_2$ 94% on RA	☐	☒
Absent right pedal pulse	☒	☐
Pale, cool, mottled right leg	☒	☐
Unable to follow commands	☐	☒

Next, review the findings that are abnormal and not expected for this particular client. These client findings are the significant cues in this clinical scenario and provide the correct responses to this test item measuring *Recognize Cues*.

Content Area: Medical-Surgical Nursing
Priority Concepts: Perfusion; Clotting
Reference(s): Ignatavicius et al., 2024, p. 743

Drag-and-Drop Test Items to Measure *Recognize Cues*

As described in Chapter 2, Drag-and-Drop test items have at least two variations: Drag-and-Drop Cloze and Drag-and-Drop Rationale. These items are similar to Drop-Down items, except for a computerized exam you would use a mouse to drag the correct responses from a list of word choices and place them in the empty blanks in one or two sentences. A test item using the Drag-and-Drop Cloze item can assess whether you are able to identify the relevant client findings that require immediate follow-up by the nurse (Sample Question 3.4).

Sample Question 3.4 — Drag-and-Drop Cloze: *Recognize Cues*

The nurse is caring for a 10-month-old infant in the pediatrician's office.

Nurses' Notes

1010: Grandparent brought baby to see the doctor because infant refused to eat or drink anything last night or this morning; vomited × 2. States that baby seems feverish with no interest in play; has had a cold with a "runny" nose and diarrhea for the past few days. Has a history of frequent upper respiratory infections. Grandparent is the baby's guardian because the infant's birthing parent is a drug addict and lives with life partner. States having to put the baby in day care last week because of going back to work to support the family. Blames self that the baby may have gotten sick from day care. Infant's current axillary temperature 103°F (39.4°C).

Complete the following sentence by selecting from the list of word choices below.

The client findings that require **immediate** follow-up are the client **had vomiting × 2**, **has diarrhea**, **has an axillary temperature of 103°F (39.4°C)**, and **refuses to eat or drink**.

Word Choices

Had vomiting × 2
Attends day care
Has diarrhea
Has a cold with a "runny" nose
Has an axillary temperature of 103°F (39.4°C)
Refuses to eat or drink
Has history of frequent upper respiratory infections

Rationale: Infants and children have a greater need for water and are very vulnerable to fluid and electrolyte imbalances. When compared with adults, infants have a lower fluid volume, therefore any loss of fluids can rapidly lead to dehydration. This infant presents with factors and assessment findings that increase the client's risk for dehydration. First, the infant lost fluid (and electrolytes) through vomiting and diarrhea. Second, the infant refuses to eat or drink, so fluids that were lost are not being replaced. The infant's temperature is elevated, which supports possible dehydration. Dehydration can lead to hypovolemic shock and if not treated could be life-threatening. These client findings require immediate follow-up. Although attending day care places the infant at risk for infections, this finding is not of immediate concern. The infant's history of frequent respiratory infections, including a current cold with "runny" nose, is of interest but does not require immediate follow up.

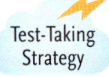

Test-Taking Strategy: The infant presents with multiple findings, including those that are consistent with possible dehydration. Dehydration in an infant can be rapidly life-threatening. Therefore client findings that support or are risk factors for dehydration would be of immediate concern to the nurse and require immediate follow-up. Use the table to determine which client findings are possibly associated with dehydration and require immediate follow-up.

Client Findings	Possibly Associated with Dehydration: Yes or No?
Had vomiting × 2	Yes
Attends day care	No
Has diarrhea	Yes
Has a cold with a "runny" nose	No
Has an axillary temperature = 103°F (39.4°C)	Yes
Refuses to eat or drink	Yes
Has history of frequent upper respiratory infections	No

Once you have competed the table, select the options in the test item for the client findings for which you responded "Yes."

Content Area: Pediatric Nursing
Priority Concepts: Fluid and Electrolyte Balance; Infection
Reference(s): Hockenberry et al., 2024, pp. 742–747

Practice Questions

Practice Question 3.1 — Multiple Response Grouping

The nurse is caring for a newborn who was born 10 minutes ago.

Nurses' Notes

1025: 35-week-old baby born via cesarean section. Weight 4.4 lb (2000 g); length 19 in. (48.3 cm). Newborn crying with limp body posture and arms and legs very relaxed. Deep reflexes diminished and skin mottled. Intermittent expiratory grunting with occasional apneic episodes and fine crackles throughout lung fields bilaterally. VS: T 96.7°F (35.9°C) axillary; HR 132 and regular; RR 54; BP 68/40. Systolic murmur heard; changes intensity when newborn moves.

For each body system listed below, select the newborn findings that require **immediate** follow-up. Each body system may support more than one relevant newborn finding.

Body Systems	Newborn Findings
Respiratory	☐ RR 54
	☐ Intermittent expiratory grunting
	☐ Fine crackles
	☐ Occasional apneic episodes
Neuromuscular	☐ Arms and legs relaxed
	☐ Crying
	☐ Limp body posture
	☐ Diminished deep reflexes
Cardiovascular/Metabolic	☐ Skin mottled
	☐ Axillary temperature 96.7°F (35.9°C)
	☐ HR 132 and regular
	☐ Presence of systolic murmur

Practice Question 3.2 — Highlight-in-Text

The nurse is caring for a 20-year-old client in the college campus health care clinic.

Highlight the findings that require **immediate** follow-up.

Nurses' Notes

1355: Client came to clinic with report of shakiness, unusual sweating, nausea, and vomiting. Is concerned about getting sick with "stomach flu" or STI during "finals week." Attended a fraternity party 3 nights ago where food and alcohol were consumed. Had "sex" for first time with college football player after the party. Nausea and vomiting started this morning but has worsened with shakiness and diaphoresis. Alert and oriented × 4. Medical history of asthma since early childhood, meningitis last year, and COVID-19 twice in the past 2 years. Most recently was diagnosed with diabetes mellitus type 1, which has been controlled by insulin and intermittent glucose monitoring. Skin cool and clammy. Breath sounds clear throughout lung fields. S_1 and S_2 present. Abdomen soft and round; BS × 4. Peripheral pulses 2+ and strong. VS: T 97.8°F (36.6°C); HR 92 and regular; RR 18; BP 106/50; SpO_2 98% on RA; FSBG 52 mg/dL (2.9 mmol/L) (Reference range 74–106 mg/dL (4.1–5.9 mmol/L).

Practice Question 3.3 — Drag-and-Drop Cloze

The nurse is caring for a 78-year-old client who was hospitalized for evacuation of a subdural hematoma.

Nurses' Notes

0730: Very drowsy this morning but can be aroused with gentle shaking. Remains oriented × 4. Does not readily respond when spoken to, but eventually answers in 1 to 2 words. Immediately after surgery a week ago, the client was alert and oriented, communicative, and continent of bowel and bladder. No adventitious or diminished breath sounds. S$_1$ and S$_2$ present; no additional heart sounds. BS hyperactive × 4 and abdomen slightly distended. Had 2 incontinent diarrheal stools during the night. Able to move all extremities, but right arm continues to be weak. Skin intact; no reddened areas noted. Plan to send to PT and OT this morning. Temperature increased from 98°F (36.7°C) last evening to 100.2°F (37.9°C) currently.

Complete the following sentence by selecting from the word choices below.

The nurse determines that the client findings that require *immediate* follow-up are [Word Choice], [Word Choice], [Word Choice], and [Word Choice].

Word Choices

Drowsiness
No adventitious or diminished breath sounds
Right arm weakness
Hyperactive BS × 4
Incontinent diarrheal stools
Speech difficulty
Elevated temperature

Practice Question 3.4 — Multiple Response Select All That Apply

The nurse is caring for a 43-year-old client in the inpatient psychiatric unit.

Nurses' Notes

1100: Admitted to unit for observation and treatment related to a suicide attempt. Attempted to cut both wrists, which are currently bandaged. Client was in a severe motor vehicle accident 5 months ago, resulting in tetraplegia. Has been living in a group home with full-time caregiver for assistance with ADLs since discharge from rehabilitation. Has no family living in the area. Has stage 3 sacral pressure injury covered with gauze dressing. Recently completed a course of antibiotics for infected sacral wound. Wears an external condom catheter and follows bowel regimen, but has frequent problems with urine leakage and bowel incontinence. Is able to transfer with supervision from bed to wheelchair using sliding board. Lost 20 lb (9.1 kg) since the accident, and describes appetite as "fair." Does not want to be here because the client is "sick of being in hospitals."

*Which of the following findings require **immediate** follow-up related to risk factors for additional or worsening pressure injuries?* **Select all that apply.**

☐ Attempted suicide
☐ Tetraplegia
☐ Current stage 3 sacral wound
☐ ADL dependent
☐ Sliding board for transfers
☐ Urinary and bowel incontinence
☐ 43 years of age
☐ Weight loss of 20 lb (9.1 kg)
☐ Fair appetite

Practice Question 3.5 — Matrix Multiple Choice

The nurse is caring for an 85-year-old client in the ED.

Nurses' Notes

1640: Client transported to ED via ambulance from skilled nursing facility. Family present and very concerned about client's condition. Client alert and oriented × 1 (person). Has difficulty talking due to shortness of breath. Reports feeling very "winded." Placed in sitting position; supplemental oxygen in place at 3 L/min. Skin warm and dry. Crackles present in both lungs; S_3 present. Abdomen slightly distended; BS present and distant × 4. Able to move all extremities. Peripheral pulses present and bounding. Cap refill >3 sec. Pitting 3+ edema in both feet. VS: T 97°F (36.1°C); HR 100 and irregular; RR 28; BP 138/76; SpO_2 92% on oxygen.

Complete the following table by selecting whether each client finding requires **immediate** *follow-up or does not require immediate follow-up.*

Client Findings	Requires Immediate Follow-Up	Does Not Require Immediate Follow-Up
Shortness of breath	☐	☐
Alert and oriented × 1	☐	☐
Crackles in both lungs	☐	☐
Bounding peripheral pulses	☐	☐
RR 28	☐	☐
BP 138/76	☐	☐
HR 100 and irregular	☐	☐
Cap refill >3 sec	☐	☐
Pitting 3+ edema both feet	☐	☐

Practice Question 3.6 — Multiple Response Select N

The nurse is caring for a 13-year-old client in the Urgent Care Center.

Nurses' Notes

0850: Newcomer parent brought child for urgent care. Reports being in the country for only 2 weeks; speaks English fluently. Reports that child started having new GI symptoms 2 days ago, which could have been "caused by something eaten at the shelter." Child started with lack of appetite and nausea but progressed to fever and vomiting with occasional diarrhea. Last night, the child went to bed earlier than usual and showed no interest in playing games or watching TV. This morning, parent noted dark urine in the toilet. Child's current temperature is 103.2°F (39.6°C). States feeling very tired and wants to go to bed.

Select the **4** *client findings that require* **immediate** *follow-up.*

☐ Anorexia
☐ Occasional diarrhea
☐ Nausea and vomiting
☐ Elevated temperature
☐ Fatigue
☐ Wants to sleep
☐ Dark urine

CHAPTER 4

Strategies for Answering NGN Questions: Analyze Cues

 THINKING SPACE

Analyze Cues is a CJ cognitive skill nurses use to examine and interpret the relevant cues recognized in a clinical scenario and establish the significance of those cues. In other words, the nurse determines what the cues mean and identifies the health problems the client is experiencing. The nurse considers the context of the clinical scenario and thinks about what could be happening. The relevant cues are analyzed to determine supporting and opposing manifestations of an evolving client condition. Then, multiple factors are considered and potential complications that could be occurring are identified for prioritization to guide subsequent planning and nursing actions. Applying the skill *Analyze Cues* is essential for making appropriate clinical judgments and is a skill that will be measured both on the NCLEX® and on your nursing course exams. When analyzing cues, focus on determining the meaning of the cues that are concerning. Connect or link these relevant cues to the client's scenario to determine the health problem(s) the client is experiencing or any evolving conditions.

How Do You Analyze Cues?

The cognitive skill *Analyze Cues* requires a prompt and comprehensive examination of client data, fitting the relevant cues into the larger picture of the overall clinical scenario, and determining what these relevant cues mean. This requires considering multiple factors about what is occurring for the client, such as the client's history of a chronic health problem, new data, or an acute condition, and narrowing them down, serving as the basis for analysis and clinical judgment. When analyzing cues, ask yourself two questions. First, ask yourself, "What do these client findings mean?" Second, ask yourself, "What is happening to this client?" Chapter 3 provides you with information about the cognitive skill *Recognize Cues*. Table 4.1 provides two examples of client findings that may be presented as part of an NGN clinical scenario. In these examples, relevant cues requiring application of the cognitive skill *Analyze Cues* are in boldface and italicized. All information in the client findings presented in these examples needs to be considered, but the relevant data are the focus to *Analyze Cues*, determine what these data mean for the client, and decide how they fit into the larger clinical picture.

 NGN TIP

Remember: Analyzing cues and determining what relevant client data mean lead to formulating client needs, prioritizing client care, planning care, and clinical decision making with implementing care.

How Does Analyzing Cues Help You Guide Client Care?

The cognitive skill *Analyze Cues* requires you to examine the relevant data in a clinical scenario, link these data to the client's clinical situation, and determine what these data mean. It is important to consider all factors presented in the clinical scenario to determine what is happening to the client. This is an important process because determining what relevant data mean tells you what is happening to the client. Once this is known, you will be able to determine what you need to prioritize, plan, and do next to meet the client's needs.

TABLE 4.1	Examples of Clinical Scenarios and How to Analyze Relevant Cues
Clinical Scenario	**Analyze Cues**
Scenario 1: A 5-week-old infant is brought by their parent to the clinic for a well-child check. The parent reports a **white coating on the tongue for the past 2 weeks.** The parent tried to clean the tongue with a washcloth, but the **coating could not be removed**. The parent reports that there is no history of a previous infection.	A white coating on the tongue of an infant could likely be milk residue or a sign of thrush. Factors to consider in analyzing these data are that there is no history of a previous infection, the finding has lasted for 2 weeks, and the coating could not be removed with a washcloth. What do these data mean? What is happening to the infant? Analysis of these data indicates new relevant cues and leads to a concern regarding the presence of thrush.
Scenario 2: A client had a vaginal birth at home. The newborn's birth weight was 7 lb 11 oz (3.2 kg), and gestational age was 38 weeks 3 days. The newborn was transferred to the hospital immediately after birth. **A heart murmur was detected at the hospital, and the newborn was scheduled for a cardiology consultation.**	A heart murmur in a newborn may be an innocent murmur, meaning that it is not a cause for concern, or it could mean that there is a congenital cardiac condition, thus the need for cardiology consultation. What do these data mean? What is happening to the newborn? Analysis of these data indicates an acute condition in the newborn and leads to a concern regarding the possible presence of a congenital cardiac condition, therefore further evaluation is required.

How Do You Analyze Cues in an NGN Clinical Scenario?

As noted in Chapter 2, NGN questions will begin with a clinical scenario presented as either a Stand-Alone item or an Unfolding Case Study. Information about the client is presented, and you need to identify the relevant data. Once these relevant data are noted, you analyze the data and link these data to the client situation to determine what the data mean and what is happening to the client. Determining what these data mean and what is happening to the client is application of the cognitive skill *Analyze Cues*. The accompanying example provides you with a medical record and client data. After reviewing information in all tabs of the medical record provided and identifying relevant cues, you then analyze the cues to determine what is happening to the client to guide client care. In this example, relevant data (cues) are in boldface and italicized. You need to analyze these data and make connections with the client situation to determine the meaning of the data. The cognitive skill *Analyze Cues* is required to ensure planning safe client care.

Example: Analyze Cues

1030: A 65-year-old client presents to the ED and reports experiencing diarrhea over the past week that is worsening.

Health History	Nurses' Notes	Vital Signs	Laboratory Results

Client reports **diarrhea 5 to 6 times daily × 1 week**. States that they get the sudden urge to have a bowel movement. Client describes it as mixed, **both watery and formed at times**. Denies melena or blood in the stool. Does not recall eating anything that would cause the symptoms. Denies associated abdominal pain or colic and has no alleviating or aggravating factors. Has not taken any medication for the symptoms. Is still able to eat and drink, and appetite is unchanged. States they "just need to stay close to a bathroom." Denies recent travel and recent antibiotic use, and states that they have no sick contacts. Current medications are reviewed, and none are associated with the complaints. The client is admitted to the observation unit for further testing.

THINKING SPACE

| Health History | Nurses' Notes | **Vital Signs** | Laboratory Results |

1030: T 98.2°F (36.8°C); **HR 110; BP 102/68;** RR 16; SpO$_2$ 98% on RA

| Health History | **Nurses' Notes** | Vital Signs | Laboratory Results |

1100: A complete blood cell count and comprehensive metabolic panel are ordered and stool culture for *Clostridium difficile*. Stool noted to be watery and tan in color. Specimen collected and sent to laboratory for testing. Some of the laboratory test results are reported.

| Health History | Nurses' Notes | Vital Signs | **Laboratory Results** |

Test and Reference Range	Result
Red blood cells (RBCs) 4.2–6.2 × 10^{12}/L (4.2–6.2 × 10^{12}/L)	4.8 × 10^{12} (4.8 × 10^{12})
White blood cells (WBCs) **5000–10,000/mm³ (5–10 × 10^9/L)**	15,000/mm³ (15 × 10^9/L)
Segmented neutrophils **62%–68% (2.5–7.5 × 10^9/L)**	75% (8.3 × 10^9/L)
Band neutrophils **0%–9% (0–1 × 10^9/L)**	10% (1.1 × 10^9/L)
Lymphocytes 20%–40% (0.1–0.4 × 10^9/L)	20% (0.1 × 10^9/L)
Monocytes 2%–8% (0.1–0.7 × 10^9/L)	2% (0.1 × 10^9/L)
Eosinophils 1%–4% (0.00–0.5 × 10^9/L)	1% (0.00 × 10^9/L)
Basophils 0.5%–1% (0.02–0.05 × 10^9/L)	1% (0.05 × 10^9/L)
Platelets 150,000–400,000/mm³ (150–400 × 10^9/L)	200,000/mm³ (200 × 10^9/L)
Hemoglobin (Hgb) 12–18 g/dL (120–180 g/L)	17 g/dL (170 g/L)
Hematocrit (Hct) 37%–52% (0.37–0.52)	46% (0.46)
Albumin 3.5–5.0 g/dL (35–50 g/L)	4.2 g/dL (42 g/L)
Blood urea nitrogen (BUN) **10–20 mg/dL (3.6–7.1 mmol/L)**	24 mg/dL (8.64 mmol/L)
Calcium 9–10.5 mg/dL (2.25–2.75 mmol/L)	10.2 mg/dL (2.7 mmol/L)
Chloride 98–106 mEq/L (98–106 mmol/L)	102 mEq/L (102 mmol/L)
Creatinine 0.5–1.2 mg/dL (44–106 μmol/L)	0.9 mg/dL (79.5 μmol/L)

Health History	Nurses' Notes	Vital Signs	**Laboratory Results**

Test and Reference Range	Result
Glucose 70–99 mg/dL (3.9–5.5 mmol/L)	87 mg/dL (4.8 mmol/L)
Potassium 3.5–5.0 mEq/L (3.5–5.0 mmol/L)	3.8 mEq/L (3.8 mmol/L)
Sodium 135–145 mEq/L (135–145 mmol/L)	142 mEq/L (142 mmol/L)
Total bilirubin 0.3–1.0 mg/dL (5.1–17 µmol/L)	0.3 mg/dL (5.1 µmol/L)
Total protein 6.4–8.3 g/dL (64–83 g/L)	6.4 g/dL (64 g/L)
Alanine aminotransferase (ALT) 4–36 U/L (4–36 U/L)	28 U/L (28 U/L)
Aspartate aminotransferase (AST) 0–35 U/L (0–35 U/L)	28 U/L (28 U/L)
Stool culture *C. difficile* toxin **Negative**	Detected

What Will You Think About to Analyze Cues in This Clinical Scenario?

To analyze cues, you will examine the relevant data and link these data to the clinical situation to interpret the data, determine what the data mean, and draw conclusions about what is happening to the client.

In this situation, the findings that are *not* within the usual or normal range include:
- Reports of frequent diarrhea; both watery and formed at times
- WBCs: 15,000/mm^3 (15 × 10^9/L)
- Segmented neutrophils 75% (8.3 × 10^9/L)
- Band neutrophils 10% (1.1 × 10^9/L)
- BUN: 24 mg/dL (8.64 mmol/L)
- HR 110
- BP 102/68
- Stool culture *C. difficile* toxin: Detected

To consider these findings in the context of the overall picture, it is important to think about why these results may be out of range and how they are connected. Reports of frequent diarrhea as the primary client problem is a good starting point to frame the analysis. It helps to start thinking about possible causes of the diarrhea. Considering the information available in the medical record, a connection can be made that the ED physician is interested in exploring *C. difficile* infection as a cause.

From there, considering why the physician might be ordering a complete blood count or comprehensive metabolic panel will help progress the analysis. Specifically, a complete blood count will provide information about signs of infection. The white blood cell (WBC) count is elevated in this case, and some components of the differential, which breaks down the number of types of WBCs in the specimen, are also abnormal. With the segmented and band neutrophils being elevated, a bacterial infection would be suspected. This is often referred to as a "shift to the left."

A comprehensive metabolic panel will provide information on hydration status, electrolyte balance, and kidney and liver function. The BUN is elevated, and in the setting of a normal creatinine level, this indicates dehydration. This fits within the clinical context

▶THINKING SPACE

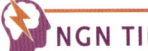

NGN TIP

Remember: Use these strategies for NGN items that measure *Analyze Cues*:
1. Examine the relevant cues or findings that are unexpected.
2. Determine the client conditions that link or connect with the client findings or cues.
3. Ask yourself, "What do these findings mean, and what is happening to the client? Are there any findings or cues that support or oppose any client conditions?"
4. Decide if any other information in the clinical situation would help establish the significance of the findings within the context of the overall clinical picture.

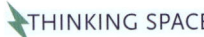

of multiple episodes of diarrhea because of suspected gastrointestinal (GI) infection. The BP is lower than normal, and the HR is elevated, also expected characteristics noted in dehydration. The potassium level and sodium level are in normal range but need to be monitored because these electrolytes are lost when a client has diarrhea. Last, detection of the *C. difficile* toxin confirms the diagnosis of *C. difficile* infection.

Which Client Findings Are Most Important When Analyzing Cues?

The cognitive skill *Analyze Cues* requires you to interpret the meaning of client findings in the context of the overall clinical picture to set the stage for making important decisions that inform and guide safe client care. All client findings are important, but those that are *not* normal or *not* expected are the most important when it comes to analyzing cues. You need to analyze these abnormal findings and ask yourself, "Is the abnormal finding acceptable or expected considering this client scenario, or is it *not* acceptable and an immediate concern for the nurse?" For example, the nurse assessing a client with an acute exacerbation of COPD would interpret *acute* shortness of breath as a manifestation of importance at this time and would determine that it requires *immediate* follow-up. However, noting a barrel chest when performing the physical assessment is relevant and abnormal, but with further analysis the nurse knows that this is a long-term manifestation of the client's chronic disease.

When Might You Need to Analyze Cues in a Clinical Situation?

The ability to effectively apply the cognitive skill *Analyze Cues* is critical and is needed when answering both traditional NCLEX®-style questions and NGN questions. As a nurse, you need to always *Analyze Cues* in a clinical situation; this is an important part of your nursing practice. Knowledge about health problems and linking this knowledge to the interpretation of history and physical assessment findings, nursing assessment findings, and diagnostic test results are required to *Analyze Cues*. Table 4.2 provides examples of common health problems and diagnostic sources that would provide relevant data that link to the listed common health problem. These data are helpful when determining what is happening to the client with the listed health problem.

Which NGN Item Types Optimally Measure *Analyze Cues*?

As noted in Chapter 2, NGN questions will begin with a clinical scenario presented as either a Stand-Alone item or an Unfolding Case Study. The types of test items and the variations that may be used to measure the cognitive skill *Analyze Cues* are presented in Table 4.3. Some of these types are presented in the Sample Questions throughout this chapter and in the Practice Questions at the end of the chapter. These test item types are discussed in Chapter 2 with additional examples. Also, visit the Evolve site for additional practice with these item types.

Drop-Down Test Items to Measure *Analyze Cues*

As mentioned in Chapter 2, Drop-Down items include Drop-Down Cloze, Drop-Down Rationale, and Drop-Down in Table. When the Drop-Down item type is used to measure *Analyze Cues,* the test taker is required to complete a sentence or blank space by choosing from a list of options. Sample Question 4.1 illustrates a Drop-Down Rationale item type. The rationale and test-taking strategy to help you derive the correct responses shown in Sample Question 4.1 are also provided.

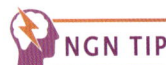

NGN TIP

Remember: In a Drop-Down Rationale test item that requires completing a rationale, there is no partial credit. You must understand the full concept and the justification through the rationale to receive credit for your answer. It is important to choose the first option correctly so the remaining option choices will be based on the correct foundation.

TABLE 4.2 Examples of Common Health Problems and Diagnostic Sources for Analyzing Cues

Common Health Problems	Diagnostic Sources
Dysrhythmias	ECG results
MI	ECG results, laboratory results (e.g., cardiac markers, troponin levels)
Heart failure	ECG results, laboratory results (e.g., B-natriuretic peptide), imaging results (chest x-ray)
Respiratory compromise	Laboratory results (e.g., arterial blood gas levels)
Pneumonia	Laboratory results (e.g., white blood cell count, inflammatory markers), imaging results (e.g., chest x-ray)
GI bleeding	Laboratory results (e.g., hemoglobin level, hematocrit level, platelets, electrolytes), imaging results (e.g., abdominal CT scan, esophagogastroduodenoscopy [EGD])
Hypotension, hypovolemia, shock	Laboratory results (e.g., blood urea nitrogen [BUN] level, creatinine level, electrolytes)
Stroke	Imaging results (e.g., CT or MRI scan of the head)
VT (DVT and PE)	Laboratory results (e.g., prothrombin time [PT], international normalized ratio [INR], partial thromboplastin time [PTT]), imaging results (e.g., Doppler ultrasound, CT scan of the lungs)
Sepsis	Laboratory results (e.g., white blood cell count, lactic acid level, glucose level)
Arterial occlusion	Imaging results (e.g., ultrasound)
Kidney dysfunction	Laboratory results (e.g., blood urea nitrogen [BUN] level, creatinine level, glomerular filtration rate [GFR]), imaging results (e.g., renal ultrasound)
Compartment syndrome	Imaging results (e.g., x-ray, MRI, compartment pressure testing)
Abdominal trauma	Laboratory results (e.g., hemoglobin level, hematocrit level, platelets), imaging results (e.g., abdominal CT scan)
Chest trauma	Laboratory results (e.g., hemoglobin level, hematocrit level, platelets), imaging results (e.g., chest CT scan)

TABLE 4.3 Test Items and Variations That Optimally Measure *Analyze Cues*

Type of Test Item	Variations
Drop-Down	Drop-Down Cloze Drop-Down Rationale Drop-Down in Table
Extended Multiple Response	Multiple Response Select All That Apply Multiple Response Select N Multiple Response Grouping
Matrix/Grid	Matrix Multiple Response Matrix Multiple Choice
Drag-and-Drop	Drag-and-Drop Cloze Drag-and-Drop Rationale
Stand-Alone	Bow-tie Trend

▸THINKING SPACE

Sample Question 4.1 — Drop-Down Rationale Item: *Analyze Cues*

1500: A client is brought to the ED by EMS, who report that the police found the client lying in an alley. The client was difficult to arouse but reported being 70 years of age and unhoused. EMS reports VS as: T 100.8°F (38.2°C), HR 110, RR 16, BP 100/52, and SpO$_2$ 91% on RA. EMS inserted an IV and NS 0.9% was infusing, and the client was receiving O$_2$ at 2 L/min on arrival to the ED. The ED physician prescribes STAT laboratory and diagnostic tests, and the nurse gathers initial assessment data on the client while awaiting test results and reviews the results as they are reported.

Health History
Client reports not really knowing current health problems. States goes to the mobile health clinic when it is in the neighborhood. Reports was given some medication for BP but ran out of the medication and never went back to the clinic for more.

Nurses' Notes
VS: T 100.8°F (38.2°C); HR 118 and irregular; RR 14; BP 106/58; SpO$_2$ 94% on O$_2$ at 2 L/min. The client was receiving O$_2$ at 2 L/min on arrival to the ED.
Weight: 110 lb (49.8 kg), reported height 5 feet 8 inches. IV NS 0.9% infusing at 100 mL/h.
Reports weakness and fatigue. States, "I have not been able to walk to the food kitchen and haven't eaten in a while. I usually hang out at the park with lots of friends, but lately I have been sleeping in the alley where the cops found me."
Dry and brittle hair, cracked lips, decreased skin elasticity, dry and scaly skin.
Conjunctiva red, tremors in hands bilaterally, muscle mass poor.
Tongue swollen, redness of oral mucosa, distended abdomen, client reports not remembering when the last BM was. Cough weak, difficulty with taking deep breaths, decreased breath sounds.

Laboratory Results

Test and Reference Range	Result
Hemoglobin (Hgb) 12–18 g/dL (120–180 g/L)	10 g/dL (100 g/L)
Hematocrit (Hct) 37%–52% (0.37–0.52)	34% (0.34)
White blood cells (WBCs) 5000–10,000/mm^3 (5–10 × 10^9/L)	11,000/mm^3 (11 × 10^9/L)
Glucose 70–99 mg/dL (3.9–5.5 mmol/L)	68 mg/dL (3.7 mmol/L)
Potassium 3.5–5.0 mEq/L (3.5–5.0 mmol/L)	5.2 mEq/L (5.2 mmol/L)
Sodium 135–145 mEq/L (135–145 mmol/L)	148 mEq/L (148 mmol/L)
Blood urea nitrogen (BUN) 10–20 mg/dL (3.6–7.1 mmol/L)	8 mg/dL (2.88 mmol/L)
Creatinine 0.5–1.2 mg/dL (44–106 µmol/L)	0.3 mg/dL (26.4 µmol/L)
Albumin 3.5–5.0 g/dL (35–50 g/L)	3.0 g/dL (30 g/L)

Diagnostic Results
Quantiferon: pending
Chest x-ray: small ill-defined shadows and nodules right lower lobe

Complete the following sentences by choosing from the lists of options provided.

The nurse determines that the client is **most likely** experiencing <u>malnutrition</u>. Assessment findings directly associated with the health problem include <u>poor muscle mass</u> and <u>albumin results</u>, and because the client reports <u>not eating in a while</u>.

Options for 1	Options for 2	Options for 3	Options for 4
Hypoglycemia	Poor muscle mass	Blood glucose result	Not remembering when the last BM was
Malnutrition	Irregular heart rate	Difficulty with taking deep breaths	Not eating in a while
Active tuberculosis	WBC result	Decreased breath sounds	Running out of BP medication
Infection	Temperature reading	Albumin results	Hanging out with lots of friends

THINKING SPACE

Rationale: Malnutrition is a deficit, excess, or imbalance of the required components of a balanced diet. This can be due to alterations in carbohydrates, proteins, fat, electrolytes, minerals, or vitamins. The clinical manifestations of malnutrition can range from mild to severe exhibiting emaciation and can lead to death. These manifestations result from numerous interactions at the cellular level. As protein intake declines, muscle wasting occurs. This leads to weakness and fatigue, anemia, and susceptibility to infection. Data from the health history and the nursing physical assessment findings reflect manifestations of malnutrition. The respiratory rate and vital capacity of the lungs is decreased, and crackles and a weak cough are characteristic. The heart rate may be increased or decreased, and the blood pressure is lower than normal. Additionally, the laboratory test results align with findings seen in malnutrition. Albumin levels would be lower than normal as well as Hgb and Hct levels, which reflect the degree of anemia. Urea and creatinine are nitrogenous end products of metabolism. Urea is the primary metabolite derived from dietary protein and tissue protein turnover, and creatinine is the product of muscle creatine catabolism; thus BUN and creatinine will be low. Electrolyte levels reflect changes between the intracellular and extracellular spaces and are often elevated; this can lead to dysrhythmias. Neurologically, the client experiences decreased or loss of reflexes, tremors, poor attention span, irritability, and confusion. The client's blood glucose is only slightly below normal, and this would be expected because of not eating. Although the client has some tremors, this is unlikely associated with hypoglycemia based on the blood glucose level. The client's chest x-ray result is most indicative of latent rather than active tuberculosis or another respiratory problem. Although the client's temperature is slightly elevated, there are no other indications of infection, and this is an unlikely problem.

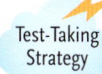
Test-Taking Strategy

Test-Taking Strategy: Focus on the client information, and think about what these data mean and what is happening to the client. Look at the health problems provided in the options and the listed assessment findings. Ask yourself if there are any findings or cues that support or oppose any health problems listed. Establish the significance of the findings within the context of the larger clinical picture. In a Drop-Down Rationale question, choosing the first option correctly is the most important part because it guides you in selecting the correct options for the remaining choices that follow. To do this, it may be helpful to look at the options for the client findings first and then pair them with the possible health problems. The health problem with the most client findings is most likely the correct answer for the first option.

To assist you in deriving the correct answers, use the approach illustrated in the table, which lists the client's assessment findings and associated health problem. Use knowledge regarding the pathophysiology of the condition to identify the findings that are directly associated with supporting the condition.

Assessment Finding	Hypoglycemia Directly Associated/Supporting Data Yes/No	Malnutrition Directly Associated/Supporting Data Yes/No	Active Tuberculosis Directly Associated/Supporting Data Yes/No	Infection Directly Associated/Supporting Data Yes/No
Irregular heart rate	No	Yes	No	No
Poor muscle mass	No	Yes	No	No
WBC result (slightly elevated)	No	No	Yes	Yes
Temp reading (slightly elevated)	No	Yes	Yes	Yes
Blood glucose result (slightly decreased)	Yes	Yes	No	No
Difficulty with taking deep breaths	No	Yes	No	No
Decreased breath sounds	No	No	No	No
Albumin results (below reference range)	No	Yes	No	No
Not remembering when the last BM was	No	Yes	No	No
Not eating in a while	Yes	Yes	No	No
Running out of BP medication	No	No	No	No
Hanging out with lots of friends	No	No	Yes	Yes

As you can visualize from this table, most assessment findings are directly associated in some way to malnutrition. Thinking about the assessment findings in this way will help with deriving the answers for all options in this question.

Content Area: Medical-Surgical Nursing
Priority Concept: Fluid and Electrolyte Balance, Tissue Integrity
Reference(s): Ignatavicius et al., 2024, pp. 1264–1272

> **NGN TIP**
>
> **Remember:** In a Drop-Down Rationale test item, it is important to choose the first option correctly so the remaining option choices are based on the correct foundation.

Matrix/Grid Test Items to Measure *Analyze Cues*

Matrix/Grid test items include Matrix Multiple Response and Matrix Multiple Choice. When the Matrix/Grid item type is used to measure *Analyze Cues,* the test taker is required to follow the question directions regarding how to select options. In a Matrix Multiple Response item, there will be response columns and rows, and each response column or row could have multiple correct responses. In a Matrix Multiple Choice item, each response row can have only one correct response. Sample Question 4.2 illustrates a Matrix Multiple Response item type. The rationale and test-taking strategy to help you derive the correct responses shown in Sample Question 4.2 are also provided.

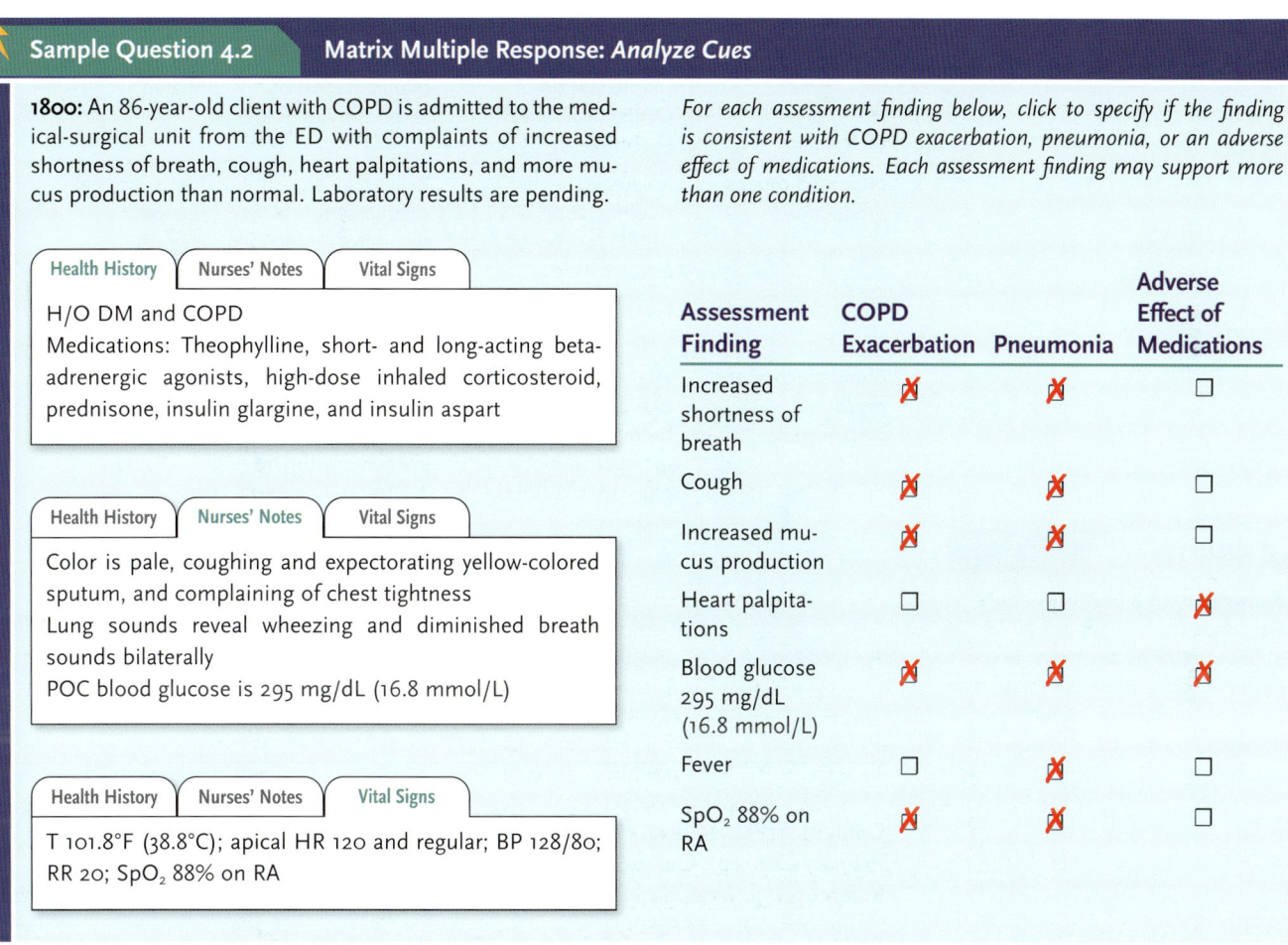

Sample Question 4.2 — Matrix Multiple Response: *Analyze Cues*

1800: An 86-year-old client with COPD is admitted to the medical-surgical unit from the ED with complaints of increased shortness of breath, cough, heart palpitations, and more mucus production than normal. Laboratory results are pending.

For each assessment finding below, click to specify if the finding is consistent with COPD exacerbation, pneumonia, or an adverse effect of medications. Each assessment finding may support more than one condition.

Health History
H/O DM and COPD
Medications: Theophylline, short- and long-acting beta-adrenergic agonists, high-dose inhaled corticosteroid, prednisone, insulin glargine, and insulin aspart

Nurses' Notes
Color is pale, coughing and expectorating yellow-colored sputum, and complaining of chest tightness
Lung sounds reveal wheezing and diminished breath sounds bilaterally
POC blood glucose is 295 mg/dL (16.8 mmol/L)

Vital Signs
T 101.8°F (38.8°C); apical HR 120 and regular; BP 128/80; RR 20; SpO₂ 88% on RA

Assessment Finding	COPD Exacerbation	Pneumonia	Adverse Effect of Medications
Increased shortness of breath	✗	✗	☐
Cough	✗	✗	☐
Increased mucus production	✗	✗	☐
Heart palpitations	☐	☐	✗
Blood glucose 295 mg/dL (16.8 mmol/L)	✗	✗	✗
Fever	☐	✗	☐
SpO₂ 88% on RA	✗	✗	☐

Rationale: Manifestations of COPD exacerbation include increased coughing, wheezing, and more severe shortness of breath than usual. Other manifestations include changes in the color, thickness, or amount of mucus. In some COPD clients, an SpO₂ of 88% could be normal, but it could also be an indication of exacerbation. In pneumonia, the client presents with fever, cough and mucus production, and shortness of breath. SpO₂ could be lower than normal because of the compromised respiratory status. Sharp or stabbing chest pain is also characteristic. The glucose level increases in the presence of infection such as pneumonia or in COPD exacerbation because the stress response in the body increases the amount of certain hormones such as cortisol and adrenaline. This leads to the body's increased production of glucose. Prednisone and other corticosteroids can increase blood glucose levels by making the liver resistant to insulin. Theophylline is a bronchodilator. Signs of toxicity are nausea, vomiting, abdominal pain, tachycardia, and muscle tremor. Heart palpitations are also a sign of toxicity.

THINKING SPACE

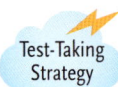

Test-Taking Strategy: For each of the client conditions asked about in this question, ask yourself, based on the findings in the Health History and Nurses' Notes data, whether the assessment findings are specifically related or not specifically related to the suspected client condition and why you are interpreting the findings in this way. You can organize your thinking process as illustrated in the table.

THINKING SPACE

Assessment Finding	COPD Exacerbation	Pneumonia	Adverse Effects of Medications
Increased shortness of breath	Related because of the added stress on the respiratory system	Related because of the added stress on the respiratory system	Not specifically related
Cough	Related as a chronic manifestation of COPD, worsened in exacerbation	Related as an acute manifestation of respiratory infection	Not specifically related
Increased mucus production	Related as a chronic manifestation of COPD, worsened in exacerbation	Related as an acute manifestation of respiratory infection	Not specifically related
Heart palpitations	Not specifically related	Not specifically related	Related to theophylline toxicity
Blood glucose 295 mg/dL (16.8 mmol/L)	High-dose inhaled and oral corticosteroid therapy can cause an increase in blood glucose; client has diabetes	Related as a manifestation of infection, especially in clients with DM	Related to prednisone
Fever	Not specifically related	Related as a manifestation of respiratory infection	Not specifically related
SpO$_2$ 88% on RA	Related as a chronic manifestation of COPD, worsened in exacerbation	Related as an acute manifestation of respiratory infection	Not specifically related

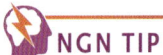

Remember: In a Matrix Multiple Response item, there will be response columns and rows, and each response column or row could have multiple correct responses.

Content Area: Medical-Surgical Nursing
Priority Concept: Gas Exchange, Perfusion
Reference(s): Ignatavicius et al., 2024, pp. 547–558; 580–585; Lilley et al., 2023, pp. 497–501, 557, 580

Drag-and-Drop Test Items to Measure *Analyze Cues*

Drag-and-Drop test items include Drag-and-Drop Cloze and Drag-and-Drop Rationale. When the Drag-and-Drop item type is used to measure *Analyze Cues*, the test taker is required to complete a sentence or fill in a blank space by choosing from a list of options and dragging that selected option to the answer space. Sample Question 4.3 illustrates a Drag-and-Drop Rationale item type. The rationale and test-taking strategy to help you derive the correct responses shown in Sample Question 4.3 are also provided.

Sample Question 4.3 — Drag-and-Drop Rationale Item: *Analyze Cues*

1400: The nurse conducts the admission assessment for a 72-year-old client admitted to the medical-surgical unit with fever and shortness of breath. The medical record reveals the following findings:

Health History | Nurses' Notes | Vital Signs | Diagnostic Results

Obesity, rheumatoid arthritis, stroke 4 years ago, type 2 DM, hyperlipidemia
Has smoked 1 pack of cigarettes per day for the past 42 years.
Lives with child; does not drive owing to problems with eyesight and has limited mobility
Medications: Aspirin 81 mg daily, metformin 1000 mg twice daily, atorvastatin 10 mg daily, azathioprine 150 mg daily, oseltamivir (3 days remaining in course)

Health History | **Nurses' Notes** | Vital Signs | Diagnostic Results

72-year-old client presents to the ED with complaints of fever and shortness of breath. Reports recent upper respiratory infection with fever and body aches diagnosed as influenza at the urgent care center 3 days ago; oseltamivir was prescribed

Health History | Nurses' Notes | **Vital Signs** | Diagnostic Results

T 101.2°F (38.4°C); HR 90; BP 168/92; RR 22; SpO$_2$ 90% on 2 L/min O$_2$ via NC
Weight: 220 lb (99.79 kg)
Height (reported): 5 feet 2 inches

Health History | Nurses' Notes | Vital Signs | **Diagnostic Results**

2-view chest x-ray: left lower lobe infiltrates

Complete the following sentence by selecting from the lists of options below.

The client is at **highest** risk for developing **VTE** due to **acute infection** and **obesity**.

Options for 1	Options for 2 and 3
Aspiration	Body aches
Heart failure	Acute infection
Dysrhythmias	Inability to drive
VTE	Prescribed medications
Acute MI	Obesity

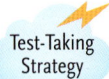

Rationale: Although the client has some risk factors for the other conditions (aspiration, heart failure, dysrhythmias, acute MI), the highest risk is for VTE. VTE history and risk are assessed at admission. Some risk factors include active cancer, previous VTE, reduced mobility, thrombophilic conditions, recent trauma or surgery, older age, cardiac and respiratory failure, acute MI, ischemic stroke, acute infection, rheumatologic disorders, obesity, and hormone treatment. Client findings consistent with these risk factors include active infection, information noted in the past medical history (obesity, rheumatoid arthritis, cardiovascular disease, such as stroke), and social factors (smoking). The presence of body aches, although consistent with infection, is nonspecific and could be related to other problems. The inability to drive is not specifically related, and the medication regimen actually decreases the client's risk for this problem.

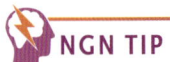

Test-Taking Strategy: First, focus on the client data, especially the relevant data and the abnormal and unexpected data, and determine what is happening to the client. Use thinking processes and determine what these data mean and how they affect the health of the client. Next, use knowledge and think about the complications that can occur with this client. Ask yourself if there are any findings or cues that support or oppose any complications. Decide which cues are of concern. In a Drag-and-Drop Rationale question, choosing the first option correctly is the most important part because it guides you in selecting the correct options for the remaining choices that follow. When answering a Drag-and-Drop Rationale item, it may be helpful to look at the options for the client findings first and then pair them with the possible complications. The complication with the most client findings is most likely the correct answer for the first option.

Client Finding	Complication
Body aches	Nonspecific to listed complications
Active infection	Risk factor for *VTE*
Inability to drive	Nonspecific to listed complications
Prescribed medications	Treatment for heart failure, dysrhythmias, acute MI, *VTE*
Obesity	Risk factor for heart failure, dysrhythmias, acute MI, *VTE*

NGN TIP

Remember: For the Drag-and-Drop Rationale item, a full understanding of "paired" information is required to answer the question correctly. The concept needs to be justified by the rationale chosen. If a question is asking about a complication and associated client findings or associated risk factors, the complication needs to be correctly identified first. Then the client findings and risk factors associated with that complication need to be determined to receive credit for the answer.

As noted, the client presents with multiple risk factors for VTE compared with the other complications listed. The client's medication regimen is preventing or treating health problems. You may need to rely on your knowledge base related to risk factors for VTE and the other conditions to some extent to answer this question correctly.

Content Area: Medical-Surgical Nursing
Priority Concept: Clotting, Perfusion
Reference(s): Ignatavicius et al., 2024, pp. 748–752

Extended Multiple Response Test Items to Measure *Analyze Cues*

Extended Multiple Response test items include Multiple Response Select All That Apply, Multiple Response Select N, and Multiple Response Grouping. When the Multiple Response item type is used to measure *Analyze Cues,* the test taker is required to follow the question directions regarding how to select options. Sample Question 4.4 illustrates a Multiple Response Select All That Apply item type. The rationale and test-taking strategy to help you derive the correct responses shown in Sample Question 4.4 are also provided.

> **NGN TIP**
>
> **Remember:** A Select All That Apply item will have at least 5 options and no more than 10 options for selection. One option or more than one option could be correct. In addition, it is possible for all options presented to be correct.

Sample Question 4.4 — Multiple Response Select All That Apply: *Analyze Cues*

A 16-year-old client reports to the nurse's office at the high school and tells the nurse about feelings of loneliness and sadness. The nurse checks the adolescent's VS, performs a psychosocial assessment, and documents in the Nurses' Notes.

Vital Signs

T 98.2°F (36.7°C); HR 90; BP 110/72; RR 18
Weight: 200 lb (90.71 kg)
Height (reported): 5 feet 3 inches

Nurses' Notes

States identifies self as a lesbian and 2 weeks ago "came out of the closet" and told parents. Reports that parents were extremely upset and stated "you are a disgrace to the family." Feeling lonely and sad.
Reports that school peers don't offer invitations to outside-of-school group events.
States that school peers laugh and giggle in a huddle when walking down school corridors.
Reports that a social media site had a school picture and the word "lesbian" was scratched across the photo.
Is afraid to go to classes and nervous because of fear of ridicule, and wants to drop out of school.
Reports feeling worthless to society.

The nurse determines that the assessment findings **most likely** *indicate which condition(s)?* **Select all that apply.**

- ☒ Rejection
- ☒ Discrimination
- ☒ Cyberbullying
- ☐ Gender self-acceptance
- ☒ Anxiety
- ☒ Clinical depression

Rationale: Rejection refers to the act of pushing someone or something away. It most frequently refers to the feelings of shame, sadness, or grief one feels when they are not accepted by others. This 16-year-old client is feeling rejection by peers in that school peers do not offer invitations to outside-of-school group events. In addition, parents tell the adolescent "…you are a disgrace to the family." Discrimination is the act of treating someone unfairly or less fairly than other groups. This adolescent is also experiencing discrimination and is being treated in a negative way by peers because of sexual orientation; the adolescent reports that school peers laugh and giggle in a huddle when walking down school corridors. Cyberbullying is bullying that takes place over digital devices and social media platforms. It includes sending, posting, or sharing negative, harmful, false, or mean content about someone else, causing embarrassment or humiliation. The adolescent reports that a

▶ THINKING SPACE

THINKING SPACE

social media site had a school picture and the word "lesbian" was scratched across the photo; this constitutes cyberbullying. Gender self-acceptance refers to how comfortable an individual is as a member of their identified gender. The nurse would need to perform further assessment of the adolescent to determine self-acceptance; however, the adolescent is afraid to go to classes because of fear of ridicule and wants to drop out of school, which are indicators that gender self-acceptance is unlikely. Anxiety is a feeling of worry, nervousness, apprehension, or uneasiness, typically about some event or something with an uncertain outcome. The adolescent displays anxiety and fear expressing being afraid to go to classes and nervous because of fear of ridicule. Depression is a mood disorder that causes a persistent feeling of sadness and loss of interest. The adolescent expresses feelings of worthlessness, loneliness, and sadness. The nurse would also further assess for feelings of self-harm due to these expressions.

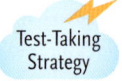

Test-Taking Strategy: The easiest way to organize your thinking processes to answer this question is to review the assessment findings and relate these findings to the characteristics of each item in the options. Create a table as illustrated below to help you organize your thoughts. Relate the assessment finding to each condition.

Assessment Finding	Rejection	Discrimination	Cyberbullying	Gender Self-Acceptance	Anxiety	Clinical Depression
Parents state "you are a disgrace to the family."	☒	☐	☐	☐	☐	☐
Feeling lonely and sad.	☐	☐	☐	☐	☐	☒
School peers do not offer invitations to outside-of-school group events.	☒	☐	☐	☐	☐	☐
School peers laugh and giggle in a huddle when walking down school corridors.	☐	☒	☐	☐	☐	☐
Social media had a picture and the word "lesbian" was scratched across the photo.	☐	☐	☒	☐	☐	☐
Afraid to go to classes and nervous because of fear of ridicule; wants to drop out of school.	☐	☐	☐	☐	☒	☐
Feeling worthless to society.	☐	☐	☐	☐	☐	☒

Content Area: Pediatric Nursing
Priority Concept: Mood and Affect, Stress and Coping
Reference(s): Halter, 2022, pp. 269, 381, 475–476; Hockenberry et al., 2024, pp. 533–534

Practice Questions

Practice Question 4.1 — Drop-Down Rationale

A 45-year-old client diagnosed with CKD requires dialysis. As a candidate for both hemodialysis and peritoneal dialysis, the client decides that peritoneal dialysis is the better option for their lifestyle. The client is hospitalized and undergoes insertion of the peritoneal dialysis catheter, and the first dialysis procedure is ordered. The nurse documents predialysis assessment data and reviews laboratory results.

Vital Signs

1100: T 98.2°F (36.8°C); apical HR 90 and regular; BP 146/98; RR 16; breath sounds clear bilaterally. Weight 160 lb (72.57 kg)

Laboratory Results

Test and Reference Range	Result
Blood urea nitrogen (BUN) 10–20 mg/dL (3.6–7.1 mmol/L)	30 mg/dL (10.8 mmol/L)
Creatinine 0.5–1.2 mg/dL (44–106 µmol/L)	6.0 mg/dL (528 µmol/L)
Glucose 70–99 mg/dL (3.9–5.5 mmol/L)	110 mg/dL (6.1 mmol/L)
Sodium 135–145 mEq/L (135–145 mmol/L)	150 mEq/L (150 mmol/L)
Potassium 3.5–5.0 mEq/L (3.5–5.0 mmol/L)	5.5 mEq/L (5.5 mmol/L)

During dialysis infusion, the nurse notes a slow inflow of the dialysate, and the client complains of pain. On assessment of the catheter, the nurse notes some fibrin clot formation in the dialysis tubing. **Complete the following sentence by choosing from the lists of options provided.**

The nurse recognizes that the slow inflow, presence of fibrin clots, and complaints of pain are **most likely** the result of 1 **[Select]** due to the 2 **[Select]**.

Options for 1	Options for 2
Peritonitis	Catheter slippage
Initial dialysis treatment	Surgical procedure
Bowel perforation	Lack of aseptic technique
Abdominal pressure	Elevated BP and laboratory results

Practice Question 4.2 — Drop-Down Rationale

An 80-year-old client who had a cholecystectomy 2 weeks ago was admitted 2 hours ago to the medical-surgical unit from the ED with acute pain located in the left upper abdomen. The client had laboratory testing and a contrast-enhanced CT scan of the abdomen. The nurse conducts an admission assessment and reviews the laboratory and diagnostic results.

Vital Signs | Laboratory Results | Diagnostic Results

1100: T 100.8°F (38.2°C); HR 90; BP 168/88; RR 24; SpO$_2$ 89% on RA; lung sounds clear but diminished to auscultation bilaterally, and breathing is nonlabored.

Vital Signs | **Laboratory Results** | Diagnostic Results

Test and Reference Range	Result
White blood cells (WBCs) 5000–10,000/mm^3 (5–10 × 10^9/L)	16,000/mm^3 (16 × 10^9/L)
Hemoglobin (Hgb) 12–18 g/dL (120–180 g/L)	16 g/dL (160 g/L)
Hematocrit (Hct) 37%–52% (0.37–0.52)	44% (0.44)
Blood urea nitrogen (BUN) 10–20 mg/dL (3.6–7.1 mmol/L)	18 mg/dL (6.48 mmol/L)
Creatinine 0.5–1.2 mg/dL (44–106 µmol/L)	0.8 mg/dL (70.6 µmol/L)
Glucose 70–99 mg/dL (3.9–5.5 mmol/L)	110 mg/dL (6.1 mmol/L)
Alanine aminotransferase (ALT) 4–36 U/L (4–36 U/L)	80 U/L (80 U/L)
Aspartate aminotransferase (AST) 0–35 U/L (0–35 U/L)	88 U/L (88 U/L)
Activated partial thromboplastin time (aPTT) 30–40 sec (30–40 sec)	32 sec (32 sec)
Prothrombin time (PT) 11–12.5 sec (11–12.5 sec)	11.4 sec (11.4 sec)
International normalized ratio (INR) 0.81–1.2 (0.81–1.2)	1.0 (1.0)
Amylase 60–120 U/L (60–120 U/L)	800 U/L (800 U/L)
Lipase 0–160 U/L (0–160 U/L)	320 U/L (320 U/L)

Vital Signs | Laboratory Results | **Diagnostic Results**

CT abdomen with contrast impression: Edema of the uncinate process of the pancreatic head, with peripancreatic fat, consistent with acute interstitial pancreatitis

Based on the assessment findings, complete the following sentence by choosing from the lists of options provided.

As a complication of acute pancreatitis, the client is at **highest** risk for developing **1 [Select]** as evidenced by **2 [Select]**.

Options for 1	Options for 2
Atelectasis	SpO$_2$ level
Bile duct calculi	PT/INR results
Pulmonary edema	CT abdomen results
Coagulation defects	BUN and creatinine levels

Practice Question 4.3 — Drag-and-Drop Cloze

A 7-year-old child is brought to the ED by a parent who reports that the child has had no energy these past few weeks and was very sleepy this morning and difficult to arouse. The nurse assesses the child, gathers data from the parent, and documents the following findings.

Nurses' Notes | Vital Signs

Child sleepy, responds to verbal stimuli and repeated commands slowly
Parent reports that the child has had no sick contacts and has been attending full days of school until today, and the child told the parent about being really tired and had a headache.
Parent reports that the child has been thirsty lately and urinating very frequently, even during the night. Parent reports thinking that the increased urination had to do with the increased fluid intake but became concerned this morning about the child because of the tiredness and feeling weak.
Child cheeks are flushed, skin dry, mucous membranes dry and crusty
Fruity, acetone-like breath odor
Reflexes diminished, muscle strength poor
Denies neck stiffness; no swelling of the neck or lymph nodes
Denies cough or difficulty breathing; lung sounds clear
Immunizations up-to-date
Allergies: No known allergies

Nurses' Notes | **Vital Signs**

Weight: 55 lb (59th percentile), parent reports that child has lost some weight over the past few weeks
Height: 49.25 inches (55th percentile)
BMI: 15.94 (58th percentile)
T: 97.9°F (36.6°C) temporal
HR: 70, pulse weak
RR: 24 deep
BP: 108/70

Complete the following sentence by choosing from the lists of options below.

Based on the assessment findings, the nurse would *most likely* suspect 1 [Select] because of 2 [Select] and 3 [Select].

Options for 1	Options for 2	Options for 3
Hyperglycemia	Flushed cheeks	Thirst and increased urination
Influenza	Fruity, acetone-like breath odor	Dry and crusty mucous membranes
Hypoglycemia	Poor muscle strength	Subnormal temperature reading
Hypothyroidism	Sleepiness	Weak pulse

Practice Question 4.4 — Drop-Down Cloze

A single parent arrives at the homeless mobile medical unit and asks to speak to a nurse about feelings experienced. The parent is holding their infant and reports that the infant was born 2 months ago. The nurse performs an assessment on the parent and documents vital signs and Nurses' Notes in the medical record.

Vital Signs | Nurses' Notes

T: 98°F (36.6°C)
HR: 68
RR: 18
BP: 188/72
SpO$_2$: 98% on RA

Vital Signs | **Nurses' Notes**

Parent holding infant; infant still and sleeping
Reports feeling a loss of interest in everything that started a few weeks before the birth of the baby and feels that symptoms are worsening
Feels as though the infant is demanding and does not feel pleasure with caring for the infant Feeling inept as a parent. Expresses fear, worthlessness, guilt, and a lack of ability to care for self and the infant because of being a single parent and unhoused
Has no appetite and has lost weight; difficulty sleeping
Breast-feeding the infant, but does not think that the infant is getting enough milk

Complete the following sentence by choosing from the list of options provided.

Based on the assessment findings, the nurse determines that the parent is *most likely* experiencing 1 **[Select]**.

Options

Bipolar disorder
Postpartum psychosis
Postpartum obsessive-compulsive disorder
Peripartum depression

Practice Question 4.5 — Multiple Choice Select All That Apply

A 45-year-old client is admitted to the ED because of frequent episodes of chest pain unrelieved by sublingual nitroglycerin. The ECG shows ST segment elevation. Troponin levels are elevated. While awaiting results of diagnostic studies and transfer to the cardiac unit, the nurse monitors the client and checks vital signs.

Vital Signs

1200: HR 88; RR 22; BP 142/86
1215: HR 92; RR 24; BP 120/82
1230: HR 106 and weak; RR 28; BP 100/62
1245: HR 120 and weak; RR 32; BP 90/58

The nurse determines that these vital sign findings most likely indicate which complication(s)? Select all that apply.

☐ Dysrhythmias
☐ Pulmonary edema
☐ Cardiogenic shock
☐ Cardiac tamponade
☐ Pulmonary embolism
☐ Dissecting aortic aneurysm

Practice Question 4.6 — Matrix Multiple Response

At 1300 hours, an 86-year-old client with altered mental status who is accompanied by their neighbor is admitted to the medical-surgical unit, and the nurse is performing an assessment. The client has an IV solution of a 1000-mL bag of 0.9% sodium chloride hung at 1200 in the ED that is infusing at 100 mL/h. At 1400 hours, 1 hour after admission, the client's neighbor calls the nurse and reports that the client has a pounding headache, is having trouble breathing, and seems scared. The nurse assesses the client, reviews the laboratory results, and documents in the Nurses' Notes.

Nurses' Notes | Vital Signs | Laboratory Results

1300: Client is weak and reports has not been able to eat or drink in the past 3 days because of anorexia.
Skin is very dry, dry mucous membranes, sleepy.
Client reports a history of heart failure, hypertension, and hyperlipidemia.
Breath sounds clear bilaterally.
Medications include lisinopril, carvedilol, and digoxin.
1400: Client is dyspneic and complaining of chest tightness, coughing, and is pale; neck vein distention is seen. Breath sounds wheezing and congestion bilaterally; 500 mL remaining in the IV bag.

Nurses' Notes | Vital Signs | Laboratory Results

1300: T 100.2°F (36.8°C); apical HR 72 and regular; BP 100/68; RR 24; SpO$_2$ 90% on RA
1400: T 100.2°F (36.8°C); apical HR 110 and regular; BP 152/98; RR 28; SpO$_2$ 89% on RA

Nurses' Notes | Vital Signs | Laboratory Results

Test and Reference Range	Result
Blood urea nitrogen (BUN) 10–20 mg/dL (3.6–7.1 mmol/L)	24 mg/dL (8.64 mmol/L)
Creatinine 0.5–1.2 mg/dL (44–106 µmol/L)	1.8 mg/dL (159.4 µmol/L)
Digoxin 0.5–2.0 ng/mL (0.64–2.56 nmol/L)	2.2 ng/mL (2.8 nmol/L)
Sodium 135–145 mEq/L (135–145 mmol/L)	148 mEq/L (148 mmol/L)
Potassium 3.5–5.0 mEq/L (3.5–5.0 mmol/L)	5.2 mEq/L (5.2 mmol/L)

*For each assessment finding below, click to specify if the finding is **most likely** consistent with dehydration, circulatory overload, or digoxin toxicity. Check one response only for each row.*

Assessment Finding	Dehydration	Circulatory Overload	Digoxin Toxicity
Anorexia	☐	☐	☐
Dry mucous membranes	☐	☐	☐
BUN and creatinine levels	☐	☐	☐
Sodium and potassium levels	☐	☐	☐
Digoxin level	☐	☐	☐
Elevation in BP and RR	☐	☐	☐
Wheezing and congestion bilaterally in lungs	☐	☐	☐
Neck vein distention	☐	☐	☐

CHAPTER 5

Strategies for Answering NGN Questions: Prioritize Hypotheses

THINKING SPACE

Prioritize Hypotheses is a clinical judgment cognitive skill nurses use to establish and rank client needs, problems, or hypotheses in order of priority. When prioritizing hypotheses, the nurse considers potential occurrences such as the likelihood of what could happen in a specific scenario, the urgency of it, and associated risks. In addition, environmental factors and individual factors need to be considered when prioritizing hypotheses. These factors are described in this chapter.

What Do Hypotheses Mean?

You may ask, "What are *hypotheses*?" A *hypothesis* (singular) or *hypotheses* (plural) are in part a prediction that you make about a clinical scenario to determine the client's priority needs. Once you interpret the relevant data in a clinical scenario and consider all possibilities or predictions about what is occurring, you then rank these predictions according to their urgency, risks, and time constraints for the client to decide on the priority needs for care. You need to determine which needs are *most immediate* and *most serious,* and why. You need to ask yourself, "Which explanations are most likely? Which explanations are least likely? Which of these explanations are the most immediate and serious?"

What Does Prioritizing Mean?

NGN TIP

Remember: When you prioritize, decide which client needs are primary and require immediate attention and which ones could be delayed until a later time because they are not urgent.

Prioritizing means that you need to rank the client's needs in order of importance. It is important to focus on all information in the clinical scenario because the order of importance may vary depending on the health problems, the environmental setting, and the client's condition. When a clinical situation is presented, you may also need to consider what the client deems a priority, which may be quite different from what you think is most important.

What to Consider When Prioritizing Hypotheses

Applying the cognitive skill *Prioritize Hypotheses* is essential for making appropriate clinical judgments and is a skill that will be measured both on the NGN and on your nursing course exams. When prioritizing hypotheses, in addition to the information in the clinical scenario, you need to consider external factors and connect or link these factors to the clinical scenario to determine priority client needs. In fact, considering external factors is important when applying every cognitive skill. The cognitive skill *Prioritize Hypotheses* involves considering all possibilities or predictions about what is occurring, ranking these predictions by their urgency and risks for the client, and deciding where to start with planning care. A description of how each external factor affects your thinking process in determining priority client needs is discussed in this chapter. See Box 5.1 for the possible external factors you may be asked about or need to consider in a clinical scenario.

BOX 5.1 External Factors to Consider When Prioritizing Hypotheses

Environmental Factors	Individual Factors
• Environment	• Knowledge
• Client observation	• Skills
• Resources	• Specialty
• Medical records	• Candidate (test-taker) characteristics
• Consequences and risks	• Prior experience
• Time pressure	• Level of experience
• Task complexity	
• Cultural considerations	

From National Council of State Boards of Nursing (NCSBN). (2019). *Next Generation NCLEX® News*, Winter 2019. <https://www.ncsbn.org/public-files/NGN_Winter19.pdf>

External Factors and Prioritizing Hypotheses

The cognitive skill *Prioritize Hypotheses* asks you to determine priority client needs in a specific clinical scenario. In doing so, you need to consider the context of any external factors presented. The NCSBN notes that there are environmental factors and individual factors that need to be considered (see Box 5.1). Following is a description of how each external factor affects your thinking process in determining priority client needs.

Environmental Factors

Environment

The *environment* refers to the setting in which client care is taking place. The environment is important to think about because you may need to reorder priority client needs and your approach to answering a question. Establishing priority client needs in the ED may be very different than how you would order these needs in a community-based clinic. For example, a client experiencing an emergent problem, such as a myocardial infarction (MI) or symptoms of acute coronary syndrome, would need to have care prioritized differently based on the resources available in the environment in which the care is taking place. In the clinic setting, the nurse would call EMS to transport the client to the hospital as a priority, whereas in the ED setting, the nurse would facilitate management of the problem, such as initiating the treatment plan, obtaining diagnostic testing, and analyzing the results.

Client Observation

The nurse's observations of the client need to be considered to establish hypotheses and then rank them in order of priority, which will be necessary to guide further client care. When your thinking process is focused on prioritizing, this guides you to the next step, generating solutions by asking, "Where do I start?" For example, when caring for a client who is in pain, the priority client need could be pain, which would guide the nurse to determine that conducting a thorough and comprehensive pain assessment is the priority. This would help the nurse generate the most appropriate solutions and interventions and allow for a connected follow-up assessment after pain medication or other pain-relieving measures are instituted.

Resources

Availability of resources will affect the way you answer a question about a clinical scenario. For example, if you were a first responder to a mass casualty site, you would triage victims differently than you would if the victims were brought to the ED because the available resources would be quite different and much more limited at the mass casualty site. Also, think about this situation: If a cardiac arrest was discovered, you would answer a question differently if you had additional personnel to assist than if you (the nurse) were the only person available.

THINKING SPACE

Medical Records

NGN test items present a medical record as part of the question; this is another external factor you need to consider before answering the question about the clinical scenario. All information provided in the medical record needs to be reviewed and critically analyzed before you determine the urgency of findings, think about explanations of those findings, and establish priority client needs. Refer to Chapter 3, which discusses the cognitive skill *Recognize Cues,* and Chapter 4, which discusses the cognitive skill *Analyze Cues*—both of which need to be applied when considering information in a medical record before applying the skill *Prioritize Hypotheses.*

Consequences and Risks

While thinking about explanations for client findings and establishing and ranking hypotheses based on the explanations, you need to think about the consequences and risks associated with the findings to guide you in priority setting. For example, the nurse caring for a client with dehydration would think about the risks and consequences associated with fluid volume deficit being left untreated or unmanaged while considering the urgency or priority of nursing actions that would be required to treat the problem. Another example may be a client with a UTI, who would be monitored for signs and symptoms of sepsis and shock as potential complications that would be a priority.

Time Pressure

Time pressure is another external factor to consider when applying the skill *Prioritize Hypotheses.* If time is part of the data presented in the question, it may be a factor to consider as you are deciding on the answer or answers to the question. As an example, a nurse taking care of a postoperative client would consider client data findings differently and consider different explanations of the findings based on whether the client just came out of surgery, has been out of surgery for 8 hours, or had the surgery several days before. Another example of time as a factor in prioritization is related to how long it may take to meet a client need. If you had a client experiencing dyspnea, for instance, you would consider elevating the head of the client's bed right away to alleviate the respiratory distress, which takes seconds to do, before listening to lung sounds, which will take more time.

Task Complexity

Task complexity is a measure of the difficulty of a task that the nurse considers and takes into account in order to complete the task. For example, with regard to prioritizing hypotheses, one factor a home care nurse would think about is how much time would be needed and how involved the client's needs are for each assigned client for the day. The nurse would organize the schedule according to the clients' needs and the complexity of the care to be provided. The nurse may have a client who needs an admission assessment completed, a client who needs a wound irrigation, and a client requiring teaching about a simple dressing change. The nurse would consider the complexity of the tasks involved with the care being provided as one factor to decide how to prioritize.

Cultural Considerations

The last environmental factor to think about is cultural considerations. If information related to the client's culture is included in the clinical scenario, it will be important to consider these factors as you are answering test questions. As an example, you may need to consider dietary preferences as they relate to culture and diversity to provide nutrition that is aligned with important values and meet the client's needs while the client is in your care. Or you may need to consider higher-risk health problems that are specific to a cultural group when you are prioritizing hypotheses.

Individual Factors

Knowledge and Skills

Nursing knowledge and skills are individual factors considered when nursing exam questions are developed for your nursing courses and for the NGN. Intuitively, exam questions will be written to test specific nursing knowledge and skills, based on expected activities performed by new graduate nurses. When caring for a client, you need to use nursing knowledge when applying all cognitive skills including *Prioritizing Hypotheses.* In your nursing program, it is critical that you *not* learn just by memorizing concepts. Learning by memorization is short-lived and is a superficial type of learning that does not require any thinking. You need to approach the learning process so you will be able to make connections from what you previously learned to a new situation you may encounter and be able to know what is most urgent when prioritizing hypotheses. This type of learning is called *deep learning,* and it requires retrieval knowledge and thinking. For example, let's say you are caring for a client who has an MI. You would need to recall many previously learned concepts and skills to prioritize hypotheses and safely care for that client. Some concepts and skills you would need to recall are the anatomic structure of the heart and coronary arteries, their function, cardiac rhythms, emergency treatments, and complications associated with an MI.

Specialty

Another individual factor is the nursing specialty. Nursing exams and NGN test items include questions about foundations of care, pharmacology, medical-surgical nursing, obstetrics nursing, or mental health nursing. As noted earlier, deep learning is important because you may, for example, need to apply previously learned physical assessment concepts or foundational concepts to a new situation. Consider this scenario when prioritizing hypotheses: An 85-year-old client is admitted to the nursing unit with weakness, confusion, an elevated temperature, tachycardia, and hypotension. You would need to consider all possibilities or predictions about what is occurring in this client, such as possible dehydration or infection. You would then rank these predictions according to their urgency and risk(s) for the client to decide on the priority need(s). You would need to determine which needs are *most immediate* and *most serious,* and why.

Candidate Characteristics, Prior Experience, and Level of Experience

Candidate characteristics, such as prior experience and level of experience, are additional individual factors considered with the application of cognitive skills and clinical judgment. As an example, a new nursing graduate may not be as skilled as an experienced nurse about actions to take when the nurse notices a change in a client's clinical condition. This skill depends on prior experience and current level of experience. However, it is important to remember that regardless of prior experience or level of experience, client safety is the priority, and the nurse needs to be able to rank priority needs swiftly if a client's condition deteriorates. Nurses with less experience can always use the guidance of more experienced nurses as an invaluable resource.

How Do You Know That You Need to Prioritize?

As a nurse, you will be prioritizing all the time; this skill is a critical one to ensure safety for each client. For example, when you receive an assignment for the nursing shift, you will need to prioritize client needs for a group of clients and determine which assigned client you will need to assess first, second, third, and so on. Look at the following scenario about prioritizing for a group of clients.

Scenario 1: The nurse is assigned the following three clients during the 0600–1400 shift. Who would the nurse assess first, second, and third?

Client 1: Client admitted to the nursing unit during the night because of difficulty breathing
Client 2: Client on IV antibiotics and due to receive a dose at 0900
Client 3: Client being discharged to home today who needs further teaching about insulin administration and diet

In addition, as a nurse, you will also need to prioritize client needs for one client. On the NCLEX®, prioritizing client needs for one client are most commonly presented. Look at the following example of prioritizing for a single client.

THINKING SPACE

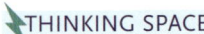THINKING SPACE

Scenario 2: The client is experiencing a sickle cell crisis. Which of the following are the client's **priority** needs? **Select all that apply.**

Client Need 1: Pain management
Client Need 2: Fluid balance
Client Need 3: Oxygenation
Client Need 4: Nutritional needs
Client Need 5: Electrolyte balance

Questions that require prioritization include strategic words or strategic phrases in the question that indicate the need to prioritize. Be sure to look for these specific words or phrases. Box 5.2 lists some common strategic words or phrases.

What Strategies Can You Use to Prioritize Hypotheses?

First and foremost, it is important to think and use your nursing knowledge. Nursing knowledge provides information that you need to process and think about critically to answer the question. Nursing knowledge is needed to answer many test items on the NCLEX®.

Three strategies you can use to assist in prioritizing client needs are the *Priority Classification System; Airway, Breathing, and Circulation;* and *Physiologic and Safety Needs.* These strategies are described in the following sections.

Priority Classification System

To start the process of priority setting, try to use the Priority Classification System and rank hypotheses as a high (top), intermediate (middle), or low (last) priority. The high-priority hypotheses then become your primary and urgent client needs. Intermediate-priority hypotheses are client needs that are less urgent but still important and can wait to be addressed. Low-priority hypotheses are client needs that are either unrelated to the client's health problem or can wait to be addressed until after attending to the high- and intermediate-priority needs. Box 5.3 provides a description of the three types of classifications.

Airway, Breathing, and Circulation

Airway, breathing, and circulation is abbreviated as the *ABCs*. You can use the ABCs to help you determine the priority client needs. Airway is always a priority in caring for any client. Think about it: If a client does not have a patent airway and breathing is ineffective

---

BOX 5.2 Common Strategic Words or Phrases

Best	Initial	Most likely
Decreased	Immediate	Most important
First	Immediately	Refute
Highest	Next	Support
Primary	Essential	
Increased	Most	

BOX 5.3 Priority Classification System

High (Top) Priority: A client need that is life-threatening or if untreated could result in harm to the client

Intermediate (Middle) Priority: A nonemergency and non–life-threatening client need that does not require immediate attention and can wait to be addressed

Low (Last) Priority: A client need that is not directly related to the client's illness or prognosis, is not urgent, and can wait until high and intermediate client needs are addressed

to oxygenate body tissues, will any other client need matter? Breathing is the next priority because breathing is needed to oxygenate tissue; again, if the airway is not patent, then the client will not be able to breathe. Finally, circulation: Circulation is critical but requires oxygenated blood to effectively oxygenate tissue. Note that there is one exception, and that is if you are prioritizing client needs in a cardiopulmonary resuscitation scenario. For these scenarios, remember to follow CAB—circulation (compressions), airway, and breathing—to prioritize. Consider the clinical scenario in which a client with chronic obstructive pulmonary disease (COPD) is experiencing difficulty breathing and the SpO_2 level is lower than the baseline level. This scenario would take high priority because the airway (and breathing and circulation as well) is involved. When ranking in the context of other client's needs, consider this clinical scenario for the client with COPD who is experiencing difficulty breathing and at the same time a postoperative client complaining of pain of 5/10 at the operative site who is asking for pain medication. Because the second clinical scenario does not involve the ABCs, the nurse would appropriately rank the client with difficulty breathing ahead of the client having pain.

Physiologic and Safety Needs

Physiologic client needs and client safety are always priorities. It is important to consider all client needs in any clinical scenario, but most likely you will need to address physiologic needs first. Remember that physiologic integrity is necessary for survival. At times, however, safety is the top priority. For example, a client who has suicidal ideation is experiencing a potentially life-threatening condition. In this case, suicide prevention is the priority for this client's care to prevent self-harm and keep the client safe.

Another example is a client who is being discharged from the hospital and needs teaching about administering insulin, so you identify teaching as a priority client need. Safety must be considered along with the teaching. However, if your client suddenly develops weakness, shakiness, and hunger, you would determine that the client is experiencing hypoglycemia. At that time, your priority client need switches from teaching to one that addresses the physiologic need of hypoglycemia, but, in addition, safety is a priority.

How Do You Prioritize Hypotheses in an NGN Clinical Situation?

As noted in Chapter 2, NGN questions will begin with a clinical scenario presented as either a Stand-Alone item or an Unfolding Case Study. Information about the client is presented, and you need to identify the relevant data. As noted in Chapter 4, once these relevant data are noted, you analyze the data and link these data to the client situation to determine what the data mean and what is happening to the client. Then, based on your judgment of what you think is happening to the client, you assign priority or urgency to those client needs, which exemplifies application of the skill *Prioritize Hypotheses*. The following example provides you with client data.

Example—Prioritize Hypotheses: A 45-year-old client is preparing for discharge following a 2-month hospitalization and will need long-term IV antibiotics. The client has a central line in place. The client has a past medical history of DM and takes insulin with meals and at bedtime. During this hospitalization, the client has become very weak and needs PT and OT to help improve functional ability. The client will be moving in with family, who will be the primary caregivers. The client will have home health support services to help manage medications. The client is anxious about going home and having to rely on others to help with care.

After reviewing information in all tabs of the medical record and once relevant cues have been identified and analyzed, you then prioritize hypotheses. You will need to determine the urgency of the identified client needs to guide the next steps in client care. The cognitive skill *Prioritize Hypotheses* is required to ensure planning safe client care. Remember to consider the external factors previously discussed when considering the priorities of care.

THINKING SPACE

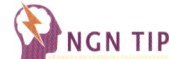

Remember: In a clinical scenario, the priority order of client needs is not static. In other words, as a client's condition changes, whether that be improvement or deterioration, the priority of needs can change.

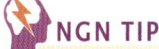

Remember: *Prioritize Hypotheses* is the cognitive skill in which you rank the urgency of client needs. This leads to formulating a plan of care based on those needs *(Generate Solutions)* and to clinical decision making with implementing care *(Take Actions)*.

THINKING SPACE

What Will You Think About to Prioritize Hypotheses in This Clinical Scenario?

To *Prioritize Hypotheses*, you would need to think about the client's needs based on the information provided in the scenario. As the nurse preparing the client for discharge, you would consider what the client will need in the first few days at home until the client's new routine is established and home health care services and other supports are in place.

Begin by considering the external factors that may be important in the scenario. Thinking about these factors before looking at the question you are being asked will help your thinking process as you answer. Consider the environment—a hospital setting. This helps frame your thinking in terms of what the role of the nurse is in providing teaching and support to the client during this time. Think about any client observation data—the client will need long-term IV antibiotics, is weak after a prolonged hospitalization, has a past medical history of DM and takes insulin, and is anxious about going home. These client needs are important to address as priorities in the discharge teaching. This scenario mentions the resources of home health care and family support. As you think about answering questions about this situation, consider these resources and how they may factor into the way the questions are answered. Other considerations as you prioritize hypotheses for this scenario may be task complexity and consequences and risks. The client will need IV antibiotics and insulin. These are important interventions in which you will need to provide very clear and understandable teaching to promote safety and mitigate risk and any unintended consequences. In this scenario, thinking also about the external factors, you would consider the following as priority hypotheses:

- Safety in the home environment
- Discharge needs
- Establishing care with home health support
- Maintaining a central line
- Administering antibiotics
- Complications of a central line
- Side effects of medications
- Client and caregiver teaching

NGN TIP

Remember: Use these strategies for NGN items that measure *Prioritize Hypotheses*:
- Examine the clinical scenario and any relevant external factors.
- Determine the urgency of the client findings as you assign priority in planning subsequent client care.
- Ask yourself, "Which needs are most immediate and most serious, and why?"
- Ask yourself, "What could explain what I am seeing with the client, and what explanations are most likely or least likely?"

Which NGN Item Types Optimally Measure *Prioritize Hypotheses*?

Three types of test items are most likely to be used to optimally measure the cognitive skill *Prioritize Hypotheses*. Variations of each type will be presented on the NGN. Table 5.1 presents these item types and their variations.

All of these test item types are discussed in Chapter 2, and some examples are provided. The following section explains the three major item types that best measure *Prioritize Hypotheses*.

TABLE 5.1 Test Items and Variations That Optimally Measure *Prioritize Hypotheses*

Type of Test Item	Variations
Drop-Down	Drop-Down Cloze Drop-Down Rationale Drop-Down in Table
Multiple Response	Multiple Response Select N Multiple Response Select All That Apply Multiple Response Grouping
Drag-and-Drop	Drag-and-Drop Cloze Drag-and-Drop Rationale

Drop-Down Test Items to Measure *Prioritize Hypotheses*

Drop-Down items include Drop-Down Cloze, Drop-Down Rationale, and Drop-Down in Table. When the Drop-Down item type is used to measure *Prioritize Hypotheses*, the test taker is required to complete a sentence or blank space by choosing from a list of options. Sample Question 5.1 illustrates a Drop-Down Rationale item type used to measure the cognitive skill *Prioritize Hypotheses*. The rationale and test-taking strategy to help you derive the correct responses in Sample Question 5.1 are also provided.

Sample Question 5.1 — Drop-Down Rationale Item: *Prioritize Hypotheses*

The nurse is caring for a 70-year-old client on the acute medical-surgical unit.

Health History | Nurses' Notes | Vital Signs | Medication Administration Record

Two days ago, the client was transported to the ED by EMS with nausea, vomiting, confusion, and right-sided weakness. The client was diagnosed with hemorrhagic stroke and was treated with surgical evacuation the same day. The client now has new-onset right-sided paralysis with garbled speech and a weak cough and swallow reflex. Past medical history includes hypertension, osteoarthritis, and type 2 diabetes mellitus.

Health History | **Nurses' Notes** | Vital Signs | Medication Administration Record

0700: Neurologic: Alert and oriented × 2, and restless. Disoriented to time and situation. Pupils are equal in size, 4 mm and round bilaterally. Left eye is brisk and reactive to light; right eye is sluggish to response to light. Right eye has paralysis of upward gaze.
Cardiovascular: Audible S1 and S2. Capillary refill is less than 2 seconds. Radial and pedal pulses are 3+ bilaterally.
Respiratory: Rhonchi auscultated in bilateral lower lung fields.
Integumentary: Incision on left temporal aspect of the skull. Dressing is dry and intact.
Gastrointestinal: Bowel sounds present × 4 quadrants. Abdomen soft, nondistended.
Musculoskeletal: Unable to push against resistance with right upper and lower extremities, muscle strength 0/5.
Metabolic: FSBG: 135 mg/dL (7.5 mmol/L). Reference range: 70–99 mg/dL (3.9–5.5 mmol/L).

Health History | Nurses' Notes | **Vital Signs** | Medication Administration Record

0715: T 100°F (37.7°C); HR 102; RR 24; BP 150/86; SpO_2 90% on RA; Pain: 5 (on a 0-to-10 pain intensity scale) decreased from 7/10 at 0630

Health History | Nurses' Notes | Vital Signs | **Medication Administration Record**

Medication	0700	1000	1130	2000
Metformin 500 mg orally daily		Due		
Insulin aspart subcutaneously per sliding scale 151–200 mg/dL (8.4–11.1 mmol/L) = 3 units 201–250 mg/dL (11.2–13.9 mmol/L) = 5 units 251–300 mg/dL (14–16.7 mmol/L) = 8 units >300 mg/dL (>16.7 mmol/L) = call physician	Due		Due	
Insulin glargine 10 units subcutaneously at bedtime				Due
Lisinopril 20 mg orally daily	Due		Due	
Morphine 4 mg IV push prn pain 7 or greater out of 10	4 mg at 0632			

Complete the following sentence by choosing from the lists of options provided.

The **most** concerning potential complication is <u>atelectasis</u> as evidenced by <u>SpO_2 on RA</u>.

Options for 1	Options for 2
Atelectasis	HR 102
Diabetic ketoacidosis (DKA)	SpO_2 90% on RA
Life-threatening dysrhythmia	FSBG 135 mg/dL (7.5 mmol/L)
Uncontrolled pain	Pain level 5/10

THINKING SPACE

Rationale: The client experienced a hemorrhagic stroke and was treated with surgical evacuation. The client is now experiencing new-onset right-sided paralysis with garbled speech and a weak cough and swallow reflex, which are likely complications from the stroke. The client is also showing additional signs of neurologic deficits as evidenced by disorientation, sluggish pupillary response, and right eye paralysis. Due to the weakness and neurologic deficits, a primary concern is atelectasis, which occurs when the alveoli in the lungs deflate, affecting gas exchange in the lower airways. The client would not likely be able to perform effective coughing and deep breathing, and the client might have difficulty following commands, increasing the risk for atelectasis. The client is showing signs of atelectasis as evidenced by the SpO_2 of 90% on RA and rhonchi auscultated in the bilateral lower lung fields. The client's FSBG is 135 mg/dL (7.5 mmol/L), so the client is not experiencing DKA. A life-threatening dysrhythmia is not the most concerning potential complication because the HR is only slightly elevated at 102, and there is no evidence of dysrhythmia. Uncontrolled pain is not the most concerning potential complication because the pain level is decreasing with morphine administration.

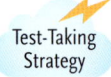

Test-Taking Strategy: Focus on the information in the scenario, and remember that with questions that require prioritizing, there may be multiple options that are pertinent, and you will need to decide which options take priority. As illustrated in the table, consider each potential complication, whether it is likely occurring or not likely occurring, and the evidence supporting each condition, and then assign priority to those conditions based on available evidence.

Client Condition	Likely Occurring/ Not Likely Occurring	High Priority/ Low Priority	Available Evidence
Atelectasis	Likely occurring	High priority	Weak cough and swallow reflex, SpO_2 90% on RA, rhonchi in bilateral lower lung fields, history of stroke with residual deficits
Diabetic ketoacidosis	Not likely occurring	Low priority	FSBG 135 mg/dL (7.5 mmol/L), taking insulin regularly, blood glucose monitored regularly, no other signs/symptoms of diabetic ketoacidosis
Uncontrolled pain	Not likely occurring	Low priority	Pain 5/10, improving with pain medication
Life-threatening dysrhythmia	Not likely occurring	Low priority	HR 102, no other signs/symptoms of dysrhythmias

This thinking process will help you answer the first part of the question: determining the complications. Life-threatening dysrhythmias and diabetic ketoacidosis are not present and can be eliminated first. Although pain is present, it is likely controlled, so this can be eliminated next. Remember that atelectasis is a primary concern for the client experiencing stroke. Once you have decided on the potential complication, look for the supporting evidence for the complication.

Content Area: Medical-Surgical Nursing
Priority Concepts: Gas Exchange; Perfusion
Reference(s): Ignatavicius et al., 2024, pp. 498, 944, 951–952, 1370; Lilley et al., 2023, p. 150

NGN TIP

Remember: In a Drop-Down Rationale test item, it is important to choose the first option correctly so the remaining option choices are based on the correct foundation.

Multiple Response Test Items to Measure *Prioritize Hypotheses*

As discussed in Chapter 2, Multiple Response test items include Multiple Response Select All That Apply, Multiple Response Select N, and Multiple Response Grouping. When the Multiple Response item type is used to measure *Prioritize Hypotheses* or other cognitive skills, the test taker is required to follow the question directions regarding how to select options. Sample Question 5.2 illustrates a Multiple Response Select All That Apply item type. The rationale and test-taking strategy to help you derive the correct responses shown in Sample Question 5.2 are also provided.

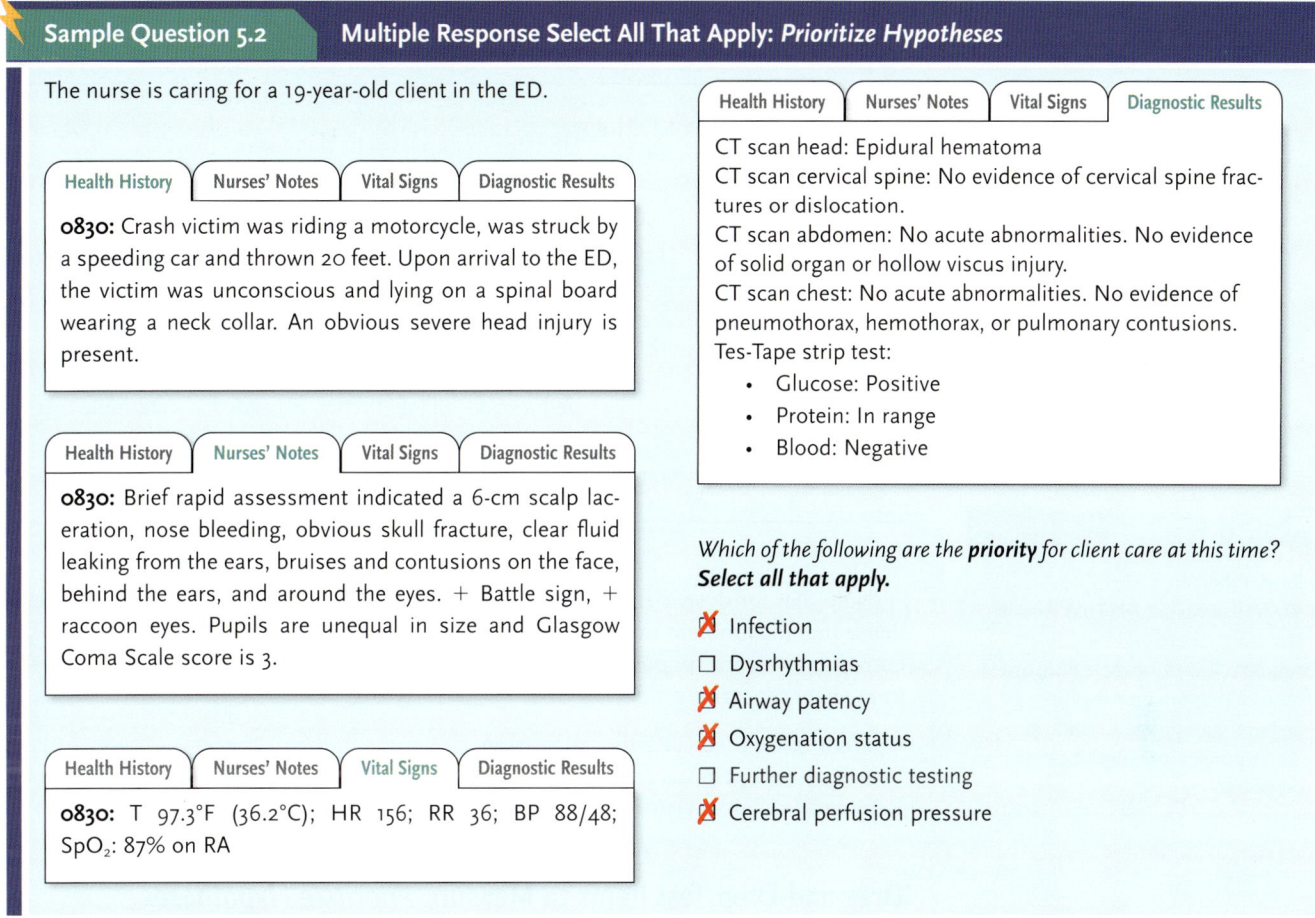

Rationale: The client is a victim of a motorcycle crash and has an obvious severe head injury. The CT scan of the head indicates an epidural hematoma, which is a potentially fatal condition that requires immediate neurosurgical intervention to relieve pressure on the brain. An epidural hematoma is usually caused by a linear fracture crossing a major artery in the dura, resulting in a tear. It can have either a venous or arterial origin. The CT scan of the cervical spine, abdomen, and chest are unremarkable. The Tes-Tape strip test indicates that the fluid leaking from the nose and ears is positive for glucose, the protein level is in range, and blood is not detected. Other findings of concern include the 6-cm scalp laceration, nose bleeding, + Battle sign and + raccoon eyes, pupillary findings, and the Glasgow Coma Scale score. The HR is elevated at 156, RR is elevated at 36, BP is decreased at 88/48, and SpO_2 is decreased at 87% on RA. Airway patency and cerebral perfusion pressure are immediate concerns with an epidural hematoma. Oxygenation status is another immediate concern, and administering supplemental oxygen will assist with oxygenation to the brain and vital organs. Because there is a skull fracture, infection of the underlying structures inside the skull is a potential complication; therefore monitoring for signs and symptoms of infection is another priority.

▸THINKING SPACE

THINKING SPACE

Further diagnostic testing is not necessary at this time and does not provide additional information to direct the client's care. The priority treatment will be emergency neurosurgery to stop the bleeding. Dysrhythmias are not an immediate concern at this time because the pulse is most likely elevated because of the low circulating blood volume from blood loss; the treatment for this will likely be to administer intravenous fluids to maintain blood volume.

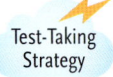

Test-Taking Strategy: Note the strategic word *immediate*. Think about the scenario and the effects of the injury. Look at each option provided, and make an association with the information presented in the medical record, as illustrated in the table.

Option	Evidence from Medical Record
Infection	Skull fracture—opening into brain
Dysrhythmias	HR 156—likely related to blood loss No specific evidence of dysrhythmias
Airway patency	Severe head injury possibly damaging respiratory center in brain
Oxygenation status	Severe head injury, low circulating blood volume, HR 156, RR 36, BP 88/48, SpO$_2$ 87% on RA
Further diagnostic testing	Assessment completed including VS; CT scan of head, cervical spine, abdomen, and chest; Tes-tape strip test performed—all information is needed to determine that emergency neurosurgical intervention is required
Cerebral perfusion pressure	Severe head injury, Glasgow Coma Scale score 3, pupillary changes, BP 88/48, overall neurologic status

Note that for dysrhythmias and further diagnostic testing, there is no specific evidence that the problem exists, or it would delay necessary emergency intervention. The correct options are supported by clear evidence and therefore would be considered the immediate concerns.

Content Area: Medical-Surgical Nursing
Priority Concepts: Gas Exchange; Perfusion
Reference(s): Ignatavicius et al., 2024, pp. 956–958, 961–962

Drag-and-Drop Test Items to Measure *Prioritize Hypotheses*

As discussed in Chapter 2, Drag-and-Drop test items include Drag-and-Drop Cloze and Drag-and-Drop Rationale items. When the Drag-and-Drop item type is used to measure *Prioritize Hypotheses*, the test taker is required to complete a sentence or blank space by choosing from a list of options or word choices. Sample Question 5.3 illustrates a Drag-and-Drop Rationale item type, and Sample Question 5.4 illustrates a Drag-and-Drop Cloze item type. The rationale and test-taking strategy to help you derive the correct responses in Sample Question 5.3 and Sample Question 5.4 are also provided.

> **NGN TIP**
>
> **Remember:** In a Multiple Response Select All That Apply test item, there will be 5 to 10 options. There may be only one correct response or multiple correct responses. In addition, all responses presented could be correct.

> **NGN TIP**
>
> **Remember:** A Drag-and-Drop Rationale test item requires full understanding of paired information and justification through a rationale. Both the concept and the rationale must be correct to earn credit.

Sample Question 5.3 — Drag-and-Drop Rationale: *Prioritize Hypotheses*

The nurse working at the outpatient dialysis center is assisting in performing hemodialysis.

Nurses' Notes

1000: Client's BP during dialysis decreased to 82/54. Reduced the temperature of the dialysate, adjusted the rate of the dialyzer blood flow, placed the client in the Trendelenburg position, and administered albumin as prescribed.

1045: BP 80/52; client reporting light-headedness.

Complete the following sentence by selecting from the lists of options below.

The client is **most** at risk for developing **myocardial injury** due to **pericardial disease**.

Options for 1	Options for 2
Hypoglycemia	Fluid shifts
Myocardial injury	DM
Infectious disease	Pericardial disease
Fluid volume imbalances	Frequent blood transfusions
Disequilibrium syndrome	Rapid reduction of electrolytes

Rationale: Certain adverse effects can occur during hemodialysis, including hypotension, disequilibrium syndrome, cardiac events, and reactions to dialyzers. Hypotension is a common complication caused by heat transfer resulting in vasodilation. Initially the nurse would reduce the temperature of the dialysate; adjust the rate of the dialyzer blood flow; place the client in Trendelenburg position; and administer a fluid bolus, albumin, or mannitol as prescribed. If these interventions do not resolve the problem and if hypotension persists, the nurse would consider myocardial injury and possible underlying pericardial disease as a cause. The other conditions noted can occur with hemodialysis; however, the client findings in this clinical scenario and the fact that the interventions were ineffective indicate a cardiac event.

Test-Taking Strategy: Note the strategic word *most,* and remember that this word indicates the need to prioritize. This likely means that some or all of the options are correct or make sense in the clinical scenario, but you need to decide which condition the client is most at risk for developing. Even though a cardiac history is not noted in the scenario, note that the actions the nurse took were ineffective; this points to pericardial disease as the underlying cause. In the table, begin by matching the condition on the left with the potential underlying cause on the right.

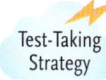

Conditions	Potential Underlying Causes
Hypoglycemia	DM
Myocardial injury	Pericardial disease
Infectious disease	Frequent blood transfusions
Fluid volume imbalances	Fluid shifts
Disequilibrium syndrome	Rapid reduction of electrolytes

From here, based on the data in the clinical scenario, you need to decide which condition the client is most at risk for developing, knowing that these are all possible with hemodialysis. Note that the nurse already reduced the temperature of the dialysate, adjusted the rate of the dialyzer blood flow, placed the client in Trendelenburg position, and administered albumin as prescribed, and the BP was still low. This will direct you to consider myocardial injury caused by pericardial disease as the priority client need.

Content Area: Medical-Surgical Nursing
Priority Concepts: Gas Exchange; Perfusion
Reference(s): Ignatavicius et al., 2024, p. 1481

Sample Question 5.4 — Drag-and-Drop Cloze: *Prioritize Hypotheses*

Health History | Laboratory Results

1000: A 38-year-old client presents to the ED complaining of severe back pain in the right flank area rated 9 (on a 0 to 10 pain intensity scale). The client has a history of hypertension, DM, hyperlipidemia, hypothyroidism, arthritis, and renal calculi. The CT scan of the abdomen shows a 10-mm renal calculus in the right kidney with hydronephrosis. The client is requesting ketorolac for the pain, stating that this has worked well in the past. Home medications include lisinopril, metformin, atorvastatin, levothyroxine, and ibuprofen. The ED physician resumes all home medications except for the ibuprofen, adds tamsulosin daily and ketorolac as needed for pain, orders laboratory testing, and arranges for a urology consultation. The urologist assesses the client and adds morphine as needed for pain to the medication regimen. The urologist also orders extracorporeal shockwave lithotripsy (ESWL) for the following day. Laboratory results return, and the nurse reviews the results.

Health History | Laboratory Results

Test and Reference Range	Result
Red blood cells (RBCs) 4.2–6.2 × 10^{12}/L (4.2–6.2 × 10^{12}/L)	5.8 × 10^{12}/L (5.8 × 10^{12}/L)
White blood cells (WBCs) 5000–10,000/mm³ (5–10 × 10^9/L)	9000/mm³ (9 × 10^9/L)
Platelets 150,000–400,000/mm³ (150–400 × 10^9/L)	200,000/mm³ (200 × 10^9/L)
Hemoglobin (Hgb) 12–18 g/dL (120–180 g/L)	17 g/dL (170 g/L)
Hematocrit (Hct) 37%–52% (0.37–0.52)	50% (0.50)
Albumin 3.5–5.0 g/dL (35–50 g/L)	3.6 g/dL (36 g/L)
Blood urea nitrogen (BUN) 10–20 mg/dL (3.6–7.1 mmol/L)	32 mg/dL (11.52 mmol/L)
Calcium 9–10.5 mg/dL (2.25–2.75 mmol/L)	10.2 mg/dL (2.7 mmol/L)
Chloride 98–106 mEq/L (98–106 mmol/L)	102 mEq/L (102 mmol/L)
Creatinine 0.5–1.2 mg/dL (44–106 μmol/L)	2.2 mg/dL (194.3 μmol/L)
Glucose 70–99 mg/dL (3.9–5.5 mmol/L)	80 mg/dL (4.45 mmol/L)
Potassium 3.5–5.0 mEq/L (3.5–5.0 mmol/L)	4.4 mEq/L (4.4 mmol/L)
Sodium 135–145 mEq/L (135–145 mmol/L)	140 mEq/L (140 mmol/L)
Urinalysis Bilirubin: Negative Glucose: Negative Blood: Negative pH: 4.6–8.0 Protein: Negative Specific gravity: 1.005–1.030	Bilirubin: Negative Glucose: Negative Blood: Positive pH: 5.0 Protein: Trace Specific gravity: 1.012

Complete the following sentence by selecting from the list of word choices below.

Word Choices

- Pain management
- Stone analysis
- Preparation for ESWL
- Administer tamsulosin

The *priority* client need would be **pain management** followed by **preparation for ESWL**.

Rationale: Calculi (also known as *stones*) are deposits of minerals that form into stones inside the urinary tract, and they can be found in the kidneys, ureters, or bladder. When the calculus moves, it can cause pain that is often described as unbearable. Medications are integral to the treatment of clients with this problem, particularly for the management of pain. Because the client is experiencing such severe pain, the priority need is pain management, and the nurse would administer prescribed pain medication as a priority. Ketorolac can be very effective for pain associated with renal calculi. It is classified as an NSAID. This medication can be problematic in the setting of impaired renal function. Because the client's BUN and creatinine levels are elevated and there is blood noted on the urinalysis, NSAIDs should be avoided, and the nurse would opt for another pain management choice, such as the prescribed morphine. Opioid analgesics are often needed for the client experiencing renal colic from calculi. The nurse would need to contact the physician to inform them of the abnormal renal function and to clarify whether the ketorolac should be discontinued as an option for pain management. Extracorporeal shock wave lithotripsy (ESWL) uses shock waves to break a kidney stone into small pieces that can more easily travel through the urinary tract and pass from the body. The nurse would prepare the client for this procedure next. Tamsulosin is classified as an alpha-adrenergic antagonist; it works by relaxing the smooth muscle in the bladder neck and thereby assists with passing the stone. This medication would be administered, but not as the priority need in this scenario. A 10-mm stone may be difficult to pass, but after ESWL the stone fragments will pass and may pass more easily if tamsulosin is part of the treatment plan. The stone then can be analyzed for composition and type, and this information will assist with determining the best treatment.

Test-Taking Strategy: Note the strategic word *priority* in this question. The ability to use judgment and prioritize client needs is needed to answer this question correctly. Considering the client's needs in the context of the health problem the client is experiencing can help you decide on priorities of care. Using a thinking process as illustrated in the table may be helpful.

Plan/Intervention	Assists With Immediate Client Need	Does Not Assist With Immediate Client Need
Pain management	☒	☐
Stone analysis	☐	☒
Preparation for ESWL	☒	☐
Administer tamsulosin	☐	☒

Once you determine that pain management and preparation for ESWL are the priorities because they assist with immediate client needs, you need to rank order these and decide which one should come first and which should follow. Focusing on the client and the client's experience will help you decide on pain management as the first priority, followed by preparation for ESWL.

Content Area: Medical-Surgical Nursing
Priority Concepts: Elimination; Inflammation
Reference(s): Ignatavicius et al., 2024, p. 1422–1426

THINKING SPACE

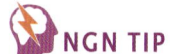
Test-Taking Strategy

NGN TIP

Remember: In a Drag-and-Drop Cloze test item, you will be asked to drag an option from a list of choices to fill in the blank in a sentence.

Practice Questions

Practice Question 5.1 — Multiple Response Grouping

A 12-year-old client visits the health care clinic for a follow-up visit after laboratory and other testing.

Health History | Nurses' Notes | Diagnostic Tests | Laboratory Results

0900: Parent states that client was diagnosed at 3 years of age with cystic fibrosis (CF).

Health History | **Nurses' Notes** | Diagnostic Tests | Laboratory Results

0900: VS: T 98.2°F (36.6°C); HR 78; RR 16; BP 118/70; SpO_2 96% on RA; denies pain.

Skin: Warm, dry, intact.

Respiratory: Dry cough. Reports sputum expectoration of thick, white mucus following respiratory treatments. Lung sounds clear to auscultation in all lung fields.

GI: Increased appetite. Reports taking pancreatic enzymes with all meals and snacks. Bowel sounds active × 4 quadrants. Regular bowel movements that are brown and fatty.

GU: Urinating more frequently than usual.

Weight: 91.5 lb (41.5 kg)

Height: 59 inches (149.8 cm)

Health History | Nurses' Notes | **Diagnostic Tests** | Laboratory Results

0930: Chest x-ray: Mild lung hyperinflation; no chest infiltrates, atelectasis, or bronchiectasis

---

Health History | Nurses' Notes | Diagnostic Tests | **Laboratory Results**

Test and Reference Range	Results
0930: Oral glucose tolerance test (OGTT) 2 hours: < 140 mg/dL (7.8 mmol/L)	240 mg/dL (13.37 mmol/L)

For each body system, select the **priority** client need to prevent a complication of the client's health problem. Each body system supports one priority client need.

Body System	Priority Client Need
Respiratory	☐ Oscillatory positive expiratory therapy (PEP)
	☐ Oxygen administration
GI	☐ Pancreatic enzyme therapy
	☐ Low-fat diet
Immune	☐ Prophylactic antibiotic therapy
	☐ Contact precautions with separation from others with CF by at least 6 feet
Endocrine	☐ Insulin administration
	☐ Recombinant human growth hormone administration
Integumentary	☐ High-sodium foods
	☐ Oatmeal baths

Practice Question 5.2 — Multiple Response Select N

A 68-year-old client complaining of chest pain is admitted to the medical-surgical nursing unit for acute coronary syndrome.

Nurses' Notes

1230: The cardiologist prescribes a continuous IV heparin infusion per protocol. The client weighs 165 lb (74.8 kg), and baseline partial thromboplastin time (PTT) is drawn. A heparin bolus is administered as prescribed, and a continuous infusion is initiated based on the protocol noted in the Medication Administration Record.

Medication Administration Record

Baseline PTT and every 6 or 12 hours after start of continuous infusion based on protocol.

Heparin 80 units/kg IV bolus prior to start of continuous infusion.

Start heparin 25,000 units in 250 mL D_5W (concentration 100 units/mL) continuous infusion 18 units/kg/h.

Adjust continuous infusion based on the following:
- PTT less than 35 seconds: IV bolus 80 units/kg, increase rate by 4 units/kg/h, PTT in 6 hours
- PTT 35–45 seconds: IV bolus 40 units/kg, increase rate by 2 units/kg/h, PTT in 6 hours
- PTT 46–70 seconds (goal): No bolus, no rate change, PTT in 12 hours
- PTT 71–90 seconds: No bolus, decrease rate by 2 units/kg/h, PTT in 12 hours
- PTT above 90 seconds: No bolus, stop infusion

0700: The next day, the oncoming nurse assigned to monitor the client assesses the client and checks laboratory results drawn 1 hour ago.

Nurses' Notes

Client states, "I feel okay; I just have a hard time sleeping since I've been in the hospital. My chest pain is better. I had a nosebleed this morning, but it stopped. I'm ready for breakfast; it should be here soon." The heparin infusion is running at 13.5 mL/h.

Laboratory Results

Test and Reference Range	Results
0600:	
PTT	
30–40 seconds	92 seconds

*Select the **3 priority** needs that are of **immediate** concern.*

☐ Appetite
☐ Chest pain
☐ Nosebleed
☐ PTT results
☐ Heparin infusion
☐ Difficulty sleeping

Practice Question 5.3 — Drag-and-Drop Rationale

A 70-year-old client had an exploratory laparotomy with colectomy due to small bowel obstruction and was transferred to the postoperative medical-surgical nursing unit 8 hours ago. The oncoming nurse receives report and assesses the client.

Nurses' Notes | Vital Signs

1900: Client received general anesthesia and has a PCA pump with hydromorphone for pain control. Client has been using the PCA pump every 10 minutes for the past 8 hours.

Skin: Warm, dry, intact.

Respiratory: RR 18, unlabored. SpO2 96% on 2 L/min O_2 via NC. Dry cough, no sputum. Lung sounds clear to auscultation in all lung fields.

Cardiovascular: Apical pulse rate 80. Heart sounds: regular rate and rhythm.

GI: Bowel sounds absent × 4 quadrants. Abdomen firm to palpation. Dressing over midline abdominal incision intact with scant amount of serosanguineous drainage noted. Dressing changed per surgeon's order, wound cleansed with normal saline, and dressing reapplied. Incision is well approximated; no redness, swelling, or tenderness at incision site. Pain at incision site rated 2 (on a 0 to 10 pain intensity scale).

Genitourinary: Unable to urinate since arrival to unit 8 hours ago.

Neurologic: Alert and oriented × 3.

Nurses' Notes | **Vital Signs**

T 98.2°F (36.7°C); HR 80; RR 18; BP 138/78; SpO$_2$ 96% on 2 L/min O$_2$ via NC; pain rated 2 (on a 0 to 10 pain intensity scale)

Based on the client findings, complete the following sentence by choosing from the lists of options below.

The client is at **highest** risk for developing **1 [Select]** as evidenced by **2 [Select]**.

Options for 1	Options for 2
Infection	Urine output
Atelectasis	Temperature
Hemorrhage	BP
Urinary retention	RR
Wound dehiscence	Drainage on dressing

Practice Question 5.4 — Multiple Response Select All That Apply

The nurse working at a psychiatric outpatient clinic is performing an intake assessment on a 28-year-old client accompanied by their parent.

Health History

1400: Parent reports that the client has been increasingly withdrawn, spending most of the time in their bedroom for the past 6 months. Parent noticed that the client seems preoccupied and is often talking to oneself. Parent reports that the client has difficulty maintaining employment due to the symptoms. Client admits to hearing voices that tell them they are worthless and others are plotting against them. Client has also been neglecting personal hygiene and refusing to eat meals with the family. Client denies substance use or history of head injury. There is no significant past medical history, and the client has never been hospitalized for psychiatric reasons. There is no known family history of psychiatric disorders. Client lives with parents and a younger sibling. Client has limited social interactions outside of the family and has no close friends.

Nurses' Notes

1400: Mental status examination:

Appearance: Disheveled and has poor hygiene.

Behavior: Appears withdrawn, avoids eye contact. Observed talking to oneself.

Speech: Tangential and disorganized.

Mood/Affect: Appears anxious and states suspicion of clinical staff. Blunted affect.

Thought Process/Content: Exhibits paranoid delusions with auditory hallucinations that are persecutory in nature.

Cognition: Demonstrates impaired concentration and memory.

Insight/Judgment: Lacks insight into condition as evidenced by denying the need for treatment.

---

*Based on the client's clinical presentation, which of the following are the **priority** concerns?* **Select all that apply.**

☐ The client is exhibiting signs of schizophrenia.

☐ The client likely has generalized anxiety disorder.

☐ The client will require long-term inpatient hospitalization.

☐ The client is primarily experiencing delusions of reference.

☐ The client's problem-solving abilities and daily functioning are intact.

☐ The client is experiencing positive, negative, and cognitive symptoms.

Practice Question 5.5 — Drop-Down in Table

A 59-year-old postmenopausal client with stage IV bilateral breast cancer had a double mastectomy. One month later, the client visits the clinic for a follow-up.

> **Nurses' Notes**
>
> **1500:** Reports experiencing some unusual symptoms.
> Reports pelvic pain, vaginal discharge, burning on urination.
> Having hot flashes, dizziness; states that left leg feels warm and tender.
> Feeling weak, and experiencing bone pain and joint stiffness.
> Has been constipated; having stomach cramps, nausea, and vomiting.
> Biopsy showed a hormone receptor–positive tumor, and the client is taking tamoxifen.

*For each body system, select the one **priority** concern specific to a complication of tamoxifen therapy.*

Body System	Priority Concern
Genitourinary	☐ Pelvic pain
	☐ Vaginal discharge
	☐ Burning on urination
Cardiovascular	☐ Hot flashes
	☐ Dizziness
	☐ Tenderness and warmth to left leg
Musculoskeletal	☐ Weakness
	☐ Bone pain
	☐ Joint stiffness
GI	☐ Constipation
	☐ Stomach cramps
	☐ Nausea and vomiting

Practice Question 5.6 — Multiple Response Select N

The nurse is caring for a 29-year-old gravida 3, para 2 (G3P2) pregnant client who came to the labor and delivery unit experiencing a precipitous labor.

> **Health History** | Nurses' Notes | Vital Signs
>
> **1500:** 29-year-old G3P2 client at 38 weeks' gestation presented to the labor and delivery unit in active labor. Reports experiencing sudden and intense contractions that started 1 hour ago. Over that time, contractions quickly increased in frequency and intensity. Reports associated pressure in lower back and pelvis, rectal pressure, and spontaneous rupture of membranes shortly after contractions started. Previously had 2 uncomplicated vaginal deliveries at 39 weeks and 38 weeks, both with active labor lasting approximately 6 to 8 hours. Reports no significant medical history and has been taking prenatal vitamins and attending prenatal appointments. Married and has 2 children; reports good social support at home.

> Health History | **Nurses' Notes** | Vital Signs
>
> **1500:** Fundal height consistent with gestational age. Uterus firm. Contractions regular. Cervix fully dilated, 2+ station. Reassuring fetal heart rate pattern.

> Health History | Nurses' Notes | **Vital Signs**
>
> **1500:**
> T 98.2°F (36.7°C); HR 96; RR 18; BP 112/78; SpO$_2$: 98% on RA

*Based on this clinical scenario, select the **5** potential complications that would be of **highest priority** to the nurse.*

☐ Placental abruption
☐ Fetal shoulder dystocia
☐ Fetal intracranial trauma
☐ Excessive uterine bleeding
☐ Inadequate fetal oxygenation
☐ Birthing parent perineal trauma

CHAPTER 6

Strategies for Answering NGN Questions: Generate Solutions

Generate Solutions is a CJ cognitive skill nurses use to create the plan of care. When generating solutions, the nurse uses knowledge of treatments and interventions that would address identified client needs and modifies these needs to meet priorities of care. The nurse needs to be able to generate the best possible evidence-based solutions to provide safe care.

What to Consider When Generating Solutions

Applying the cognitive skill *Generate Solutions* is essential for planning and making appropriate clinical judgments and is a skill that will be measured both on the NGN and on your nursing course exams. When generating solutions, you will need to consider the information in the clinical scenario and connect appropriate actions to your ranked hypotheses (client needs). You will use the hypotheses to identify interventions that would achieve an expected client outcome. Because the cognitive skill *Generate Solutions* is a skill that involves thinking through several care options to create the plan of care, you will need to decide which actual or potential interventions are acceptable in the scenario and which are potentially harmful and therefore need to be avoided. See Box 6.1 for examples of acceptable and contraindicated interventions in a plan of care for a client with heart failure exacerbation with fluid volume overload.

The Plan of Care and Generating Solutions

The cognitive skill *Generate Solutions* asks you to determine outcome criteria based on priority client needs while planning care. In doing so, you will need to think about appropriate interventions, consider the evidence that will help determine whether the client has met outcomes and to what extent, and then communicate and document the plan of care.

How Do You Know That You Need to Generate Solutions?

As a nurse, you will be problem solving and using your nursing knowledge to create evidence-based plans of care based on previous client data and presenting hypotheses. For example, when you assume care for your assigned clients, you will look at the previously established plan of care and consider current hypotheses to determine the appropriateness of the interventions in the plan of care. You may need to revise a plan of care based on evolving client needs. As the nurse, you need to think about what you would plan to do as well as what you would plan not to do to meet the client's needs. Ask yourself, "What are the desirable outcomes for this client? What interventions will achieve these outcomes? What interventions need to be avoided?" Box 6.2 lists some important considerations related to *Generate Solutions* that will help you to effectively apply this cognitive skill.

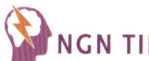

Remember: When you *Generate Solutions,* you are using your nursing knowledge of evidence-based practice to decide which interventions or actions need to be taken in a clinical scenario to meet the client's needs.

THINKING SPACE

THINKING SPACE

BOX 6.1 Heart Failure Exacerbation With Fluid Overload: Examples of Acceptable and Contraindicated Interventions

Acceptable Interventions	Contraindicated Interventions
Monitor for edema	Provide sodium in the diet
Monitor daily weight	Encourage fluid intake
Monitor I&O	Administer IV fluids
Monitor labs (B-natriuretic peptide [BNP], electrolytes)	Maintain the same position in bed
Assess lung and heart sounds	Promote high activity level
Administer diuretics	Maintain bedrest
Encourage activity as tolerated	
Place client in the upright position	
Assess VS	

Data from Ignatavicius, D. D., Rebar, C. R., and Heimgartner, N. M. (2024). *Medical-surgical nursing: Concepts for clinical judgment and collaborative care* (11th ed.). St. Louis: Elsevier, p. 691.

BOX 6.2 Considerations Related to Generate Solutions

- Use known client data and prioritized hypotheses.
- Decide on expected outcomes of safe client care.
- Create a list of multiple actual and potential interventions—not just the best intervention.
- Remember that actual and potential interventions could be actions or collecting more information.
- Communicate and document expected outcomes clearly.
- Revise interventions as client needs evolve.

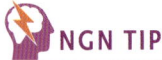

NGN TIP

Remember: Generating solutions requires the nurse to identify expected outcomes by using established hypotheses and priorities to define a set of interventions that will achieve outcomes.

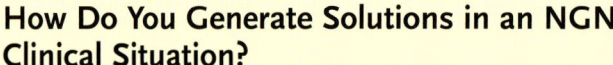

How Do You Generate Solutions in an NGN Clinical Situation?

As noted in Chapter 2, NGN questions will begin with a clinical scenario presented as either a Stand-Alone item or an Unfolding Case Study. Chapter 3 discusses the cognitive skill *Recognize Cues* in which information about the client is presented and you need to identify the relevant data. As discussed in Chapter 4, once these relevant data are noted, you analyze the data and link these data to the client situation to determine what the data mean and what is happening to the client. Then, as stated in Chapter 5, based on your judgment of what you think is happening to the client, you identify client needs and assign priority or urgency to those needs. At this point, you are ready to begin thinking about outcome criteria and developing a plan of care consisting of evidence-based nursing interventions, applying the skill *Generate Solutions*. The following example provides you with a clinical scenario in which you use client data to *Generate Solutions*. Remember to consider both acceptable and contraindicated interventions as you apply this cognitive skill.

Example: Generate Solutions

An 88-year-old client is admitted to the medical-surgical nursing unit from the ED with acute confusion.

| History and Physical | Nurses' Notes |

0900: Client's children brought client to the ED when the client wasn't making sense on the phone one evening. Children report that when arriving at the client's home, the client was in disarray, was very weak, and was speaking incoherently. Client has a history of stroke 2 years ago and type 1 diabetes mellitus (DM). Spouse died from breast cancer in the past year.

CHAPTER 6 Strategies for Answering NGN Questions: Generate Solutions

| History and Physical | Nurses' Notes |

1100: Client arrives to the nursing unit diagnosed with acute delirium related to hypoglycemia. Client's appetite is very poor. Prescribed IV fluids $D_{10}W$ at 75 mL/h are administered.

▸THINKING SPACE

What Will You Think About to Generate Solutions in This Clinical Scenario?

To generate solutions, you need to think about the client's problem based on the information provided in the scenario. As the nurse caring for the client, you would consider what client outcome data would demonstrate improvement in the acute confusion and what interventions you would need to perform to promote attainment of this goal.

Begin by considering the outcome data. What would tell you that the acute confusion is improving? It would be important to know this client's cognitive baseline. You could ask the children if the client has any confusion at baseline or if the client is normally alert and oriented. Next, you could consider outcome criteria based on level of consciousness and cognition. Perhaps a return to the client's baseline cognition would be an appropriate outcome to consider in the plan. Another appropriate outcome would be for the client to remain safe and free from injury. With these outcomes in mind, you would think about the nursing interventions or actions that will assist in achieving these goals. Remember that some interventions may be focused on assessment and others on actions. Nursing interventions to consider for the plan of care in this clinical scenario might be:

- Perform a mental status assessment during every shift.
- Assess for hypoglycemia and hyperglycemia, and treat accordingly with available prescribed interventions.
- Identify contributing factors, such as medications, hypoglycemia, infection, or other problems that may result in acute confusion.
- Promote adequate hydration, nutritional intake, and sleep.
- Facilitate sensory awareness, and use sensory aids as appropriate, such as glasses and hearing aids.
- Provide orientation to surroundings as often as needed.
- Encourage visitation from family and support persons.
- Assist with toileting needs frequently.
- Communicate and document changes in cognition.

Which NGN Item Types Optimally Measure *Generate Solutions*?

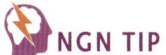
NGN TIP

Remember: With NGN item types that measure *Generate Solutions*, you could be asked about planning assessment-related interventions and action-related interventions.

Four types of test items are most likely to be used to optimally measure the cognitive skill *Generate Solutions*. Variations of each type will be presented on the NGN. Table 6.1 presents these item types and their variations. All of these test item types are discussed in Chapter 2, and some examples are provided. The following section describes the four major item types that best measure *Generate Solutions* and provides a sample test item.

TABLE 6.1	Test Items and Variations That Optimally Measure *Generate Solutions*
Type of Test Item	**Variations**
Drag-and-Drop	Drag-and-Drop Cloze
	Drag-and-Drop Rationale
Drop-Down	Drop-Down Cloze
	Drop-Down Rationale
	Drop-Down in Table
Extended Multiple Response	Multiple Response Select N
	Multiple Response Select All That Apply
	Multiple Response Grouping
Matrix/Grid	Matrix Multiple Choice
	Matrix Multiple Response

THINKING SPACE

Drag-and-Drop and Drop-Down Test Items to Measure *Generate Solutions*

As discussed in Chapter 2, Drag-and-Drop items include Drag-and-Drop Cloze and Drag-and-Drop Rationale, and Drop-Down items include Drop-Down Cloze, Drop-Down Rationale, and Drop-Down in Table. When the Drag-and-Drop item type is used to measure *Generate Solutions,* the test taker is required to drag words from a list of choices to fill in the blank of a sentence or sentences. When a Drop-Down item type is presented, the test taker is required to select words from a drop-down menu to fill in the blank of a sentence or sentences. Sample Question 6.1 illustrates a Drag-and-Drop Cloze item type. The rationale and test-taking strategy to help you derive the correct responses shown in Sample Question 6.1 are also provided.

Sample Question 6.1 — Drag-and-Drop Cloze Item: *Generate Solutions*

A 32-year-old client G2P1 is admitted to the labor and delivery unit, and the nurse assigned to care for the client reviews the health history.

History and Physical | Nurses' Notes | Vital Signs

0900: 32-year-old G2P1. First delivery was vaginal and uncomplicated. Has a history of uncomplicated mitral valve stenosis that is currently being monitored. No other medical history. No prescribed medication taken except for prenatal vitamins. Uterine ultrasound done 1 week ago showed normal progression of pregnancy, and examination revealed 100% effacement with 4-cm dilation.

History and Physical | **Nurses' Notes** | Vital Signs

1400: Client delivers a 7 lb 4 oz (3.35 kg) baby via an uncomplicated vaginal delivery. Postdelivery the client is breast-feeding/chest-feeding the baby.

1500: Client's spouse calls the nurse because the client is complaining of abdominal cramping and complains that the peri-pad feels wet. The nurse checks the pad and finds that it is saturated with blood. The nurse assesses the fundus while another nurse checks VS. The fundus is soft and 4 fingerbreadths above the umbilicus and deviated to the right.

History and Physical | Nurses' Notes | **Vital Signs**

1400: T 98.6°F (36.0°C); HR 92; RR 20; BP 132/78; SpO$_2$ 95% on RA.
1500: HR 120; RR 24; BP 98/62; SpO$_2$ 92% on RA.

Complete the following sentence by selecting from the lists of options below.

To meet the client's needs, the nurse would ***immediately*** plan for **uterine massage** and **IV infusion of oxytocin**.

Options for 1	Options for 2
Uterine massage	Hysterectomy
Rapid administration of blood	Uterine tamponade
Administration of methylergonovine	Oxygen administration
Manual exploration of the uterine cavity	IV infusion of oxytocin

Rationale: The initial actions in management of excessive postpartum bleeding focus on interventions to contract the uterus and stop the bleeding. Immediate interventions if the bleeding is due to uterine atony include firm massage of the uterine fundus, expression of any clots in the uterus, elimination of bladder distention, and continuous IV infusion of oxytocin. It may be necessary to insert an indwelling urinary catheter to prevent bladder distention and to monitor urine output as a measure of renal perfusion to vital organs. Laboratory studies will be monitored and usually include a complete blood cell count with platelet count, fibrinogen, fibrin split products, prothrombin time, and partial thromboplastin time. Blood type and antibody screen are done if not previously performed. Rapid administration of crystalloid solutions or blood products or both may be necessary to restore intravascular volume, but this is not the immediate intervention. Methylergonovine is a medication that is administered intramuscularly to produce sustained uterine contractions; however, this medication is contraindicated in the presence of hypertension or cardiovascular disease because it can induce vasoconstriction. Therefore this is not a safe option for this client because of the history of mitral valve stenosis. Oxygen may be administered by nonrebreather facemask to enhance oxygen delivery to the cells, but this is not the immediate intervention. In addition, the SpO_2, although lower than the previous reading, is still a normal value. If the uterus does not become firm and bleeding persists, the obstetrician may perform manual exploration of the uterine cavity for retained clots or placental fragments. If treatment measures are ineffective, uterine tamponade or surgical management may be necessary, and a hysterectomy may be needed.

Test-Taking Strategy: First, it is important to note the word *immediately* in the question. This tells you that some or all of the options may be correct, and you need to select the option for each blank area that would be a first action. Retrieving your knowledge on the causes of postpartum bleeding, think about what would be immediate or primary actions as part of the plan of care in this particular clinical scenario, as illustrated in the table. Note that in the first column, you are presented with a set of actions. You need to decide if each listed action is primary for the client in this question, or if there are any data in the client's history that would make any of the actions unsafe actions and contraindicated.

Nursing Action	Primary	Contraindicated
Uterine massage	Yes	No
Rapid administration of blood	No	No
Administration of methylergonovine	Yes	Yes
Manual exploration of the uterine cavity	No	No
Hysterectomy	No	No
Uterine tamponade	No	No
Oxygen administration	No	No
IV infusion of oxytocin	Yes	No

For those options that are primary and not contraindicated, these are the actions you would consider as being the correct answers to this question. If an action is not a primary action, but rather a later action if other interventions were unsuccessful, or if the action is contraindicated, then these are probably not the correct answers to this question.

Content Area: Obstetrics-Newborn Nursing
Priority Concepts: Perfusion, Reproduction
Reference(s): Lowdermilk et al., 2024, p. 728

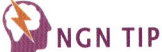

NGN TIP

Remember: In a Drag-and-Drop Cloze item, the maximum score is equivalent to the number of targets for answer boxes, and partial credit is given for correct responses.

Multiple Response Test Items to Measure *Generate Solutions*

As discussed in Chapter 2, Multiple Response test items include Multiple Response Select All That Apply, Multiple Response Select N, and Multiple Response Grouping. When the Multiple Response item type is used to measure *Generate Solutions* or other cognitive skills, the test taker is required to follow the question directions regarding how to select options. Sample Question 6.2 illustrates a Multiple Response Select All That Apply item type. In this item type, the test taker needs to select all responses that apply to the clinical scenario. The rationale and test-taking strategy to help you derive the correct responses shown in Sample Question 6.2 are also provided.

Sample Question 6.2 | **Multiple Response Select All That Apply:** *Generate Solutions*

A 68-year-old client presents to the ED complaining of numbness and tingling of the left side of the face and the left arm that started 2 hours ago.

History and Physical | Vital Signs | Physician's Orders | Diagnostic Results

1100: No known past medical history, and does not take any medications on a routine basis.
Numbness and tingling began 2 hours ago. Focal neurologic deficits on the left side of the body.

History and Physical | **Vital Signs** | Physician's Orders | Diagnostic Results

1100: T 97.5°F (36.4°C); HR 98; RR 20; BP 152/84; SpO₂ 96% on RA.

History and Physical | Vital Signs | **Physician's Orders** | Diagnostic Results

1100: Stat CT scan of the brain.

History and Physical | Vital Signs | Physician's Orders | **Diagnostic Results**

1145: CT scan: ischemic stroke affecting the middle cerebral artery.

Which of the following actions would the ED nurse plan for the client? **Select all that apply**.

☒ Complete a swallow screen.
☐ Allow thickened liquids only.
☒ Administer fibrinolytic therapy.
☒ Obtain an electronic infusion pump.
☒ Perform a cardiovascular assessment.
☐ Insert an indwelling urinary catheter.
☐ Administer IV antihypertensive medication.
☒ Perform frequent neurologic assessments.

THINKING SPACE

Rationale: An ischemic stroke is caused by a blockage of a cerebral or carotid artery. Multiple interventions are needed to ensure safety for the client experiencing a stroke. The client with an ischemic stroke may experience impaired swallowing as a complication of the stroke. The nurse needs to complete a swallow screen per agency protocol to determine if there are any impairments with swallowing. This action will prevent complications such as pneumonia from aspiration. The nurse needs to keep the client NPO until the appropriate diagnostic testing is completed, such as a video fluoroscopic swallow study, which is usually performed by a speech-language pathologist; therefore thickened liquids would not be given at this time until this workup has been performed. The nurse would anticipate a prescription to administer fibrinolytic therapy. This is the standard of practice for clients experiencing ischemic stroke who meet specified criteria. Exclusionary criteria include more than 4.5 hours from onset of symptoms, age older than 80 years, anticoagulant use, ischemic injury to greater than one-third of the brain, significant neurologic impairment, and history of both stroke and DM. This client does not meet any of these exclusionary criteria and therefore would be considered a candidate for fibrinolytic therapy. To safely administer this therapy, the nurse needs to use an electronic infusion pump and double-check the dose with another licensed nurse. A cardiovascular assessment is important to assess for heart murmurs, dysrhythmias such as atrial fibrillation, and hypertension. With an ischemic stroke, a BP of approximately 150/100 is needed to maintain cerebral perfusion. With a BP of 152/84, an IV antihypertensive medication would not be indicated. For a client receiving fibrinolytic therapy, invasive tubes such as indwelling urinary catheters should not be placed for at least 24 hours or until the client is stable to prevent bleeding. Frequent neurologic assessments per agency protocol are important for early detection of further clinical deterioration in clients with ischemic stroke and for clients receiving fibrinolytic therapy.

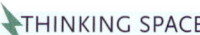

THINKING SPACE

Test-Taking Strategy: Note that the question is asking about nursing actions to plan care for the client experiencing an ischemic stroke. Think about the scenario and the potential effects of these interventions on the health problem presented. Look at each option provided, and make an association with the information presented in the medical record, as illustrated in the table.

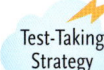

Test-Taking Strategy

Intervention	Potential Effects on Ischemic Stroke
Complete a swallow screen.	Ensures safety in the event of dysphagia as a complication of the stroke.
Allow thickened liquids only.	Is unsafe and could result in aspiration; need to wait until further workup and consultation are performed.
Administer fibrinolytic therapy.	Would promote a more favorable outcome for a client with ischemic stroke meeting criteria.
Obtain an electronic infusion pump.	Needed to safely administer fibrinolytic therapy.
Perform a cardiovascular assessment.	Important information such as heart sounds and BP are needed to monitor for complications in a client with ischemic stroke.
Insert an indwelling urinary catheter.	No indication that this is necessary, and it could pose a risk for UTI and bleeding.
Administer IV antihypertensive medication.	A BP of 150/100 is needed to maintain cerebral perfusion; BP is not high enough for an IV antihypertensive medication.
Perform frequent neurologic assessments.	Assists in early detection of clinical deterioration.

The correct options are those that ensure safety, monitor for complications or clinical deterioration, or promote a more favorable outcome of care. The options that are unsafe and could result in additional complications or that do not have the data to support the interventions are the incorrect options.

Content Area: Medical-Surgical Nursing
Priority Concepts: Perfusion; Tissue Integrity
Reference(s): Ignatavicius et al., 2024, pp. 944–956

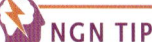

NGN TIP

Remember: In a Multiple Response Select All That Apply item, credit is given for correct responses, and credit is deducted for incorrect responses.

Sample Question 6.3 illustrates a Multiple Response Select N item type, in which the test taker is presented with a clinical scenario and asked to select a specified number of correct options from a list of several options. The rationale and test-taking strategy to help you derive the correct responses shown in Sample Question 6.3 are also provided.

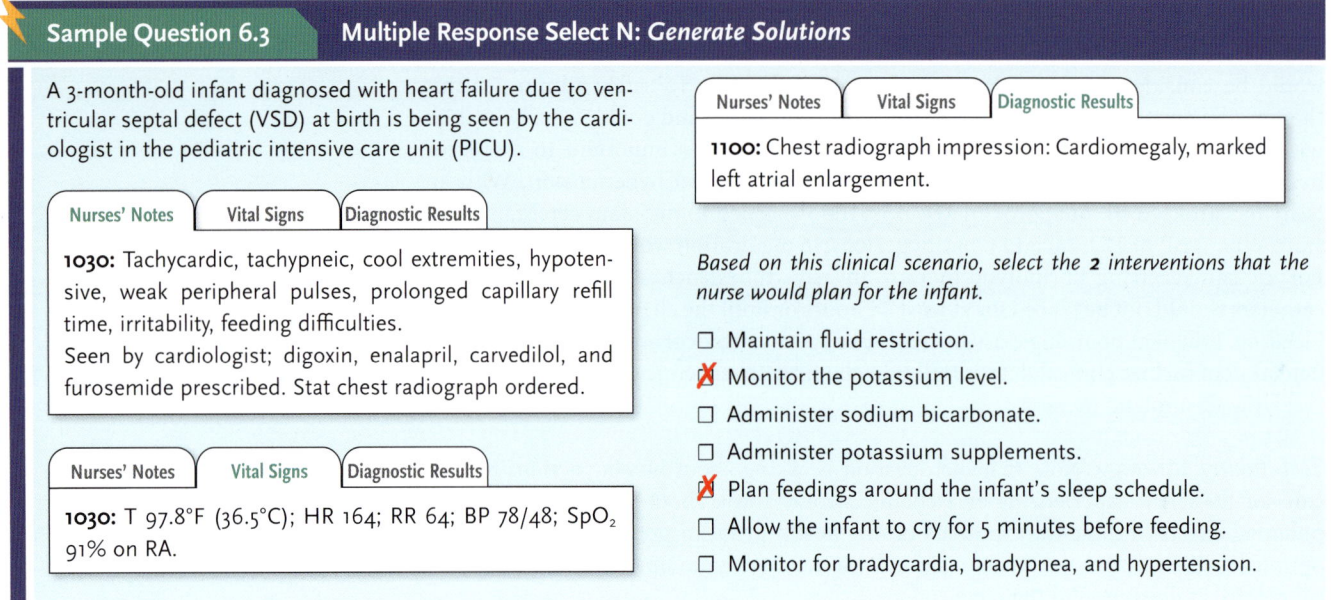

Sample Question 6.3 — Multiple Response Select N: *Generate Solutions*

A 3-month-old infant diagnosed with heart failure due to ventricular septal defect (VSD) at birth is being seen by the cardiologist in the pediatric intensive care unit (PICU).

Nurses' Notes | Vital Signs | Diagnostic Results

1030: Tachycardic, tachypneic, cool extremities, hypotensive, weak peripheral pulses, prolonged capillary refill time, irritability, feeding difficulties.
Seen by cardiologist; digoxin, enalapril, carvedilol, and furosemide prescribed. Stat chest radiograph ordered.

Nurses' Notes | **Vital Signs** | Diagnostic Results

1030: T 97.8°F (36.5°C); HR 164; RR 64; BP 78/48; SpO₂ 91% on RA.

Nurses' Notes | Vital Signs | **Diagnostic Results**

1100: Chest radiograph impression: Cardiomegaly, marked left atrial enlargement.

*Based on this clinical scenario, select the **2** interventions that the nurse would plan for the infant.*

☐ Maintain fluid restriction.
☒ Monitor the potassium level.
☐ Administer sodium bicarbonate.
☐ Administer potassium supplements.
☒ Plan feedings around the infant's sleep schedule.
☐ Allow the infant to cry for 5 minutes before feeding.
☐ Monitor for bradycardia, bradypnea, and hypertension.

▸THINKING SPACE

Rationale: Heart failure is the inability of the heart to pump an adequate amount of blood to the rest of the body to meet metabolic demands. Heart failure can occur as a consequence of congenital heart disease, such as VSD. Clinical manifestations of heart failure may include tachycardia, tachypnea, cool extremities, hypotension, weak peripheral pulses, prolonged capillary refill time, irritability, and feeding difficulties, among other findings. Even though fluid volume overload is a problem with heart failure, fluid restriction is often not needed in infants because of their feeding difficulties. Medication therapy is a mainstay of heart failure management for an infant with congenital heart disease. Medications that improve cardiac function include digoxin, angiotensin-converting enzyme inhibitors such as enalapril, and beta blockers such as carvedilol. In management of heart failure exacerbation, diuretics such as furosemide may be prescribed. Monitoring the potassium level is very important for anyone taking furosemide because it is a potassium-wasting diuretic. Often, potassium supplementation is needed; however, for the infant being given enalapril, potassium supplementation is usually not needed, even when the infant is taking furosemide, because the enalapril also blocks the action of aldosterone, which can lead to hyperkalemia, especially if potassium supplementation is given. Sodium bicarbonate is a medication used in chronic kidney disease; although renal impairment can occur with heart failure, sodium bicarbonate is not part of the treatment regimen for heart failure. An important part of care for the infant with heart failure is maintaining nutritional status. The metabolic rate for these infants is greater because of poor cardiac function, therefore their caloric needs are higher. Feeding difficulties occur because of lack of energy related to the cardiac problem. Feedings need to be planned around the infant's sleep schedule so energy can be conserved for feedings and feedings can be most effective. The infant needs to be fed soon after awakening so energy is not depleted from crying.

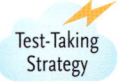
Test-Taking Strategy

Test-Taking Strategy: Note that this question asks you to select 2 correct options. The ability to use clinical judgment and determine whether listed interventions would be safe and effective is needed to answer this question correctly. Using a thinking process as illustrated in the table may be helpful.

Intervention	Assists With Health Problem	Indicated	Not Indicated
Maintain fluid restriction.	No	☐	☒
Monitor the potassium level.	Yes	☒	☐
Administer sodium bicarbonate.	No	☐	☒
Administer potassium supplements.	No	☐	☒
Plan feedings around the infant's sleep schedule.	Yes	☒	☐
Allow the infant to cry for 5 minutes before feeding.	No	☐	☒
Monitor for bradycardia, bradypnea, and hypertension.	No	☐	☒

For each intervention, decide whether it would be indicated or not indicated in this scenario. To decide that, think about whether the intervention assists with the health problem. If so, then it would be indicated. If not, it would be not indicated.

Content Area: Pediatric Nursing
Priority Concept: Gas Exchange; Perfusion
Reference(s): Hockenberry et al., 2024, pp. 959–967

Matrix/Grid Test Items to Measure *Generate Solutions*

As discussed in Chapter 2, Matrix/Grid test items include Matrix Multiple Choice and Matrix Multiple Response. When the Matrix/Grid item type is used to measure *Generate Solutions,* the test taker is required to select a single option (Matrix Multiple Choice) or more than one option (Matrix Multiple Response) from a list of several options in a table with rows. Sample Question 6.4 illustrates a Matrix Multiple Choice item type. The rationale and test-taking strategy to help you derive the correct responses shown in Sample Question 6.4 are also provided.

Sample Question 6.4 — Matrix Multiple Choice: *Generate Solutions*

A client who is 5 days postoperative following a right colectomy to remove a bowel tumor calls the nurse and reports feeling a popping sensation in the incision after an episode of forceful coughing.

Nurses' Notes

1400: Client reports feeling a popping sensation in the incision after an episode of forceful coughing. Abdominal dressing removed. Incision open, and wound layers are separated; a portion of the bowel is protruding from the wound.

Select whether the following potential interventions are indicated or not indicated for the client at this time.

Potential Intervention	Indicated	Not Indicated
Place the client with the head and body flat and with the hips and knees bent.	☐	☒
Place a sterile, warm, saline-soaked dressing over the open wound.	☒	☐
Don sterile gloves, and gently reinsert the protruding bowel into the wound.	☐	☒
Provide the client with small amounts of water or juice to stay hydrated.	☐	☒
Notify the surgeon.	☒	☐
Prepare the client for surgery.	☒	☐
Assess VS every 5 to 10 minutes.	☒	☐

Rationale: Evisceration is total separation of wound layers and protrusion of internal organs through the wound. It usually occurs between the fifth and tenth days after surgery. The separation of wound layers occurs most often in clients who have diabetes, are obese, are malnourished, have an immune deficiency, or use steroid medication. Evisceration is a surgical emergency, and the nurse would stay with the client and have another nurse notify the surgeon and/or Rapid Response Team immediately and bring any needed supplies. The nurse would provide reassurance to the client and position the client in the supine position with the hips and knees bent and with the head of the bed at 15 to 20 degrees. This position prevents stretching of the abdominal tissues and prevents pressure on the incision line, which would worsen the condition. Using sterile technique, the nurse would apply one to two large abdominal dressings saturated with warm normal saline to the wound. This will prevent hypothermia and provide moisture to the tissues and protruding organ. The nurse would not attempt to reinsert the protruding organ because this could cause trauma. The nurse would monitor the client's VS every 5 to 10 minutes until the surgeon arrives and would monitor for signs of shock. The client is not allowed to have anything by mouth to decrease the risk of aspiration if surgery is necessary.

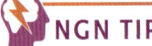

Remember: In a Matrix Multiple Choice item type, you will be asked to select one option per row, and there can be up to 10 rows in an item.

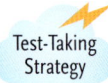

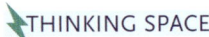

Test-Taking Strategy: Note that this question is asking about interventions that are either indicated or not indicated based on the clinical scenario involving evisceration. Using a thinking process as illustrated in the table, you can decide whether each option would be part of a safe and effective plan of care for a client in this situation and then think about what the outcome of that action might be.

Potential Intervention	Safe and Effective	Potential Outcome
Place the client with the head and body flat and with the hips and knees bent.	No	Lying flat could cause further tissue disruption from pressure on the incision line.
Place a sterile, warm, saline-soaked dressing over the open wound.	Yes	Will prevent hypothermia and provide moisture to the affected organs and tissues.
Don sterile gloves, and gently reinsert the protruding bowel into the wound.	No	Could cause trauma.
Provide the client with small amounts of water or juice to stay hydrated.	No	Aspiration could occur in the event surgery is needed.
Notify the surgeon.	Yes	Obtain additional orders; determine details for likely surgery.
Prepare the client for surgery.	Yes	Repair the surgical site.
Assess VS every 5 to 10 minutes.	Yes	Monitor for clinical deterioration, early detection of shock.

Organizing the information in this way will allow you to then decide whether these potential interventions are indicated or not indicated in this clinical scenario. You will need to rely on your nursing knowledge of the care involved with this postoperative complication to answer this question correctly.

Content Area: Medical-Surgical Nursing
Priority Concept: Perfusion; Tissue Integrity
Reference(s): Ignatavicius et al., 2024, pp. 183, 187

Practice Questions

Practice Question 6.1 — Multiple Response Grouping

A 58-year-old client is recovering on the medical-surgical nursing unit from an L4–L5 spinal fusion completed 3 hours ago.

Medication Administration Record

Hydromorphone via PCA, 0.2 mg every 10 minutes, with a 4-mg lock-out dose in 4 hours.

For each body system, specify the potential intervention that would be appropriate for the initial plan of care to monitor for or prevent adverse effects of hydromorphone. **Each body system may support more than one potential nursing intervention.**

Body System	Potential Nursing Intervention
Renal	☐ Assess renal function.
	☐ Monitor I&O.
	☐ Maintain fluid restriction.
Respiratory	☐ Assess RR frequently.
	☐ Ensure that naloxone is available.
	☐ Place the PCA on hold if RR is less than 18.
Cardiovascular	☐ Encourage brisk walking.
	☐ Instruct the client to change positions slowly.
	☐ Assess BP and HR frequently.
Gastrointestinal	☐ Administer methylnaltrexone.
	☐ Administer ondansetron as indicated.
	☐ Ensure adequate intake of fluids and fiber.
Urinary	☐ Assess the bladder frequently.
	☐ Prompt the client to void every 4 hours.
	☐ Perform straight catheterization every 4 hours.

Practice Question 6.2 — Multiple Response Select N

An unhoused 72-year-old client is brought to the ED by EMS. The client was found sleeping on a park bench by a jogger who reported that the client had a foul smell and an excessive amount of wetness on a pant leg.

History and Physical | Nurses' Notes | Physician's Orders

0600: Client reports history of peripheral vascular disease and has not received follow-up care.
Has an arterial leg ulcer that is open and draining copious amounts of drainage.
Physician in to see client.

History and Physical | **Nurses' Notes** | Physician's Orders

1600: Client requiring multiple dressing changes through the day owing to the excessive drainage.
1630: Seen by the wound care team.

History and Physical | Nurses' Notes | **Physician's Orders**

0630: Admit to medical-surgical unit for wound care management.
Wound culture.
Pack the wound with sterile, saline-moistened gauze, and then cover with a dry, sterile dressing, with daily dressing changes and as needed.
1700: Begin negative-pressure wound therapy (NPWT).

Which **5** interventions would the nurse include in the plan of care for the client to maintain and ensure a good seal during NPWT?

☐ Identify air leaks using a stethoscope.
☐ Shave the hair on the skin around the wound.
☐ Make sure the periwound skin surface area is dry.
☐ Avoid wrinkles when applying the transparent film.
☐ Fill uneven skin surfaces with a skin barrier product.
☐ Frame the periwound area with a hydrocolloid dressing.
☐ Cut the transparent film to extend 1/2 inch beyond the wound perimeter.
☐ Use as many additional dressing layers as needed for identified air leaks.

Practice Question 6.3 — Drag-and-Drop Rationale

A 44-year-old postoperative client returned to the nursing unit from the PACU following a bilateral mastectomy.

Nurses' Notes | Vital Signs | Physician's Orders

1300: Alert and oriented. Reports incisional pain rated 2/10 (on a 0–10 pain scale).
Bilateral incisions on the chest covered with a dry, sterile dressing; clean, dry, and intact.
Lung sounds clear to auscultation bilaterally. S1S2, no S3S4. +2 peripheral pulses, no edema.
4 Jackson-Pratt drains from the incisional areas: #1 with 5 mL of sanguineous drainage, #2 with 10 mL of sanguineous drainage, #3 with 5 mL of sanguineous drainage, #4 with 10 mL of sanguineous drainage, compressed for suction.

Nurses' Notes | **Vital Signs** | Physician's Orders

1300: T 98.2°F (36.8°C); HR 70; RR 20; BP 146/72; SpO_2 97% at 3 L/min O_2 via NC; Pain rated 2/10.

Nurses' Notes | Vital Signs | **Physician's Orders**

1300:
Monitor VS per agency protocol.
Titrate oxygen to maintain SpO_2 greater than 92%.
Monitor incision site for signs of bleeding.
Monitor and maintain surgical drains.
Enoxaparin 40 mg subcutaneously daily.
Apply sequential compression devices (SCDs) below the knee bilaterally for venous thrombosis prevention.
Pain management via PCA pump.
Clear liquids advance to regular as tolerated.
Incentive spirometry per unit protocol.
Ondansetron 4 mg IV every 4 hours as needed for nausea.

Based on the client findings, complete the following sentence by choosing from the lists of options below.

To ensure client safety, the nurse plans to **first** 1 **[Select]** to address 2 **[Select]**.

Options for 1	Options for 2
Administer enoxaparin	Pain
Administer pain medication	Infection
Increase supplemental oxygen	Hypoxemia
Empty and compress surgical drains	Thrombus risk

Practice Question 6.4 — Multiple Response Select All That Apply

A 22-year-old client presents to the outpatient mental health clinic.

History and Physical | Nurses' Notes

1000: Reports no previous history of mental health problems or a family history.

History and Physical | Nurses' Notes

1000: Reports feeling "down" and having difficulty maintaining responsibilities with school. States experiencing a hard time finding friends, that peers in class don't think the client is smart, and that they make fun of the client behind the client's back. Reports not speaking to parents and that the only support system is the client's partner. States "putting myself through school." Describes not being able to meet assignment deadlines and thinks about considering quitting school. Counseling at the psychological center and group therapy discussed with the client.

Based on this scenario, which of the following interventions would the mental health nurse plan for the client? **Select all that apply.**

☐ Set realistic goals for behavior modification.
☐ Reward the client for practicing new behaviors.
☐ Provide positive regard for adaptive behaviors only.
☐ Encourage the client to practice behavior modification.
☐ Help the client identify negative qualities and experiences.
☐ Help the client identify their own behaviors needing change.
☐ Reinforce self-worth with time and attention by giving one-on-one time.

Practice Question 6.5 — Matrix Multiple Choice

A 32-year-old client is hospitalized in the neurologic unit after sustaining a head injury after falling from a ladder while working in the garage.

Nurses' Notes

0800: Client unresponsive and unable to take in food or fluids. Prepared for central line insertion and total parenteral nutrition (TPN) as prescribed for nutritional support.

Select whether the following potential interventions are indicated or not indicated for the client at this time.

Potential Intervention	Indicated	Not Indicated
Administer insulin.	☐	☐
Assess for diaphoresis.	☐	☐
Monitor the IV site.	☐	☐
Follow Droplet Precautions.	☐	☐
Monitor blood glucose level every 6 hours.	☐	☐
Discontinue the infusion if the bag is empty while waiting for the next TPN bag to become available.	☐	☐

Practice Question 6.6 — Multiple Response Select N

A 46-year-old client is visited by a home health nurse following discharge from the hospital with a diagnosis of new-onset diabetes mellitus.

Nurses' Notes

1000: Discharged from the hospital with a diagnosis of new-onset diabetes mellitus (DM). Admitted to the hospital after reporting increased thirst, increased hunger, and increased urination for 7 days. Client's blood glucose level was significantly elevated on admission, and the client was treated for DKA. After being stabilized, the client was discharged to home with a diagnosis of new-onset DM. Teaching started on self-management and measures to prevent hospitalization. Client reports often feeling hungry, irritable, shaky, and weak as well as having a headache.

Based on the client's reported symptoms, which **5** *measures would the home care nurse plan to teach this client to implement when these symptoms occur?*

☐ Eat 6 saltine crackers.
☐ Eat 3 graham crackers.
☐ Drink 120 mL of fruit juice.
☐ Drink 240 mL of skim milk.
☐ Consume 6 to 10 hard candies.
☐ Consume 4 tablespoons of honey.
☐ Drink 120 mL of a diet soft drink.
☐ Decrease carbohydrate intake.
☐ Administer insulin based on a sliding scale.

CHAPTER 7

Strategies for Answering NGN Questions: Take Actions

Take Actions is a CJ cognitive skill that is activity oriented and involves the nurse performing appropriate and necessary interventions based on the client's situation and generated solutions. Thus this cognitive skill involves the nurse undertaking an action or multiple actions. Necessary nursing actions can be those interventions that prevent health problems, maintain client stability, improve the client's condition, prevent complications of a health problem, or manage an emergency, such as a complication or deterioration in a client's condition. Taking actions can also involve client teaching and assessment or reassessment of the client. The ability to use clinical judgment to make decisions about essential actions to take in a clinical situation is a crucial nursing responsibility to ensure safe client care.

The cognitive skill *Take Actions* requires using nursing knowledge about the clinical event encountered, thinking about generated solutions, determining necessary actions to meet desired outcomes, understanding the rationale for such actions, and implementing these actions. Ask yourself, "What will I do? Why do I need to do this? What support do I need? How do I accomplish this?" Sometimes you need to think and make quick decisions about immediate actions to take, and this is why nursing knowledge is so important. As a nurse, you need to know what action(s) are appropriate and necessary, which actions address the highest priorities of care, and how the actions will be performed. Therefore the CJ cognitive skill *Take Actions* is essential to meet the client's needs and ensure client safety and high-quality care. This ability will be measured both on the NCLEX® and by your instructors during classroom activities, on course exams, and in the laboratory and clinical settings.

▸THINKING SPACE

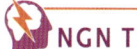

NGN TIP

Remember: Focus on the needs of the client, and think about what you will do to meet these needs. Ask yourself, "What action(s) will I take?"

How Do You Know What Actions to Take?

Implementing care after deciding what actions to take is the focus of the CJ cognitive skill *Take Actions*. Once you have identified possible interventions that will resolve or manage the client's priority health problems, think about other factors that may have an impact on the actions you take. Some factors are as follows, along with questions to ask yourself.

Clinical scenario: What is happening to the client? What are the priority needs? What will I do to address and meet these needs? What are the expected outcomes of care? What will I do to stabilize the client and/or prevent complications and clinical deterioration in the client?

Nursing knowledge: What have I previously learned about these assessment findings and this clinical scenario? Which nursing interventions have I learned are necessary in the care of a client with these assessment findings and this health problem?

Clinical experiences: Have I cared for a client in the past with similar health problems or client needs? What actions did I take in caring for a client with similar needs?

Scope of practice: What necessary actions must I take in my role? What necessary actions can be performed by someone in another health care role?

THINKING SPACE

How Will Nursing Actions Be Tested?

Taking a nursing action is the same as implementing nursing care. Much of what you will do as a nurse involves taking actions to care for a client and meeting that client's needs. Therefore you can expect to be frequently tested on nursing actions. Beginning with your first nursing course, you were tested on actions you would take in a variety of clinical scenarios. Sometimes testing required you to identify the actions you need to take; other times you were tested on how the actions would be performed. As a basic example, you may have been presented with a scenario in which a client is experiencing constipation and asked about which actions you would take to alleviate this health problem. Or you may have been asked about which actions you would take if a client experienced cramping during administration of an enema to alleviate constipation. As a more complex example, you may have been presented with a scenario in which a client with heart failure is experiencing dyspnea and asked about which actions you would take. Or you may have been asked about which actions you would take to prevent complications of heart failure such as pulmonary edema or what you would do if a client with heart failure were to develop pulmonary edema.

Which NGN Item Types Optimally Measure *Take Actions*?

As noted in Chapter 2, NGN questions will begin with a clinical scenario presented as either a Stand-Alone item or an Unfolding Case Study. The types of test items and the variations that may be used to measure the cognitive skill *Take Actions* are presented in Table 7.1. Some of these types are presented in the Sample Questions throughout this chapter and in the Practice Questions at the end of the chapter. These test item types are discussed in Chapter 2 with additional examples. Also, refer to the Evolve site for additional practice with these item types.

Drop-Down Test Items to Measure *Take Actions*

Drop-Down items include Drop-Down Cloze, Drop-Down Rationale, and Drop-Down in Table. When the Drop-Down item type is used to measure *Take Actions*, the test taker is required to complete a sentence or blank space by choosing from a list of options or word choices. Sample Question 7.1 illustrates a Drop-Down Rationale item. The rationale and test-taking strategy to help you derive the correct responses shown in Sample Question 7.1 are also provided.

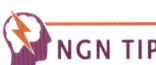NGN TIP

Remember: A Drop-Down Rationale item provides you with a scenario and data about the client. It may include a *Take Actions* sentence in which you need to select the correct action to take and the rationale for that action from the drop-down menus. It is important to choose the first option correctly so the remaining option choices are based on the correct foundation.

TABLE 7.1 Test Items and Variations That Optimally Measure *Take Actions*	
Type of Test Item	**Variations**
Drop-Down	Drop-Down Cloze Drop-Down Rationale Drop-Down in Table
Extended Multiple Response	Multiple Response Select All That Apply Multiple Response Select N Multiple Response Grouping
Matrix/Grid	Matrix Multiple Response Matrix Multiple Choice
Drag-and-Drop	Drag-and-Drop Cloze Drag-and-Drop Rationale

Sample Question 7.1 — Drop-Down Rationale: *Take Actions*

The nurse is caring for a 79-year-old unhoused client at a mobile health clinic.

Nurses' Notes

1100: Client was discharged from the hospital 1 week ago for treatment of heart failure.
Reports beginning the prescribed exercise regimen of walking one block 3 times weekly, but feeling extremely fatigued the day after walking. Reports has avoided walking this week because of feeling so tired. Lung sounds clear bilaterally, no peripheral edema. Reports sleeping well at a shelter with 2 pillows for head elevation. Up to bathroom to void once nightly.

Vital Signs

T 98.6°F (37°C); HR 68; RR 20; BP 112/68; SpO$_2$ 92% on RA

Complete the following sentence by selecting from the list of options provided.

The nurse would **advise the client to slow down on the exercising** because **tolerance to increased activity needs to be built up and takes time**.

Options for 1	Options for 2
Advise the client to slow down on the exercising.	The heart needs to contract efficiently, and exercise is one treatment measure to accomplish this.
Inform the client to maintain the same exercise regimen.	An additional dose of the prescribed diuretic needs to be taken before exercising.
Instruct the client to check the amount of ankle edema before exercising.	Tolerance to increased activity needs to be built up and takes time.

Rationale: The client with heart failure would be encouraged to stay as active as possible and to maintain a regular exercise regimen such as a walking program. However, the client must be taught not to overexert. The nurse would teach the client to try to walk at least 3 times a week and slowly increase the time walked over several months. Tolerance to the increased activity needs to be built up and takes time. If chest pain or severe dyspnea occurs while exercising or the client is fatigued the next day, the client is probably advancing the activity too quickly and should slow down. Telling the client to maintain the same exercise regimen is incorrect and could be harmful. Checking the amount of ankle edema before exercising may be a helpful action but is not related to the exercise and the fatigue. The nurse would not advise a client to take an additional dose of the prescribed diuretic because prescribing medications is not part of a nurse's scope of practice and because this action does not specifically address the problem or concern. The heart does need to contract efficiently, and exercise is one component of the treatment program, but this is not related to the action the nurse would take to assist the client with alleviating the extreme fatigue experienced. The client's vital signs and other findings are not abnormal for a client with this health problem. The heart rate and blood pressure may be lower than normal range, but this is expected due to the medication usually prescribed to treat heart failure. The need to void during the night is expected because of the diuretic therapy normally prescribed to treat heart failure.

Test-Taking Strategy: Focus on the information in the scenario, and note that the client feels extremely fatigued the day after walking. Think about the pathophysiology associated with heart failure and the healing process of the heart in this condition. Use your knowledge about heart failure to determine that the findings noted in the Nurses' Notes are expected. Organize your thinking process as illustrated in the table, and think about the possible effect on the heart and subsequent fatigue with each action.

THINKING SPACE

NGN TIP

Remember: Before taking a nursing action, you need to consider what is relevant in the client scenario, what is happening to the client, what the priority client needs are, and the expected outcomes of care.

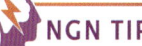
Test-Taking Strategy

Nursing Action	Possible Effect on Heart and Fatigue
Advise the client to slow down on the exercising.	Allows the heart to recover while also benefiting from exercise, which should help with fatigue
Inform the client to maintain the same exercise regimen.	May cause overexertion of the heart, worsening fatigue
Instruct the client to check the amount of ankle edema before exercising.	May help promote early detection of problems, but is not specifically related to fatigue

Think about what the nurse would do. Once you have determined the action to take, think about the reason for that action. Maintaining the same exercise regimen could be harmful, so eliminate that option. Checking the amount of edema in the ankles is not an incorrect measure, but it is unrelated to the information in the scenario. Therefore your action would be to advise the client to slow down on exercising. Next, think about why you are taking this action. Remember that the heart needs to heal, and this takes time and involves building up tolerance.

Content Area: Medical-Surgical Nursing
Priority Concept: Mobility, Perfusion
Reference(s): Ignatavicius et al., 2024, pp. 59, 704–705

Extended Multiple Response Test Items to Measure *Take Actions*

Extended Multiple Response test items include Multiple Response Select All That Apply, Multiple Response Select N, and Multiple Response Grouping. When the Multiple Response item type is used to measure *Take Actions,* the test taker needs to follow the question directions regarding how to select options. Sample Question 7.2 illustrates a Multiple Response Select N item type. A Multiple Response Select N question will tell you how many options you need to select. The rationale and test-taking strategy to help you derive the correct responses shown in Sample Question 7.2 are also provided.

Sample Question 7.2 — Multiple Response Select N: *Take Actions*

1000: A 72-year-old client presents to the ED at the veteran's hospital accompanied by the spouse.

History and Physical | Nurses' Notes

1000: Client was diagnosed with PTSD at 35 years of age. Client served as a sergeant in the military and was a prisoner of war for 10 years. Client reports experiencing persistent symptoms of increased arousal, hypervigilance, and flashbacks. Treatment includes trauma-focused psychotherapy and sertraline.

History and Physical | Nurses' Notes

1000: Spouse reports that the client has been extremely anxious and not able to sleep. Client is unkempt in appearance. Wearing wrinkled and stained clothes. Hair is not combed, and client is unshaved. Client reports experiencing extreme anxiety over the past week. Has had difficulty sleeping and constant flashbacks about the torture as a prisoner of war. Client reports "not wanting to do anything at all" and "feeling an enormous amount of guilt because I could not get my military troop out in time." Client states "I haven't gone to any of my psychotherapy sessions but have been taking my medication. I don't know why, but I just wish I were dead."

*Select the **3 initial** actions the nurse would take at this time.*

☐ Provide illness teaching about PTSD.
☒ Provide ongoing surveillance of the client.
☐ Ask the ED physician to order a sedative.
☒ Use a direct, nonjudgmental approach in discussing suicide.
☒ Ask the client about an intent to commit suicide and if the client has a plan to do so.
☐ Develop a schedule for the client's attendance to the trauma-focused psychotherapy sessions.

Rationale: PTSD in adults is characterized by persistent re-experiencing of a highly traumatic event that is outside the range of a usual event. This traumatic event involves actual or threatened death or serious injury. Responses of intense fear, helplessness, or horror are felt. For this client, the PTSD-inducing event was the military and prisoner of war experience. The major features of PTSD include re-experiencing the trauma through flashbacks; avoiding stimuli associated with the trauma; experiencing persistent symptoms of increased arousal evidenced by irritability, difficulty sleeping, difficulty concentrating, and hypervigilance; and experiencing alterations in mood such as chronic depression or a lack of interest in social activities. On assessment, the nurse would gather information about the time of onset of re-experiencing the events, their frequency and severity, and the level of distress. Further assessment for suicidal or violent ideation, insomnia, social withdrawal, functional impairment, family and social supports, and past medical and psychiatric history are indicated. The client's health history indicates a diagnosis of PTSD. The Nurses' Notes reflect the characteristics of PTSD, but of priority concern is that the client states, "I wish I were dead." This alerts the nurse to suicidal ideation in the client, and initial nursing actions would focus on this priority. The nurse would provide ongoing surveillance with one-on-one monitoring to ensure safety. The nurse would discuss suicide with the client using a nonjudgmental approach to show respect of the client's situation. The nurse would ask the client about an intent to commit suicide and if there is a plan to do so; this validates the seriousness and acuteness of the situation and the need for further actions. Although providing illness teaching about PTSD and developing a schedule for the client's attendance to the trauma-focused psychotherapy sessions are important, they are not initial actions and can be addressed later. Medication is usually a last intervention and would not be a helpful initial action in this situation.

NGN TIP

Remember: A Multiple Response Select N item provides you with a scenario and data about the client and includes answer options. The item will tell you the number of options (N) that need to be selected. You will not be allowed to select more options than the N specifies. You can select fewer options than the N specifies, but then you will lose some credit. So be sure to follow the directions for these item types.

Test-Taking Strategy: The focus of the question is on *initial* nursing actions to take when a client verbalizes a statement that indicates a risk for suicide. The word *initial* indicates time pressure in that some actions could be correct but can be performed later. Note also that you need to select three actions. Read each option, and think about which actions relate to suicide risk. Organize your thinking process as illustrated in the table, and you can decide whether each nursing action directly addresses suicide risk and would directly promote safety related to this risk.

Test-Taking Strategy

 THINKING SPACE

Nursing Action	Directly Addresses Suicide Risk	Directly Promotes Safety Related to Suicide Risk
Provide illness teaching about PTSD.	No	No
Provide ongoing surveillance of the client.	Yes	Yes
Ask the ED physician to order a sedative.	No	No
Use a direct, nonjudgmental approach in discussing suicide.	Yes	Yes
Ask the client about an intent to commit suicide and if the client has a plan to do so.	Yes	Yes
Develop a schedule for the client's attendance to the trauma-focused psychotherapy sessions.	No	No

Content Area: Mental Health Nursing
Priority Concept: Mood and Affect, Stress and Coping
Reference(s): Halter, 2022, pp. 299–302

Matrix/Grid Test Items to Measure *Take Actions*

Matrix/Grid test items include Matrix Multiple Response and Matrix Multiple Choice. When the Matrix/Grid item type is used to measure *Take Actions,* the test taker is required to follow the question directions regarding how to select options. In a Matrix Multiple Response item, there will be response columns and rows, and each response column or row could have multiple correct responses. In a Matrix Multiple Choice item, each response row can have only one correct response. Sample Question 7.3 illustrates a Matrix Multiple Choice item type. The rationale and test-taking strategy to help you derive the correct responses shown in Sample Question 7.3 are also provided.

Sample Question 7.3 — Matrix Multiple Choice: *Take Actions*

The nurse is caring for a 28-year-old client who is 3 weeks postpartum and admitted to the hospital with endometritis.

Select whether the following potential nursing actions are indicated or not indicated for the client at this time.

Nurses' Notes

0900: Client is 3 weeks postpartum and reports is breast-feeding the infant. Client reports chills and malaise, loss of appetite, abdominal pain and cramping, and foul-smelling vaginal drainage that is purulent. Severe uterine tenderness is noted on palpation. Blood drawn for WBCs, lactic acid, and blood cultures. Urine obtained through straight cath and sent to lab. IV saline lock inserted, antibiotic started after lab draws and urine was obtained.
T 102°F (38.8°C); HR 110; RR 24; BP 100/52; SpO$_2$ 94% on RA

Orders

0830:
Stat labs: WBCs, lactic acid, blood cultures
IV saline lock
Straight catheterization for urine culture and sensitivity
O$_2$ at 2 L/min via NC
Ceftriaxone 1 g IV every 12 hours
Acetaminophen 650 mg orally every 4–6 hours for discomfort and fever

Laboratory Results

0930:

Test and Reference Range	Results
WBC 5000–10,000/mm^3 (5–10 × 10^9/L)	20,000/mm^3 (20 × 10^9/L)
Lactic acid 5–20 mg/dL (0.6–2.2 mmol/L)	22 mg/dL (2.42 mmol/L)

Potential Nursing Actions	Indicated	Not Indicated
Assist the client to the left side-lying flat position.	☐	☒
Administer the IV antibiotic.	☒	☐
Place the client on transmission-based Contact Precautions.	☐	☒
Administer acetaminophen 650-mg oral dose.	☒	☐
Restrict fluids to 1000 mL daily.	☐	☒
Provide heat to the abdomen.	☒	☐
Inform the client that breast-feeding will need to be stopped and the infant will need to switch to bottle feeding.	☐	☒

Rationale: Endometritis is inflammation and/or infection of the lining of the uterus. It is usually caused by normal inhabitants of the vagina and cervix but can be caused by other organisms such as *Chlamydia trachomatis*. The client with endometritis looks and feels sick. Major signs and symptoms are fever of 100.4°F (38°C) or higher, chills, malaise, anorexia, abdominal pain and cramping, uterine tenderness, and purulent foul-smelling lochia. Tachycardia and subinvolution can also be present. Laboratory data reveal an elevated WBC count. Elevated lactic acid levels can be present if hypoperfusion occurs. A blood culture and catheterized urine specimen may be obtained to identify the bacteria present. Administration of IV antibiotics is the initial treatment with the goal of confining the infection to the uterus and would be initiated as soon as possible after laboratory specimens are obtained. Other medications may include antipyretics for fever and oxytocics to increase drainage of lochia and promote involution. The client would be placed in the Fowler position to promote lochia drainage; lying flat would not accomplish these goals. Medication such as acetaminophen is given for discomfort and to reduce fever. Standard precautions are appropriate and sufficient. Transmission-based precautions such as Contact Precautions are not necessary; endometritis is not usually a contagious disease except for certain sexually transmitted organisms. Fluids are encouraged to maintain hydration. Comfort measures such as a warm blanket or heating pad are provided. Endometritis is not a contraindication to breast-feeding. If the client is breast-feeding the infant and will be separated from the infant during hospitalization, the client will need to pump the breasts to establish and maintain lactation.

Test-Taking Strategy: Focus on the client's diagnosis, and think about the pathophysiology and manifestations of this health problem. Next, look at the assessment data to determine the actions necessary in the care of a client with endometritis. Select the answers recalling that endometritis is inflammation and/or infection of the lining of the uterus. Organize your thinking process as illustrated in the table, and think about what measures would treat inflammation and infection and provide comfort to the client and the rationale for the action.

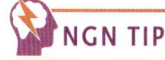

NGN TIP

Remember: A Matrix Multiple Choice item provides you with a scenario and data about the client and includes two or three options columns. There will be at least four rows that present nursing actions or other data in the first column. You need to select one response per row for each item listed in the first column.

Test-Taking Strategy

THINKING SPACE

Nursing Action	Treats Infection/ Inflammation/ Promotes Comfort	Rationale
Assist the client to the left side-lying flat position.	No	This position will not promote the drainage of lochia. Lochia drainage is necessary to prevent stasis, exacerbating the condition.
Administer the IV antibiotic.	Yes	Administering IV antibiotics is the initial treatment with the goal of confining the infection to the uterus. They need to be started as soon as possible following the collection of prescribed laboratory specimens.
Place the client on transmission-based Contact Precautions.	No	Endometritis is not usually a contagious disease except for certain sexually transmitted organisms. Standard precautions are sufficient.
Administer acetaminophen 650-mg oral dose.	Yes	The client has a temperature of 102°F (38.8°C), warranting the need for an antipyretic.
Restrict fluids to 1000 mL daily.	No	Fluids are needed to maintain hydration. This will also help promote lochia drainage.
Provide heat to the abdomen.	Yes	Provides comfort because the client is experiencing abdominal pain and cramping.
Inform the client that breast-feeding will need to be stopped and the infant will need to switch to bottle feeding.	No	There is no reason to stop breast-feeding because the condition is not contagious.

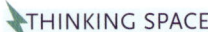 THINKING SPACE

Content Area: Obstetrics-Newborn Nursing
Priority Concepts: Inflammation, Infection
Reference(s): Lowdermilk et al., 2024, p. 739

Extended Multiple Response Test Items to Measure *Take Actions*

Extended Multiple Response test items include Multiple Response Select All That Apply, Multiple Response Select N, and Multiple Response Grouping. When the Multiple Response item type is used to measure *Take Actions*, the test taker is required to follow the question directions regarding how to select options. Sample Question 7.4 illustrates a Multiple Response Select All That Apply item type. With a Multiple Response Select All That Apply test item, you need to do exactly as the item type describes, select all options that apply. The rationale and test-taking strategy to help you derive the correct responses shown in Sample Question 7.4 are also provided.

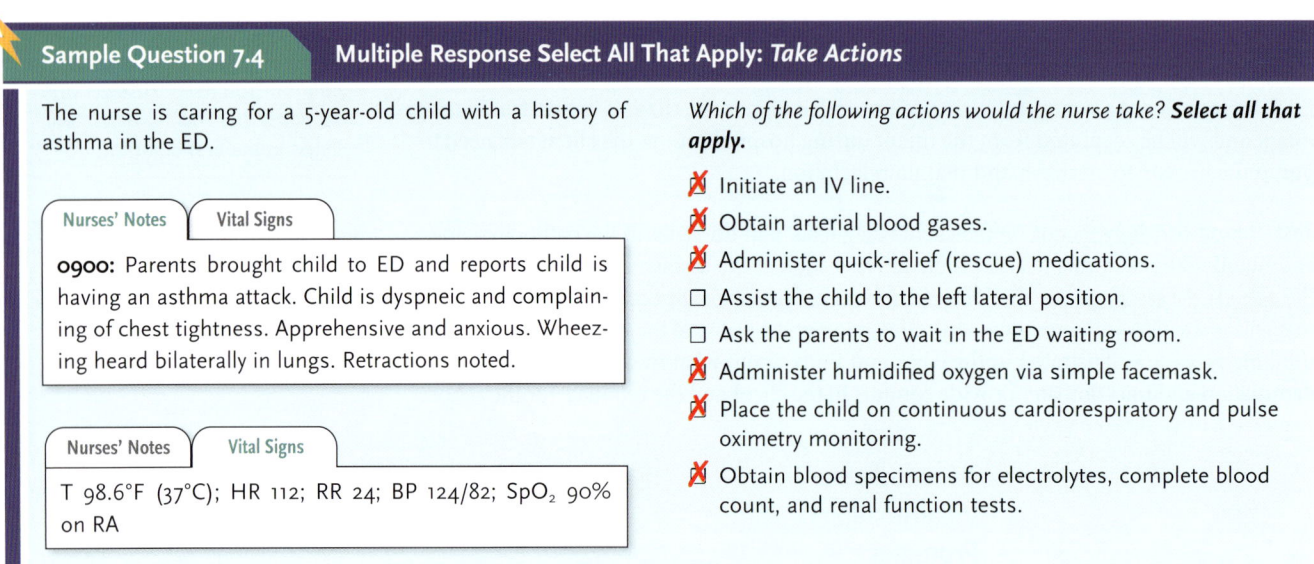

Sample Question 7.4 — Multiple Response Select All That Apply: Take Actions

The nurse is caring for a 5-year-old child with a history of asthma in the ED.

Nurses' Notes
0900: Parents brought child to ED and reports child is having an asthma attack. Child is dyspneic and complaining of chest tightness. Apprehensive and anxious. Wheezing heard bilaterally in lungs. Retractions noted.

Vital Signs
T 98.6°F (37°C); HR 112; RR 24; BP 124/82; SpO$_2$ 90% on RA

Which of the following actions would the nurse take? **Select all that apply.**

- ☒ Initiate an IV line.
- ☒ Obtain arterial blood gases.
- ☒ Administer quick-relief (rescue) medications.
- ☐ Assist the child to the left lateral position.
- ☐ Ask the parents to wait in the ED waiting room.
- ☒ Administer humidified oxygen via simple facemask.
- ☒ Place the child on continuous cardiorespiratory and pulse oximetry monitoring.
- ☒ Obtain blood specimens for electrolytes, complete blood count, and renal function tests.

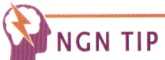 **NGN TIP**

Remember: A Multiple Response Select All That Apply item provides you with a scenario and data about the client and a list of options. You will need to select one or more answer options as they apply to the scenario. There may be only one correct option or multiple correct options. There will be at least 5 options with no more than 10 options, but all 10 options could be correct.

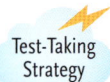 Test-Taking Strategy

Rationale: For a child with an acute asthma exacerbation, the nurse would monitor airway, breathing, and circulation closely via continuous cardiorespiratory and pulse oximetry in the event that supportive measures are needed. Pulse oximetry is monitored as well to ensure an oxygen saturation level above 90% and to ensure adequate oxygenation of tissues. Humidified oxygen via simple facemask is administered to improve SpO$_2$ levels and to avoid drying secretions. Oxygen via NC will dry secretions. Dyspnea, chest tightness, wheezing, and retractions are indicators of respiratory compromise. The child with an acute asthma exacerbation is usually very apprehensive and anxious and needs to be comforted. It is important to reassure the child that the child will not be left alone and to allow the parents to remain with the child. The child is allowed to assume a position of comfort that will promote maximum ventilation function. Placing the child in the left lateral position would not enhance breathing and ventilation. An IV line is necessary for administration of fluids and IV medications if needed. Quick-relief (rescue) medications usually via inhalation are given to open constricted airways and allow air exchange and to enhance tissue oxygenation. Laboratory studies and arterial blood gases are performed to obtain a baseline and to determine the need for additional and more aggressive intervention. The elevated heart rate, respiratory rate, and blood pressure are expected to return to normal range once treatment is provided.

Test-Taking Strategy: Focus on the information in the scenario and note the child's problem, an acute asthma exacerbation. You need to use knowledge about the pathophysiology of an acute asthma exacerbation to assist in answering correctly. Think about what is expected in this event to determine nursing actions. Recalling that the primary goals of care are to provide oxygenation and to implement measures that will ensure adequate ventilation will assist in answering correctly. Also recall that anxiety and apprehension exacerbate a problem with airway and oxygenation, so ensuring psychosocial support is important. You can also use a thinking process as illustrated in the table to answer this question.

▶ THINKING SPACE

Nursing Action	Helpful/Likely to Address the Problem	Not Helpful/Not Likely to Address the Problem
Initiate an IV line.	☒	☐
Obtain arterial blood gases.	☒	☐
Administer quick-relief (rescue) medications.	☒	☐
Assist the child to the left lateral position.	☐	☒
Administer humidified oxygen via simple facemask.	☒	☐
Ask the parents to wait in the ED waiting room.	☐	☒
Place the child on continuous cardiorespiratory and pulse oximetry monitoring.	☒	☐
Obtain blood specimens for electrolytes, complete blood count, and renal function tests.	☒	☐

Content Area: Pediatric Nursing
Priority Concept: Gas Exchange, Perfusion
Reference(s): Hockenberry et al., 2024, pp. 928–931; Ignatavicius et al., 2024, p. 540–548

Practice Questions

Practice Question 7.1 — Multiple Response Select All That Apply

An occupational nurse employed at a toy factory is called for emergency assistance to a 42-year-old victim of an accident.

Nurses' Notes | Vital Signs

1400: Victim is sitting on the floor leaning against a wall. Victim's index and middle finger were completely severed by a machine saw. The fingers are seen on the floor 2 feet away from the victim.

Nurses' Notes | Vital Signs

1400: T 98.2°F (36.7°C); HR 120; RR 22; BP 132/84; SpO₂ 95% on RA

Which of the following actions would the nurse take? **Select all that apply.**

☐ Call 911 (EMS).
☐ Elevate the affected hand above the victim's heart level.
☐ Place the fingers in a waterproof, sealed plastic bag.
☐ Check the victim for airway or breathing problems.
☐ Place the waterproof, sealed bag containing the fingers on ice.
☐ Apply direct pressure to the amputation sites with layers of dry gauze.
☐ Remove the dry gauze after 10 minutes to check the status of the bleeding.
☐ Ensure that the amputated fingers are transported to the hospital with the victim.

Practice Question 7.2 — Drop-Down Rationale

A client who is 4 weeks postpartum presents to the clinic with excessive vaginal bleeding.

Nurses' Notes | Vital Signs

1000: Client is 4 weeks postpartum and reports excessive vaginal bleeding with occasional spurts of excessive blood. Reports pelvic pain and feelings of pelvic heaviness, backache, fatigue, and persistent malaise.

Nurses' Notes | **Vital Signs**

1000: T 98.9°F (37.1°C); HR 100; RR 20; BP 110/70; SpO₂ 95% on RA

Complete the following sentence by selecting from the lists of options provided.

The nurse would **1 [Select]** because the client is *most* likely experiencing **2 [Select]**.

Options for 1	Options for 2
Contact the obstetrician.	Infection
Instruct the client to apply a heating pad on a low setting to the abdomen.	Septic shock
Teach the client about the warning signs of postpartum complications.	Subinvolution of the uterus

Practice Question 7.3 — Matrix Multiple Response

A 65-year-old client was hospitalized and treated for symptoms of heart palpitations and extreme shortness of breath. On admission, diagnostic studies were performed.

Diagnostic Studies

ECG: atrial fibrillation
CT of the lungs: negative for embolism
Chest x-ray: enlarged left ventricle

The nurse is preparing the client for discharge and provides teaching about prescribed medications. For each medication listed, select the teaching point the nurse would provide to the client. Each teaching point may support more than one medication.

Teaching Point	Amiodarone	Metoprolol	Warfarin
Routine laboratory monitoring	☐	☐	☐
Monitor and report signs of bleeding	☐	☐	☐
Monitor and report shortness of breath	☐	☐	☐
Monitor BP and HR	☐	☐	☐
Consume consistent amounts of green, leafy vegetables	☐	☐	☐

Practice Question 7.4 — Matrix Multiple Choice

A parent brings a 6-month-old child to the ED.

Health History

1830: Parent reports that the child has been coughing and sneezing, seems to be "breathing funny," and feels warm. Parent reports being single and unhoused. Reports "living on the street, but sleeps in a shelter with the child most nights." Parent states that the child does not have a pediatrician and has not received any child care since birth. Reports still breast-feeding as the child's primary nutritional intake, but child has been refusing to feed.

Nurses' Notes

1830: T 102°F (38.8°C); HR 176; RR 80; SpO$_2$ 91% on RA
Coughing, sneezing with runny nose
Copious secretions
Color pale, no cyanosis, listless, retractions noted, wheezes noted at lung bases bilaterally
Weight 12.8 lb (5.8 kg), length 22 inches

Orders

1900:
Rapid RSV antigen test
Heated high-flow oxygen 1 L/min via NC
Insert IV, and administer 0.9% NS 25 mL/h
Admit to pediatric unit

Laboratory Results

1930:

Test and Reference Range	Result
RSV antigen test negative	Positive

The physician admits the child to the hospital, and the admitting pediatric nurse reviews the ED notes. Select whether the following potential nursing actions are indicated or not indicated for the child at this time.

Potential Nursing Actions	Indicated	Not Indicated
Monitor weight.	☐	☐
Administer oral fluids.	☐	☐
Perform a well-baby assessment.	☐	☐
Suction the airway and nares as needed.	☐	☐
Restrict the parent from holding the child.	☐	☐
Monitor airway status and vital signs.	☐	☐
Assist the parent to pump breast milk.	☐	☐
Institute Contact Precautions and Droplet Precautions.	☐	☐
Contact social services for consultation.	☐	☐
Institute chest percussion and chest physiotherapy for drainage.	☐	☐

Practice Question 7.5 — Multiple Response Select All That Apply

The nurse is caring for a 48-year-old client following a laparoscopic cholecystectomy on the surgical outpatient unit.

Nurses' Notes | Vital Signs

1100: Alert and oriented. Dressing dry and intact. IV 5% dextrose/lactated Ringer's infusing at 100 mL/h. Has not voided.

Nurses' Notes | **Vital Signs**

1100: T 99.2°F (37.3°C); HR 92; RR 16; BP 118/72; SpO_2 97% on RA. Reports pain rated 4/10 (on a 0–10 pain scale)

Which of the following actions would the nurse take in managing this client's care in the **immediate** postoperative period? **Select all that apply.**

☐ Keep the head of the bed flat.
☐ Assist the client to the bathroom to void.
☐ Assess the incision sites frequently.
☐ Administer antiemetics as needed.
☐ Maintain strict NPO status.
☐ Administer pain medication.
☐ Encourage use of the incentive spirometer.

Practice Question 7.6 — Drop-Down Rationale

The nurse is caring for a hospitalized 70-year-old client who has cellulitis on both lower extremities caused by methicillin-resistant *Staphylococcus aureus* (MRSA) and is being treated with IV vancomycin.

Vital Signs | Laboratory Results

1100: T 100.8°F (38.2°C); HR 88; RR 18; BP 110/72; SpO_2 96% on RA; Reports pain rated 3/10 (on a 0–10 pain scale)

Vital Signs | **Laboratory Results**

1100:

Test and Reference Range	Result
Vancomycin trough level 10–20 mcg/mL (10.3498–13.7998 μmol/L)	16 mcg/mL (11.3981 μmol/L)
White blood cells (WBCs) 5000–10,000/mm³ (5–10 × 10⁹ /L)	11,000/mm³ (11 × 10⁹ /L)
Blood urea nitrogen (BUN) 10–20 mg/dL (3.6–7.1 mmol/L)	20 mg/dL (7.1 mmol/L)
Creatinine 0.5–1.2 mg/dL (44–106 μmol/L)	0.6 mg/dL (53 μmol/L)

The next dose of vancomycin is due now, and the nurse checks the laboratory results. Complete the following sentence by selecting from the lists of options provided.

The nurse would **1 [Select]** because **2 [Select]**.

Options for 1	Options for 2
Hold the next dose.	The WBC count is slightly elevated.
Administer a lower dose.	The trough level is normal.
Administer the next dose orally.	The creatinine level indicates toxicity.
Administer the next dose as prescribed.	The BUN level is high but not toxic.

CHAPTER 8

Strategies for Answering NGN Questions: Evaluate Outcomes

Evaluate Outcomes is a CJ cognitive skill that involves examining outcomes and measuring client progress toward meeting those outcomes in the plan of care. It is an ongoing and continuous process that compares actual client outcomes with the expected outcomes in a clinical scenario. It provides a basis for determining the need to modify the plan of care. As an iterative process, this skill involves revisiting the clinical scenario and examining the application of the CJ cognitive skills *Recognize Cues, Analyze Cues, Prioritize Hypotheses, Generate Solutions,* and *Take Actions*. Thus the cognitive skill *Evaluate Outcomes* involves looking back and making necessary revisions or modifications to provide safe and effective client care.

A nurse always needs to determine the effectiveness of the plan of care. In addition to determining the effectiveness of the plan of care, the CJ cognitive skill *Evaluate Outcomes* requires communicating client findings as well as documenting and reporting the client's response to treatment and care. As a nurse, you need to ask yourself, "Did my actions help? Are things improved? Are things worse; has the client's condition declined? Are things unchanged?" Based on your evaluation findings, you will need to think about how to move forward and what changes may be necessary to achieve the outcomes of care. Therefore the CJ cognitive skill *Evaluate Outcomes* is essential to meet the client's needs and ensure client safety and high-quality care. This ability will be measured both on the NGN and by your instructors during classroom activities, on course exams, and in the laboratory and clinical settings.

> **THINKING SPACE**

How Do You Evaluate Outcomes?

Determining the effectiveness of the care provided is the focus of the CJ cognitive skill *Evaluate Outcomes*. Once you have completed a phase of care or an aspect of care, think about what information you need to determine if the care was effective and to what degree. You may determine that expected outcomes have been met, unmet, or partially met. You will likely need to think about factors influencing the care and subsequent outcomes so you can decide what needs to happen next to move toward the outcomes. Questions to ask yourself as you apply this CJ cognitive skill may include:

- Based on previous assessments and interventions, what is happening to the client now?
- Are there ongoing or new client needs? If so, which ones are the priority?
- What must I do to address and meet these needs?
- Are the outcomes of care the same, or do they need to be revised?
- What else do I need to do to promote achievement of client outcomes?

How Will *Evaluate Outcomes* Be Tested?

In every client interaction, you will evaluate outcomes of the plan of care. Therefore you can expect that you will be tested on your ability to accurately evaluate the outcomes of care provided and determine the necessary follow-up based on that evaluation.

NGN TIP

Remember: Focus on the outcomes of client care, and think about what you need to consider as possible revisions to the plan of care. Ask yourself, "What else needs to be done and what needs to change to meet the expected outcomes?"

⚡ THINKING SPACE

Beginning with your first nursing course, you were asked about interpreting the outcomes of care in a variety of clinical scenarios. Sometimes testing required you to determine which follow-up assessments you need to conduct; other times you were tested on follow-up nursing actions you need to take to meet established outcomes. For example, you may have been presented with a clinical scenario in which a client was administered a unit of packed red blood cells because of a gastrointestinal hemorrhage. In this scenario, evaluating assessment findings including laboratory results after administration of the blood product to determine the outcome of that intervention was likely a focus of the question or questions. Or maybe you were asked about interpreting vital signs and conducting a follow-up pain assessment after administering pain medication to a postoperative client.

NGN Question Stems Addressing *Evaluate Outcomes*

Test question stems will give you clues in the wording if the aim is to determine your ability to *Evaluate Outcomes*. Box 8.1 provides a list of examples of NGN question stems that will help you know that this thinking process is being addressed.

Which NGN Item Types Optimally Measure *Evaluate Outcomes*?

Four item types optimally measure the CJ cognitive skill *Evaluate Outcomes*. Variations of each item type will most likely be presented on the NGN. Table 8.1 presents these item types and their variations. The Sample Questions that follow illustrate some of these types. The rationale and test-taking strategy to help you derive the correct responses are also provided.

Matrix Multiple Choice Test Items to Measure *Evaluate Outcomes*

In a Matrix Multiple Choice item, you will be presented with columns and rows. You will need to select one response item for each row. Sample Question 8.1 illustrates a Matrix Multiple Choice item type to measure *Evaluate Outcomes*. The rationale and test-taking strategy to help you derive the correct responses in Sample Question 8.1 are also provided.

NGN TIP

Remember: When you *Evaluate Outcomes*, you need to determine if expected outcomes have been met, unmet, or partially met. If outcomes are unmet or partially met, then you need to examine the application of the CJ cognitive skills *Recognize Cues, Analyze Cues, Prioritize Hypotheses, Generate Solutions,* and *Take Actions.* Then you need to determine what needs to be changed, revised, or added to the plan of care for outcomes to be met.

Sample Question 8.1 — Matrix Multiple Choice: *Evaluate Outcomes*

A 38-year-old client (gravida 6, para 6) at 40 weeks' gestation is admitted to the labor and delivery unit for a scheduled labor induction.

Nurses' Notes

1200: Vaginal examination reveals cervix is 80% effaced, 4 cm dilated. Client reports is not experiencing contractions. Oxytocin infusion started per obstetrician prescription and per agency protocol. Fetal monitor applied.

For each assessment finding, select whether the finding is consistent with a therapeutic outcome or an adverse outcome of oxytocin.

Assessment Finding	Therapeutic Outcome	Adverse Outcome
Altered mental status	☐	☒
Adventitious lung sounds	☐	☒
Contractions every 3–5 minutes lasting 45 seconds each	☒	☐
Sudden pain between contractions	☐	☒
Decelerations on the fetal monitor	☐	☒
Pain intensifying gradually with contractions	☒	☐

BOX 8.1 NGN Question Stems Addressing *Evaluate Outcomes*

- Which of the following client/caregiver statement(s) indicates the *need for further teaching*? *Select all that apply.*
- Highlight the findings that indicate the client is *not progressing as expected.*
- Complete the sentence by selecting from the word choices a complication and an associated client finding that indicates the client's *condition has worsened.*
- Highlight the findings that indicate the client's health problem is *not yet resolved.*
- Select whether the client/caregiver statement/observation indicates that the home care instruction is *understood* or *requires further teaching.*
- For each body system, select the finding that indicates *progression toward expected outcomes.*
- After assessment and teaching, which 4 findings are *unexpected and therefore require additional follow-up?*
- Which of the following findings are *consistent with a therapeutic outcome or an adverse outcome* of the prescribed medication? *Select all that apply.*
- For each client statement, select if the statement indicates that the *treatment plan is effective or ineffective.*
- Select 4 findings that indicate a *therapeutic outcome* of medication therapy.

TABLE 8.1 Test Items and Variations That Optimally Measure *Evaluate Outcomes*

Type of Test Item	Variations
Highlight	Highlight-in-Text Highlight-in-Table
Extended Multiple Response	Multiple Response Select All That Apply Multiple Response Select N Multiple Response Grouping
Matrix/Grid	Matrix Multiple Response Matrix Multiple Choice
Drag-and-Drop	Drag-and-Drop Cloze Drag-and-Drop Rationale
Drop-Down	Drop-Down Cloze Drop-Down Rationale Drop-Down in Table

Rationale: Oxytocin is a hormone that is produced naturally by the posterior pituitary gland. Oxytocin produces uterine contractions during pregnancy and can be administered to induce labor for a term pregnancy. Additional therapeutic outcomes include milk ejection and control of postpartum hemorrhage. When given for labor, the client will experience intensifying contractions, including intensifying pain as the labor progresses, until eventually the contractions are occurring every 3 to 5 minutes and lasting 45 seconds each. Because oxytocin exerts an antidiuretic effect, water intoxication is an adverse outcome of oxytocin. Assessment findings related to water retention may be noted, such as altered mental status, adventitious lung sounds, and peripheral swelling. Another adverse outcome that can occur is uterine rupture. Sudden pain between contractions, excessive vaginal bleeding, and decelerations on the fetal monitor would be noted with this complication. The client with higher parity, specifically more than five pregnancies, is at higher risk for uterine rupture when given oxytocin.

Test-Taking Strategy: Note that this question is asking you to evaluate assessment findings and decide whether they are consistent with a therapeutic or adverse outcome of oxytocin. The question is asking about the use of oxytocin for the induction of labor, therefore you need to think about the findings in the context of normal labor progression. Any finding that is not specifically related to or associated with normal labor progression should be classified as an adverse outcome. Using a table format to organize your thoughts may be helpful.

THINKING SPACE

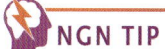

Remember: In a Matrix Multiple Choice question, each row must have only one response item selected. If you do not select a response item for each row, you will not be able to move on to the next item on the exam.

Test-Taking Strategy

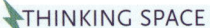
THINKING SPACE

Assessment Finding	Associated With Normal Labor Progression	Not Associated With Normal Labor Progression
Altered mental status	☐	☒
Adventitious lung sounds	☐	☒
Contractions every 3–5 minutes lasting 45 seconds each	☒	☐
Sudden pain between contractions	☐	☒
Decelerations on the fetal monitor	☐	☒
Pain intensifying gradually with contractions	☒	☐

Altered mental status, adventitious lung sounds, sudden pain *between* contractions, and decelerations on the fetal monitor are not normal findings and are not specifically related to normal labor progression.

Content Area: Obstetric-Newborn Nursing
Priority Concepts: Perfusion, Reproduction
Reference(s): Lilley et al., 2023, pp. 539–540

Highlight-in-Table Test Items to Measure *Evaluate Outcomes*

In a Highlight-in-Table item, you will be presented with client information in table format. Sample Question 8.2 illustrates a Highlight-in-Table item type to measure *Evaluate Outcomes* and presents a table with body systems and associated assessment findings in addition to a lab table. The rationale and test-taking strategy to help you derive the correct responses in Sample Question 8.2 are also provided.

Sample Question 8.2 — Highlight-in-Table: *Evaluate Outcomes*

An 86-year-old client was hospitalized 4 days ago because of multiple episodes of severe watery diarrhea, anorexia, and weakness.

History and Physical | Orders | Vital Signs

0800: Client arrives at ED reporting multiple episodes of severe watery diarrhea, anorexia, and weakness with crampy abdominal pain and exhibiting signs of severe dehydration. Client's spouse reports that the client had not eaten much for 4 days prior and complained of thirst but had not been able to "hold anything down."

History and Physical | **Orders** | Vital Signs

0830: IV NS with 40 mEq potassium chloride at 100 mL/h
Ondansetron 4 mg IV stat
Laboratory studies per protocol
Stool and blood cultures

History and Physical | Orders | **Vital Signs**

0815: T 98.9°F (37.1°C); HR 96; RR 20; BP 100/70; SpO$_2$ 95% on RA

On day 4 of hospitalization, the nurse assesses the client and reviews the laboratory results drawn in the morning.

Highlight the client findings that indicate the client's health problem is not yet resolved.

Assessment	Findings
Gastrointestinal	Tolerating clear liquids and soft foods. States has an appetite. ==Had two episodes of brown, watery diarrhea at 0700 and 0800. Reports cramping abdominal pain currently rated 4/10== (on a 0–10 pain scale).
Genitourinary	Urine output 240 mL during the night. Voided 100 mL at 0800, yellow and ==concentrated urine.==
Vital signs	==T 101.2°F (38.4°C)==; HR 90; RR 20; BP 118/80; SpO$_2$ 95% on RA.

Test and Reference Range	Result
White blood cells (WBCs) 5000–10,000/mm^3 (5–10 × 10^9/L)	10,000/mm^3 (10 × 10^9/L)
Blood urea nitrogen (BUN) 10–20 mg/dL (3.6–7.1 mmol/L)	==22 mg/dL (7.92 mmol/L)==
Creatinine 0.6–1.2 mg/dL (53–106 µmol/L)	0.9 mg/dL (79.5 µmol/L)
Potassium 3.5–5.0 mEq/L (3.5–5.0 mmol/L)	==3.3 mEq/L (3.3 mmol/L)==
Sodium 135–145 mEq/L (135–145 mmol/L)	==148 mEq/L (148 mmol/L)==
Stool culture Negative	Negative
Blood cultures Negative	Negative

Rationale: The client has been treated for severe dehydration. Although the nurse is not provided with much baseline information about the client, there are abnormal data that indicate that the client's health problem has not resolved. The client had multiple episodes of diarrhea, and although the cause of the diarrhea is unknown, it has led to severe dehydration. The client had two episodes of brown, watery diarrhea at 0700 and 0800 on day 4 of hospitalization, 1 hour apart, and also reports cramping abdominal pain rated 4/10 (on a 0–10 pain scale). This indicates that the client is still experiencing the health problem. Although the urine output is minimally adequate, the urine is concentrated, indicating insufficient body fluid. In addition, a deficit of normal body fluid can cause hyperthermia, and this client is exhibiting an elevated temperature at 101.2°F (38.4°C). Because the stool and blood cultures are negative and the WBC count is within the reference range, infection is not likely, and the temperature elevation is probably associated with dehydration. In dehydration, some electrolytes are lost, specifically potassium. The client's potassium level is low, known as *hypokalemia*. The sodium level is elevated (known as *hypernatremia*), and this is an indicator of dehydration and that the health problem is not resolved. In hypernatremia, the body contains too little water for the amount of sodium, therefore the sodium level in the blood becomes abnormally high when water loss exceeds sodium loss. The BUN is slightly elevated at 22 mg/dL (7.92 mmol/L), and in the setting of a normal creatinine level, this indicates dehydration.

Test-Taking Strategy: Note that the question is asking you to evaluate assessment findings that indicate that the client's health problem has not yet resolved. Focus on the information in the scenario, and note that the client is severely dehydrated. Use knowledge of the pathophysiology associated with dehydration and its manifestations. Look for abnormal data in the findings that indicate a dehydrated state. Using a table format to organize your thoughts may be helpful.

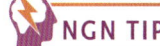

NGN TIP

Remember: In a Highlight-in-Table question, you will select from a table pieces of information that are significant to the question being asked. The table may display part of a medical record, such as history and physical, nurses' notes, vital signs, flow sheet data, orders, or laboratory results.

Test-Taking Strategy

THINKING SPACE

Related to or Consistent With Dehydration	Unrelated to or Inconsistent With Dehydration
• Had two episodes of brown, watery diarrhea at 0700 and 0800 • Reports cramping abdominal pain currently rated 4/10 (on a 0–10 pain scale) • Concentrated urine • Temperature 101.2°F (38.4°C) • BUN: 22 mg/dL (7.92 mmol/L) • Potassium: 3.3 mEq/L (3.3 mmol/L) • Sodium: 148 mEq/L (148 mmol/L)	• Tolerating clear liquids and soft foods • States has an appetite • Urine output 240 mL during the night • Yellow urine • HR 90 • RR 20 • BP 118/80 • SpO$_2$ 95% on RA • WBCs: 10,000/mm^3 (10 × 10^9/L) • Creatinine: 0.9 mg/dL (79.5 μmol/L)

Note that questions requiring you to evaluate assessment findings specific to such things as body systems, vital signs, or laboratory results may ask about those indicating that the problem has resolved or has not yet resolved. Be sure to consider all findings in the assessment when evaluating outcomes.

Content Area: Medical-Surgical Nursing
Priority Concepts: Elimination; Fluid and Electrolyte Balance
Reference(s): Ignatavicius et al., 2024, pp. 255–258

Multiple Response Select All That Apply Test Items to Measure *Evaluate Outcomes*

In a Multiple Response Select All That Apply item, you will be asked to select all responses that apply to what the question is asking. Sample Question 8.3 illustrates a Multiple Response Select All That Apply item type to measure *Evaluate Outcomes*. The rationale and test-taking strategy to help you derive the correct responses in Sample Question 8.3 are also provided.

Sample Question 8.3 — Multiple Response Select All That Apply: *Evaluate Outcomes*

A hospitalized 68-year-old client undergoes a procedure in which a biventricular pacemaker is placed in the right subclavicular area.

Nurses' Notes | Vital Signs

1300: Returned to nursing unit. Alert and oriented × 4. Assisted to void. Voided 250 mL clear, yellow urine. Reports pain at the level of the diaphragm rated 5/10 (on a 0–10 pain scale). Muscle contractions are noted over the diaphragm that correspond to the HR. Dressing over the pacemaker site is clean, dry, and intact. Client hiccupping. Teaching about pacemaker care initiated.

Nurses' Notes | Vital Signs

1300: T 98.8°F (37°C); HR 80; RR 20; BP 116/70; SpO₂ 96% on RA

Which of the following findings noted after postprocedure assessment and teaching are unexpected and therefore require additional follow-up? **Select all that apply.**

- ☒ The client reports pain at the level of the diaphragm.
- ☒ The client is hiccupping and reports it is uncomfortable and will not stop.
- ☐ The dressing over the pacemaker site is clean, dry, and intact.
- ☐ The client uses the left ear when talking on the cell phone.
- ☒ The client performs right-shoulder range-of-motion exercises.
- ☐ The client states will avoid lifting more than 10 lb using the affected side.
- ☒ Muscle contractions are noted over the diaphragm that correspond to the HR.

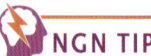

NGN TIP

Remember: In a Multiple Response Select All That Apply question, you will need to select all options that are correct. There will be at least 5 options to select from and no more than 10 options for selection. There may be only one correct response or multiple correct responses, or all options listed could be correct. If you select fewer than the number of correct options, you will not receive full credit. With a Multiple Response Select N item, you need to select the exact number of options that the instructions indicate. You can select fewer than the number of options provided, but not more. However, if you do select fewer than the number (N) indicated in the question, you will not receive full credit.

Rationale: A permanent pacemaker may be needed for a client who experiences cardiac conduction disorders that do not improve with other measures. The pacemaker is placed in a subcutaneous pocket in the right or left subclavicular area of the shoulder. Complications of pacemaker placement include pericardial effusion, pericardial tamponade, and diaphragmatic pacing. Client reports of pain at the level of the diaphragm along with muscle contractions noted over the diaphragm that correspond to the heart rate may indicate diaphragmatic pacing, which occurs when the pacemaker is malpositioned or one of the leads is dislodged, and would require additional follow-up. Although some shoulder movement should be encouraged to prevent stiffness, the client needs to avoid lifting the arms over the head, therefore additional follow-up is needed if the client is performing range-of-motion shoulder exercises. In addition, the client should avoid lifting anything more than 10 lb on the affected side because this could dislodge the pacemaker wire. Signs of pacemaker malfunction, including difficulty breathing, dizziness, fainting, chest pain, weight gain, and prolonged hiccupping, need to be reported to the cardiologist. The dressing should be clean, dry, and intact, and the pacemaker implantation site should be free from redness, swelling, and drainage. The client needs to avoid sources of electromagnetic fields and telecommunications transmitters because these could disrupt the pacemaker settings, therefore the client should use the left ear to talk on the cell phone if the pacemaker site is on the right side.

Test-Taking Strategy: Note that this question is asking you to determine which assessment findings require additional follow-up. Using a thinking process as illustrated in the table, consider whether each option is normal or expected and therefore not likely to cause harm or whether it is abnormal or unexpected and has the potential for harm. Any option that has the potential for harm would be selected because this would require additional follow-up.

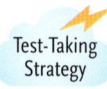

THINKING SPACE

Assessment Finding	Normal/ Expected/ Not Likely to Cause Harm	Abnormal/ Unexpected/ Potential for Harm
The client reports pain at the level of the diaphragm.	☐	☒
The client reports hiccupping that is uncomfortable and will not stop.	☐	☒
The dressing over the pacemaker site is clean, dry, and intact.	☒	☐
The client uses the left ear when talking on the cell phone.	☒	☐
The client performs right-shoulder range-of-motion exercises.	☐	☒
The client states will avoid lifting more than 10 lb on the affected side.	☒	☐
Muscle contractions are noted over the diaphragm that correspond to the HR.	☐	☒

The client reporting pain at the level of the diaphragm, the client performing right-shoulder range-of-motion exercises, the client reporting hiccupping that is uncomfortable and will not go away, and muscle contractions noted over the diaphragm that correspond to the heart rate are all abnormal, unexpected, and/or have the potential to cause harm and therefore require additional follow-up. Therefore these are the correct answers to the question.

Content Area: Medical-Surgical Nursing
Priority Concepts: Perfusion; Tissue Integrity
Reference(s): Ignatavicius et al., 2024, pp. 671–673, 678

Multiple Response Grouping Test Items to Measure *Evaluate Outcomes*

In a Multiple Response Grouping item, the options are presented in a table, and the table can have a minimum of 2 groupings and a maximum of 5 groupings.

Each grouping has a minimum of 2 options and a maximum of 4 options, and the number of options for each grouping will be the same. You need to select at least one response from each grouping category to answer the question. However, more than one response from each grouping category could be correct. Sample Question 8.4 illustrates a Multiple Response Grouping item type. The rationale and test-taking strategy to help you derive the correct responses in Sample Question 8.4 are also provided.

Sample Question 8.4 — **Multiple Response Grouping:** *Evaluate Outcomes*

A 35-year-old veteran who sustained a severe hip injury during military service returns to the postoperative unit following open reduction with internal fixation of the left hip, and the nurse performs an initial assessment.

Nurses' Notes | Vital Signs

1300: Drowsy, arousable and responsive to stimuli. Pupils equal, round, and reactive to light. Lung sounds clear on auscultation bilaterally. Peripheral pulses 2+ bilaterally. Sensation intact in bilateral lower extremities. Bowel sounds hypoactive in all quadrants. Felt the urge to void and asked for the urinal; voided 10 mL clear yellow urine, no odor. No redness over pressure point areas. No petechiae or rashes throughout the skin. Surgical dressing saturated with bright-red blood. IV 1000 mL lactated Ringer's solution infusing at 100 mL/h; IV dressing dry and intact, no swelling or redness.

Nurses' Notes | **Vital Signs**

1300: T 98.6°F (37°C); HR 120; RR 8; BP 90/56; SpO$_2$ 93% on 3 L/min O$_2$ via NC

For each body system, select the assessment finding(s) consistent with expected postoperative outcomes. Each body system may support more than one assessment finding.

Body System	Assessment Finding
Respiratory	☐ RR 8
	☒ SpO$_2$ 93% on 3 L/min O$_2$ via NC
	☒ Lung sounds clear on auscultation bilaterally
Cardiovascular	☐ BP 90/56
	☐ HR 120
	☒ Peripheral pulses 2+ bilaterally
Neurologic	☒ Drowsy, arousable, and responsive to stimuli
	☒ Pupils equal, round, and reactive to light
	☒ Sensation intact in bilateral lower extremities
Gastrointestinal/ genitourinary	☒ Bowel sounds hypoactive in all quadrants
	☐ Urine output 10 mL voided
	☒ Urine yellow, clear, no odor
Integumentary	☐ Surgical dressing saturated with bright-red blood
	☒ No redness over pressure point areas
	☒ No petechiae or rashes throughout the skin

Rationale: A respiratory rate of 8 indicates a problem with the airway or respiratory system and is not consistent with an expected postoperative finding. The normal pulse oximetry range in the postoperative period is 92% to 100%, so an SpO$_2$ of 93% is acceptable; in addition, the client is on supplemental oxygen at this time. Lung sounds should be clear. Blood pressure should be at or above baseline and could be elevated owing to pain. This client's blood pressure is low, which is an unexpected postoperative finding and could indicate a problem with perfusion or bleeding. The heart rate may be elevated above baseline because of pain; however, if it is substantially elevated, such as a heart rate of 120, this may be due to a problem with perfusion or bleeding. Peripheral pulses 2+ bilaterally is a normal and expected progression. In the postoperative period, it is expected for the client to be drowsy but arousable and responding to stimuli. Pupils should be round, equal, and reactive to light. Sensation should be intact in the extremities. Hypoactive bowel sounds in all quadrants are expected in the postoperative period because of the effects of anesthesia. Clear, yellow urine without odor is normal and expected. Urine output of 10 mL may indicate a potential postoperative problem due to the effects of anesthesia or renal impairment and could also be associated with perfusion problems; this is not an expected outcome. A surgical dressing saturated with bright-red blood likely indicates bleeding from the incision site and is not an expected outcome. No redness over pressure point areas is important to note as the operating room table can cause pressure injuries; this finding is normal and expected. No petechiae or rashes throughout the skin is also a normal and expected progression for the client in the postoperative period.

Test-Taking Strategy: Begin to answer this question by looking at each assessment finding and considering whether it would require continued monitoring versus additional or immediate action or follow-up. If the evaluation necessitates additional or immediate action or follow-up, then it would not be consistent with expected or normal outcomes in the postoperative period. Organize your thinking process as illustrated in the table.

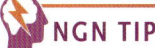

NGN TIP

Remember: In a Multiple Response Grouping item, there will be a maximum of four selections in each row or grouping. You need to select at least one response from each grouping category to answer the question.

Test-Taking Strategy

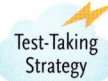

THINKING SPACE

Assessment Finding	Continue to Monitor	Requires Additional or Immediate Action/Follow-up
RR 8	☐	☒
SpO₂ 93% on 3 L/min O₂ via NC	☒	☐
Lung sounds clear on auscultation bilaterally	☒	☐
BP 90/56	☐	☒
HR 120	☐	☒
Peripheral pulses 2+ bilaterally	☒	☐
Drowsy, arousable, and responsive to stimuli	☒	☐
Pupils equal, round, and reactive to light	☒	☐
Sensation intact in bilateral lower extremities	☒	☐
Bowel sounds hypoactive in all quadrants	☒	☐
Urine output 10 mL	☐	☒
Urine yellow, clear, no odor	☒	☐
Surgical dressing saturated with bright-red blood	☐	☒
No redness over pressure point areas	☒	☐
No petechiae or rashes throughout the skin	☒	☐

Recall that questions that *Evaluate Outcomes* require you to examine outcome data provided. Depending on what the question is asking, you need to determine whether the data are expected, unexpected, or unrelated. Then you need to think about additional actions or follow-up that may be necessary based on the conclusions you have made.

Content Area: Foundations of Nursing
Priority Concepts: Clotting; Perfusion
Reference(s): Potter et al., 2023, pp. 1440–1453

Practice Questions

Practice Question 8.1 — Matrix Multiple Choice

A 68-year-old client was transferred from the hospital to a rehabilitation center 2 weeks ago following treatment for a right cerebral stroke. The nurse is preparing the client for discharge to home and reviews the admission notes.

Nurses' Notes | Vital Signs | Physician's Orders

1300: Transferred from the hospital. Client is accompanied by spouse, who will be the primary caregiver when the client returns home. Alert and oriented and understands about receiving rehabilitative therapy before returning to home. States does not really have "much to rehab" and is fine, but will do what the doctor says to get home. Has left-sided weakness, and seems impulsive with movements. Able to move right arm and leg with adequate strength noted. Has difficulty focusing, and attention span is short; spouse is assisting with answering questions. Spouse notes that client's judgment is impaired and is concerned about client's safety because of the client's impulsivity. Client exhibits left-sided neglect; lacks proprioception. Has homonymous hemianopsia.

Nurses' Notes | Vital Signs | Physician's Orders

1300: T 98.6°F (36°C); HR 92; RR 20; BP 132/78; SpO$_2$ 95% on RA

Nurses' Notes | Vital Signs | Physician's Orders

1300:
PT and OT evaluation and initiate a treatment plan as needed
Low-fat diet
Out of bed as much as tolerated
Begin to prepare client and spouse for discharge to home
Referral to case manager to plan discharge
Clopidogrel 75 mg oral daily
Carvedilol 3.125 mg oral twice daily
Docusate 100 mg oral daily
Simvastatin 20 mg oral daily

Collaboration with the client and spouse and the case manager reveals that the spouse will need assistance with the client's personal needs and activities of daily living and with ambulation and physical therapy. A home care aide is scheduled to visit the client for 3 hours daily, and physical therapy is planned for home visits 3 times weekly. The nurse implements a teaching plan and assesses readiness for discharge.

For each client or spouse statement/observation, select whether the home care instruction is either understood or requires further teaching.

Client or Spouse Statement/Observation	Understood	Requires Further Teaching
Client places the right arm into the shirt sleeve first when putting the shirt on.	☐	☐
Spouse states, "It will help vision if I approach my spouse from the right side."	☐	☐
Spouse states, "I will talk to the home care aides when they come to be sure they get all of the care done during the first hour after they arrive."	☐	☐
Client turns the head to the right and then to the left before taking on an activity.	☐	☐
Client states, "I know that I need to call for help if I need to use the bathroom."	☐	☐
Client states, "I can skip the stool softener medication if I have a bowel movement."	☐	☐
Client picks up a washcloth with the left hand to wash the face.	☐	☐

Practice Question 8.2 — Multiple Response Grouping

The nurse performs an admission assessment of a 16-year-old client being admitted to the mental health residential treatment center.

Nurses' Notes

1500: Client is accompanied by parent. Parent consistently interrupts client during the interview. Parent states that client is compulsive and always has to have everything in perfect order or becomes anxious. Parent states, "I was just like my child when I was that age and always had to look perfect and be perfect with everything that I did. I know my child is very skinny, but that is how I was when I was a teenager. I had to starve myself to keep my hourglass figure." Client reports not socializing much because of being too busy exercising and reports constant exercising all day long, at least 10 times a day for 1 hour each session. Reports the need to burn calories and stay in control of weight. States hardly eats because of feeling fat and appearing fat to others. Is very fearful of gaining weight; describes restrictive eating patterns. Loves to collect food recipes and cookbooks and prepare huge meals for other people, but does not eat with them. Denies alcohol or drug misuse. Denies suicidal ideation. Denies food binging and purging or use of laxatives or enemas. Reports amenorrhea for the past 3 months. Face is hollowed with sunken eyes. Skin is pale; hair is dry and thin. Growth of lanugo on skin; skin is yellow tinged. Complains of dizziness and skipped heartbeats.

Vital Signs

1500: T 96.4°F (35.7°C); HR 40; RR 16; BP 88/48; SpO$_2$ 92% on RA
Height: 5 ft 6 in
Weight: 88 lb (40 kg)
BMI: 15.99 kg/m^2

An interdisciplinary treatment approach was instituted to treat the client's eating disorder and included nutritional consultation, weight restoration therapy, and intensive psychotherapy and counseling and family therapy. After 70 days of treatment, the interdisciplinary team meets to discuss the client's readiness for discharge to home and use of outpatient support services.

The nurse evaluates for acceptable outcome criteria indicating readiness for discharge. For each factor below, select if the finding indicates readiness for discharge. **Each factor may support more than one finding.**

Factor	Finding
Physiologic	☐ Weight: 102 lb (46.3 kg)
	☐ Eating 80% of each of the 3 meals delivered by the dietary department and 2 snacks
	☐ **Laboratory Results:**

Test and Reference Range	Result
Potassium 3.5–5.0 mEq/L (3.5–5.0 mmol/L)	3.2 mEq/L (3.2 mmol/L)
Sodium 135–145 mEq/L (135–145 mmol/L)	130 mEq/L (130 mmol/L)
Chloride 98–106 mEq/L (98–106 mmol/L)	95 mEq/L (95 mmol/L)

Factor	Finding
Psychological	Client states:
	☐ "I really need to walk around the nursing unit 10 times a day and do 45 laps each time. I was doing 50 laps each time, but I cut down to 45."
	☐ "I counted the calories I ate for the day, and it came to 950. I think that's more than enough, but I need to keep counting the calories to be sure."
	☐ "I am clear about what triggers my disruptive eating patterns, and I know what alternative behaviors I need to take to help this."
Social	Client states:
	☐ "My best friend asked if I would go to lunch with some of our friends, but I'm not going to go because I have nothing to wear that makes me look good. All my clothes are too tight."
	☐ "My parent is taking me and my siblings to that new movie that just came out; it'll be fun. I'm really looking forward to sharing a big box of popcorn and drinking a cola!"
	☐ "I have no interest in going to my prom this year. I've gained this weight, and people in my class are definitely going to notice that."
Family support	☐ Parent states will be sure that the child eats at least 3 full meals a day and 2 snacks and will remove and throw away any "teen magazines" or other distracting books or magazines that are in the child's bedroom.
	☐ Parent states that all of the children are going to take a 15-minute walk every evening after dinner.
	☐ Parent states, "My child seems to want to stay close to home, but I'm encouraging my child to spend some time with friends from school. I think these peer relationships are important."
Follow-up	☐ Parent states that family therapy sessions are not necessary because the problem is with the one child "and not the family."
	Client states:
	☐ "I have an appointment with the nutrition person in 2 weeks, but I'm thinking that if I maintain my weight and eat like I'm supposed to, then I can cancel it."
	☐ "The nurse at my school says there is a support group for students with eating problems and that they meet weekly. Do you think this will help me?"

Practice Question 8.3 — Multiple Response Select N

A 68-year-old unhoused client was brought to the ED by EMS, who reports that the client was found lying in an alley. The client is diagnosed with atrial fibrillation and rapid ventricular response. Intravenous amiodarone is prescribed to treat the dysrhythmia.

History and Physical

1215: A 68-year-old unhoused client is brought to the ED by EMS. Reports "heart fluttering" and shortness of breath that started this morning. Associated with fatigue and dizziness; worsened by activity. No alleviating factors; symptoms are constant. Denies chest pain, losing consciousness, and difficulty breathing while lying down. Reports past medical history of hypertension, hyperlipidemia, and type 2 diabetes mellitus. States that family history is negative for cardiac events. Speaks in short sentences; appears short of breath while talking. Skin is warm, dry, and intact throughout. Rapid, irregular HR, 120–140 on auscultation. Lung sounds clear on auscultation in all fields. No peripheral edema.

Nurses' Notes

1215: Client admitted to ED. Received orders for IV amiodarone.

1230: Admission assessment completed. Amiodarone started. Continuous VS monitoring and cardiac monitor in place. Cardiac monitor shows shortened PR interval, narrowed QRS complex, and atrial fibrillation with an irregular rate of 120–140.

1300: Follow-up VS and assessment completed. Client reports tremors, light sensitivity, lack of appetite with nausea, vomiting × 1 undigested food, no hematemesis. HR 102 and regular; BP 90/56. Cardiac monitor shows prolongation of previously shortened PR interval, widening of previously narrowed QRS complex, atrial fibrillation converted to sinus rhythm. 2+ pitting peripheral edema.

Vital Signs

1215: T 98.8°F (37.1°C); HR 120–140 and irregular; RR 22; BP 128/76; SpO$_2$ 95% on RA

1230: HR 120–140 and irregular; RR 22; BP 128/76; SpO$_2$ 95% on RA

1300: HR 102 and regular; RR 22; BP 90/56; SpO$_2$ 95% on RA

Select the **4** client findings that indicate a therapeutic outcome of medication therapy.

☐ Reports of tremors
☐ Reports of photosensitivity
☐ BP 90/56
☐ HR 102 and regular
☐ Prolonged PR interval
☐ Widened QRS complex
☐ 2+ peripheral edema pitting bilaterally
☐ Reports of anorexia, nausea, and vomiting
☐ Atrial fibrillation converted to sinus rhythm

Practice Question 8.4 — Matrix Multiple Choice

A 39-year-old client is being seen in the outpatient pain management clinic for follow-up evaluation.

History and Physical

0900: Client sustained an injury to the cervical and lumbar spine in a motor vehicle accident 1 year ago and has been experiencing neck and back pain since the injury. Client has tried conservative measures, including ice and heat, massage, and PT. Client has also tried acetaminophen, NSAIDs, muscle relaxants, and opioid analgesics, and the pain has become intolerable again, even with these measures. Client was seen in clinic 1 month ago, and amitriptyline was added to the treatment plan. Visit to the clinic today for a 1-month follow-up evaluation.

Vital Signs

0900: T 98.8°F (37.1°C); HR 80; RR 22; BP 138/92; SpO$_2$ 95% on RA; reports pain rated 2/10 (on a 0–10 pain scale)

For each client statement/observation, select whether the statement/observation indicates that treatment with amitriptyline is effective or ineffective.

Statement/Observation	Effective	Ineffective
Client states, "My back and neck are sore after PT."	☐	☐
Client states, "I have been walking a mile each day before going to work."	☐	☐
Client states, "I need to wear my neck collar all the time because I need it for added support."	☐	☐
Client ambulates to the examination room and is limping and leaning a hand on the wall while walking.	☐	☐
Client states, "I know that new medication is used for depression, but it has helped my pain too."	☐	☐

Practice Question 8.5 — Drop-Down Cloze

A 58-year-old client is admitted to the medical-surgical unit from the ED with abdominal pain, fatigue, dizziness, and bright-red blood in the stool and is diagnosed with gastrointestinal hemorrhage.

History and Physical | Physician's Orders | Nurses' Notes | Lab Results

0600: History of diabetes mellitus, osteoarthritis, and depression. Smokes cigarettes 1 pack per day for 10 years, drinks 3 glasses of wine nightly, denies other recreational drug use. Medications include metformin 500 mg twice daily, ibuprofen 800 mg three times daily for joint pain, citalopram 10 mg daily

History and Physical | Physician's Orders | Nurses' Notes | Lab Results

0700:
Complete blood count (CBC)
Prothrombin time (PT)
Partial thromboplastin time (aPTT)
International normalized ratio (INR)
Type and crossmatch
1 unit PRBCs if hemoglobin is less than 8.0 g/dL (80 g/L), repeat hemoglobin and hematocrit level 2 hours after transfusion is complete
Bowel preparation (polyethylene glycol as directed) for colonoscopy
Obtain consent for colonoscopy
Pantoprazole 40 mg IV every 8 hr
Bowel rest, NPO
Normal saline IV maintenance fluids at 125 mL/h
Hydromorphone 1 mg IV push every 3 hr as needed for pain
GI specialist consultation

History and Physical | Physician's Orders | Nurses' Notes | Lab Results

0630: T 98.8°F (37.1°C); HR 100; RR 20; BP 102/68; SpO$_2$ 93% on RA; reports pain 5/10.

0800: Received and reviewed laboratory results. Started blood transfusion per protocol. Administering 1 unit PRBCs. Client reports continued abdominal pain, fatigue, dizziness. VS stable.

1200: 1 unit PRBCs completed. VS stable throughout transfusion. Client reports abdominal pain is unchanged. States no longer feels dizzy and feels less fatigued.

1400: Hemoglobin and hematocrit result updated. T 98.8°F (37.1°C); HR 82; RR 18; BP 122/74; SpO$_2$ 95% on RA

History and Physical | Physician's Orders | Nurses' Notes | Lab Results

0745:

Test and Reference Range	Result
Red blood cells (RBCs) 4.2–6.2 × 10^{12}/L (4.2–6.2 × 10^{12}/L)	4.5 (4.5 × 10^{12})
White blood cells (WBCs) 5000–10,000/mm^3 (5–10 × 10^9/L)	8000/mm^3 (8 × 10^9/L)
Platelets 150,000–400,000/mm^3 (150–400 × 10^9/L)	180,000/mm^3 (180 × 10^9/L)
Hemoglobin (Hgb) 12–18 g/dL (120–180 g/L)	7.6 g/dL (76 g/L)
Hematocrit (Hct) 37%–52% (0.37–0.52)	32% (0.32)
aPTT 30–40 seconds	32 seconds
PT 11–12.5 seconds	12.5 seconds
INR 0.81–1.2	1.0
Occult blood Negative	Detected
Type and crossmatch	O positive No antibodies detected

1400:

Test and Reference Range	Result
Hemoglobin (Hgb) 12–18 g/dL (120–180 g/L)	10.0 g/dL (100 g/L)
Hematocrit (Hct) 37%–52% (0.37–0.52)	39% (0.39)

Based on the client findings, complete the following sentence by selecting from the lists of options provided.

The nurse determines that the **1 [Select]** was effective, as evidenced by the **2 [Select]** and the **3 [Select]**.

Options for 1	Options for 2	Options for 3
Pantoprazole	Hemoglobin and hematocrit level	Vital signs
Hydromorphone	Coagulation studies result	Abdominal pain
Blood transfusion	Fecal occult blood test result	Report about fatigue and dizziness

Practice Question 8.6 — Highlight-in-Text

A 3-day-old newborn is seen at the outpatient pediatric clinic for a posthospital follow-up appointment.

Highlight the findings that indicate the need for follow-up in the 3-day-old newborn.

History and Physical | Nurses' Notes | Vital Signs | Lab Results

0800:
Infant born full-term via vaginal delivery. No labor or birth complications.
Birth weight: 7 lb 5 oz (3.4 kg)
Birth length: 19 in

History and Physical | **Nurses' Notes** | Vital Signs | Lab Results

0800: Breast-feeding every 2 to 3 hours without difficulty. Parents report infant urinates 12 to 15 times per day and has a bowel movement 5 to 6 times per day. They report that stool is greenish brown to yellowish brown, thin, and less sticky in consistency than it has been. Newborn skin is tan in color, and the sclera of the eyes is yellow. Parents state that the tan skin and yellow eyes first appeared this morning. Blood specimen sent to lab for evaluation of bilirubin level.

History and Physical | Nurses' Notes | **Vital Signs** | Lab Results

0800: T 99.6°F (37.5°C) axillary; apical HR 180 and regular; RR 70; weight 7 lb 5 oz (3.4 kg)

History and Physical | Nurses' Notes | Vital Signs | **Lab Results**

Test and Reference Range	Result
0800, Birth day 2:	
Bilirubin	
0.2–1.4 mg/dL	3.1 mg/dL
(3.4–23.8 μmol/L)	(52.7 μmol/L)
0900, Birth day 3:	
Bilirubin	
0.2–1.4 mg/dL	4.8 mg/dL
(3.4–23.8 μmol/L)	(81.6 μmol/L)

CHAPTER 9

Stand-Alone Items and Unfolding Case Studies: The Role of Contextual Factors in Making Clinical Judgments

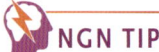
THINKING SPACE

Case studies provide the foundation for the NGN test items. There are two types of case studies used on the NGN: the Stand-Alone items and the Unfolding Case Study. Although there are some differences between the two types of case studies, both types present a realistic clinical situation commonly encountered in practice by the new nursing graduate. This chapter describes the differences between the Stand-Alone items and the Unfolding Case Study. Samples of each type of case and accompanying NGN items are illustrated throughout the chapter along with rationales and test-taking strategies.

The NCSBN Clinical Judgment Measurement Model (NCJMM) identifies the six clinical judgment cognitive (thinking) skills that the nurse applies when caring for a client and making a clinical decision to ensure safety and high-quality care (Box 9.1). The model also identifies contextual factors that influence the ability of the nurse to make appropriate clinical judgments. Benner et al. (2009) notes that the context of the clinical situation, the immediate history or the most urgent concerns, the reason the concerns are urgent, and the acknowledgment of salient factors in the case are important components of nursing practice. The context helps you see the entire situation and is built through formation in the nursing role (Benner et al., 2009). The addition of contextual factors (known as *individual factors* and *environmental factors* in the NCJMM) on the NGN is an intentional departure from the previous "sterile" traditional-style items and more effectively mirrors the realities of clinical practice and the intricacies of the nursing role. Both categories of contextual factors are considered in the daily care of a client. Environmental factors focus on the client and the environment. Individual factors are those related to the nurse caring for the client. Table 9.1 provides a list of these environmental and individual factors. Illustrating the environmental and individual factors is a focus of this chapter. As case studies are presented throughout this chapter, these environmental and individual factors are identified with color shading to distinguish them and illustrate how they are represented in a case study. Also, refer to Chapter 5 for a description and examples of how each external factor affects your thinking process in making clinical judgments.

> **NGN TIP**
>
> **Remember:** *Environmental factors* and *individual factors* are the external factors considered in the daily care of a client. Environmental factors focus on the client and the environment, and individual factors are those related to the nurse caring for the client. These factors influence your thinking process in making clinical judgments.

BOX 9.1 Cognitive Skills of the NCJMM
Recognize Cues
Analyze Cues
Prioritize Hypotheses
Generate Solutions
Take Actions
Evaluate Outcomes

TABLE 9.1 Environmental and Individual Factors That Influence Clinical Judgment

Environmental Factors	Individual Factors
Client observation	Candidate (test-taker) characteristics
Consequences and risks	Knowledge
Cultural considerations	Level of experience
Environment	Prior experience
Medical records	Skills
Resources	Specialty
Task complexity	
Time pressure	

From National Council of State Boards of Nursing (NCSBN). (2019). *Next Generation NCLEX® News,* Winter 2019. https://www.ncsbn.org/public-files/NGN_Winter19.pdf

THINKING SPACE

What Are Stand-Alone Items?

Stand-Alone items present two to three sentences of client information. These item types may present a diagnosis or an implied diagnosis and include clinical information for a specific client. The client information will most likely be presented in the form of a medical record such as Nurses' Notes, medical history, physician orders, vital signs, intake and output, or laboratory and diagnostic tests. There are two types of Stand-Alone items used on the NGN: the Bow-tie item and the Trend item. Both item types provide information that requires you to make one or more clinical decisions. Thus these item types can measure more than one CJ cognitive skill.

Bow-tie Item

The Bow-tie item can address all six cognitive skills in the NCJMM and provides a clinical scenario that includes client data at *one point in time.* Using drag-and-drop technology, the responses to the item are dragged and placed into three areas (categories) of a "figure" that looks like a bow-tie. The Bow-tie item has headers identifying each of the three areas. The options are provided in addition to specific directions as to how to answer the item. Samples of Bow-tie items are presented in Sample Question 9.1 and Sample Question 9.2. These samples provide client data in the form of a medical record.

> **NGN TIP**
>
> **Remember:** According to the NCSBN, the response options in a Bow-tie item are known as *tokens,* and the placeholders for the response items are known as *targets.* In order to move forward in the exam, all targets must be filled with the tokens, which are found directly below the Bow-tie in labeled columns.

> **NGN TIP**
>
> **Remember:** For the Bow-tie item, you need to read the information in the scenario and recognize which findings are relevant *(Recognize Cues),* make connections to determine what these relevant findings mean and what condition the client may be experiencing *(Analyze Cues),* and identify the client's immediate problem(s) *(Prioritize Hypotheses).* Then you need to identify possible solutions to address the client's needs *(Generate Solutions),* the appropriate actions to take *(Take Actions),* and parameters to monitor once actions have been taken *(Evaluate Outcomes).*

> **NGN TIP**
>
> **Remember:** To answer a Bow-tie item, select from the middle well first, which may be the *Potential Condition.* To make the correct selection, you need to identify the relevant data and organize these data to determine what the client's condition is in the clinical scenario. Then review the choices under *Potential Conditions,* and select the one that best matches your analysis. After selecting or dragging the client condition into the middle section of the Bow-tie figure, decide on the Nursing Actions that would be appropriate to manage the client condition and the Parameters that a nurse would need to monitor to determine if those actions were effective.

Sample Question 9.1 — Sample Bow-tie Item

A 53-year-old client undergoes a right lung wedge resection to remove a tumor.

History and Physical

1100: Biopsy results are pending, but the tumor has caused moderate to severe pain in the right lung area. The client has no history of cancer and reports no history of cancer in the family. The client reports working as a visiting nurse at a home health agency. Medical history includes hyperlipidemia and taking atorvastatin 40 mg daily. No other medical or surgical history reported.

Nurses' Notes

1100: Client admitted to medical-surgical unit from recovery unit following right wedge resection with one chest tube attached to a three-chamber closed chest tube drainage system. Dressing covering chest tube insertion site is occlusive, dry, and intact. 50 mL bloody drainage in the collection chamber, intermittent bubbling in the water-seal chamber, and gentle bubbling in the suction control chamber. Arousable and oriented, 2 L/min O_2 via NC, head of bed at 30 degrees. VS: T 98.6°F (37°C); HR 80; RR 20; BP 118/70; SpO_2 95% on 2 L/min O_2 via NC. Pain at right chest tube insertion site rated 3/10, increases with deep breathing and coughing.

1200: Nurse notes that client has dyspnea and reports an increase in pain to 5/10. Drainage in collection control chamber is at 100 mL of bloody drainage; there is continuous vigorous bubbling in the water-seal chamber and gentle bubbling in the suction control chamber.

HIGHLIGHT KEY

Environmental Factors
- Client observation
- Environment
- Medical records

Individual Factors
- Specialty

Complete the diagram by selecting from the choices below to specify what potential condition the client is likely experiencing, **2** nursing actions the nurse would **immediately** take to address the condition, and **2** parameters the nurse would monitor to assess the client's progress.

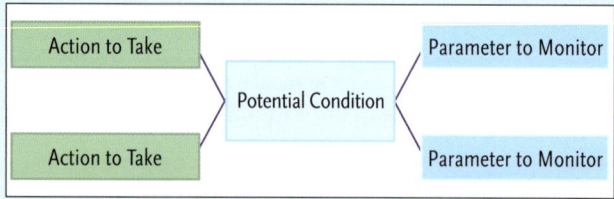

Actions to Take	Potential Conditions	Parameters to Monitor
Clamp the tubing, and determine the location of the problem	Bleeding	Chest x-ray
Apply pressure to the chest tube insertion site	Air leak in the drainage system	Hemoglobin, hematocrit, platelets, red blood cells
Check for subcutaneous emphysema	Displacement of the chest tube in the pleural space	Respiratory status, heart rate, respiratory rate, blood pressure, SpO_2
Disconnect and submerge the chest tube in a bottle of sterile water	Lung re-expansion	Fluctuation and bubbling in the water-seal chamber
Notify the surgeon		Drainage amount in the collection chamber

Answers

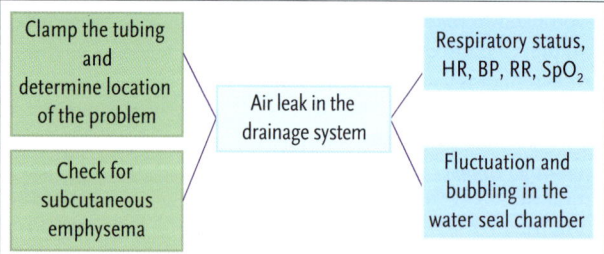

Rationale: A chest tube is a catheter inserted through the rib cage into the pleural space to remove air, fluid, or blood; prevent air or fluid from re-entering the pleural space; or re-establish normal intrapleural pressure after trauma or surgery to promote lung re-expansion. After a chest tube is inserted, it is attached to a drainage system. A traditional chest drainage system has three chambers: one for collection of drainage, one for maintaining a water seal, and one for suction control. The nurse measures the fluid in the collection chamber hourly for the first 24 hours after insertion by marking the drainage level in the collection chamber with a piece of tape or per agency protocol. Unless otherwise specified by the surgeon, drainage amounts greater than 70 to 100 mL/h are a concern. Bloody drainage is expected following lung resection, but if a change in color to bright red or a sudden increase in drainage occurs, the nurse would suspect bleeding and notify the surgeon immediately. The water-seal chamber prevents air from re-entering the pleural space. Fluctuation of the water in the water-seal chamber (moves up as the client inhales and moves down as the client exhales) is expected. Intermittent bubbling in this chamber may be noted and indicates air leaving the pleural space.

If the lung has re-expanded, the nurse would note that the fluctuation has stopped. Absence of fluctuation is also a sign of a displaced chest tube. A chest x-ray would confirm either situation. However, continuous and vigorous bubbling indicates a leak in the drainage system or the presence of a pneumothorax. If this occurs, the nurse would immediately assess the system and the client to determine the location and extent of the leak. Leaks can occur outside the client's body (e.g., within the drain or tubing connections) or within the body (e.g., at the tube insertion site or inside the chest cavity). To determine the location of the leak, the nurse would clamp the tubing as close as possible to the client. If bubbling continues, this indicates an air leak in the tubing or damage to the drainage device. If bubbling disappears when the tube is clamped, the air leak is likely at the insertion site or within the chest wall. With a significant internal air leak, the nurse would palpate subcutaneous emphysema or "crackling" (also known as *crepitus*) under the skin around the insertion site. If the leak is at the insertion site, the nurse would apply petroleum gauze and a sterile occlusive dressing to seal it off. If the air leak is due to a cracked drainage system, the nurse would replace the system following agency protocol.

Whatever its source, an air leak needs to be addressed and resolved because of the risk of tension pneumothorax; this can result in cardiac tamponade—a life-threatening emergency. Once the nurse locates the air leak and takes actions to resolve it, the surgeon is notified. The nurse monitors the client's respiratory status, heart rate, blood pressure, respiratory rate, and SpO_2 level. The nurse would also closely monitor the status of the water-seal chamber, looking for fluctuations and the absence of continuous vigorous bubbling. If bleeding is suspected, depending on its location, the nurse may need to apply pressure to the insertion site and monitor the drainage amount. In addition, the nurse would monitor laboratory values such as hemoglobin, hematocrit, platelets, and red blood cells to assess blood loss and the need for blood administration or surgical intervention. If a chest tube is disconnected from the system, it would be submerged in a bottle of sterile water to maintain the water seal until the system could be re-established.

Test-Taking Strategy: To begin answering this question, organize your thought process into three parts. This question is asking you to decide on the potential condition based on data provided in the clinical scenario. Think about each assessment finding, and decide if it is consistent with the condition listed, as illustrated in the table.

Supportive Assessment

Finding	Potential Condition
Vital signs	N/A, WNL
Dyspnea	Bleeding, air leak in the drainage system, displacement of the chest tube in the pleural space
Increased pain	Bleeding, air leak in the drainage system, displacement of the chest tube in the pleural space
100 mL of bloody drainage in the collection control chamber	N/A, expected
Vigorous bubbling in the water-seal chamber	Air leak in the drainage system
Gentle bubbling in the suction control chamber	N/A, expected

N/A, Not applicable; *WNL,* within normal limits.

THINKING SPACE

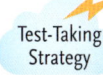
Test-Taking Strategy

THINKING SPACE

The vital signs are within normal limits and therefore are not related to any of the potential conditions. The dyspnea could be related to bleeding, an air leak in the drainage system, or displacement of the chest tube in the pleural space. Increased pain could be related to bleeding, an air leak in the drainage system, or displacement of the chest tube in the pleural space. The 100 mL of bloody drainage in the collection control chamber is an expected finding, as is gentle bubbling in the suction control chamber. Vigorous bubbling in the water-seal chamber is consistent with an air leak in the drainage system. Considering that most of the supportive assessment findings relate to an air leak in the drainage system, you would choose this as the potential condition. After you have identified the most likely potential condition, the second part of your thought process will be to decide on the most appropriate nursing actions for the care of the client with an air leak. To decide on the two interventions the nurse would immediately take, think about whether there are data to support performing each intervention, as illustrated in the table.

Immediate Action to Take	Supporting Data
Clamp the tubing.	Yes
Apply pressure to the chest tube insertion site.	No
Check for subcutaneous emphysema.	Yes
Disconnect and submerge the chest tube in a bottle of sterile water.	No
Notify the surgeon.	No

The dyspnea, increased pain, and vigorous bubbling in the water-seal chamber are the data that support clamping the tubing to further assess for an air leak in the drainage system. There are no data to support applying pressure to the chest tube insertion site. Because an air leak is suspected based on the assessment, there are data to support checking for subcutaneous emphysema. There are no data to support disconnecting and submerging the chest tube in a bottle of sterile water because the chest tube has not been dislodged from the chest. There are no data to support contacting the surgeon yet, until further assessment data are gathered. Next, you need to decide on additional parameters to monitor based on the actions you decided on. To help you with this, decide whether each listed parameter is directly related to either the condition or the nursing actions to assist in selecting the correct options, as illustrated in the table.

Parameter to Monitor	Related to Condition or Action
Chest x-ray	No—assesses for displacement of the chest tube in the pleural space and if the lung has re-expanded
Hemoglobin, hematocrit, platelets, red blood cells	No—assesses for bleeding
Heart rate, respiratory rate, blood pressure, SpO_2	Yes
Fluctuation and bubbling in the water-seal chamber	Yes
Drainage amount in the collection chamber	No—expected finding

The chest x-ray is not specifically related to an air leak in the chest drainage system and is a distractor because this would be useful in assessing for displacement of the chest tube in the pleural space and also in assessing if the lung has re-expanded. The hemoglobin, hematocrit, platelets, and red blood cells are also a distractor because this would be useful in assessing for bleeding. The heart rate, respiratory rate, blood pressure, and SpO_2 are important parameters to monitor for an air leak as this information would enable the nurse to detect any complications of this problem. Fluctuation and bubbling in the water-seal chamber is directly related as this provides information about the functionality of the chest drainage system. The drainage amount in the collection chamber is an expected finding in this clinical scenario and therefore is not a parameter that needs to be monitored specific to the air leak.

Content Area: Medical-Surgical Nursing
Priority Concept: Gas Exchange; Perfusion
Reference(s): Ignatavicius et al., 2024, pp. 565–567; Potter et al., 2023, pp. 999–1000; 1028–1034

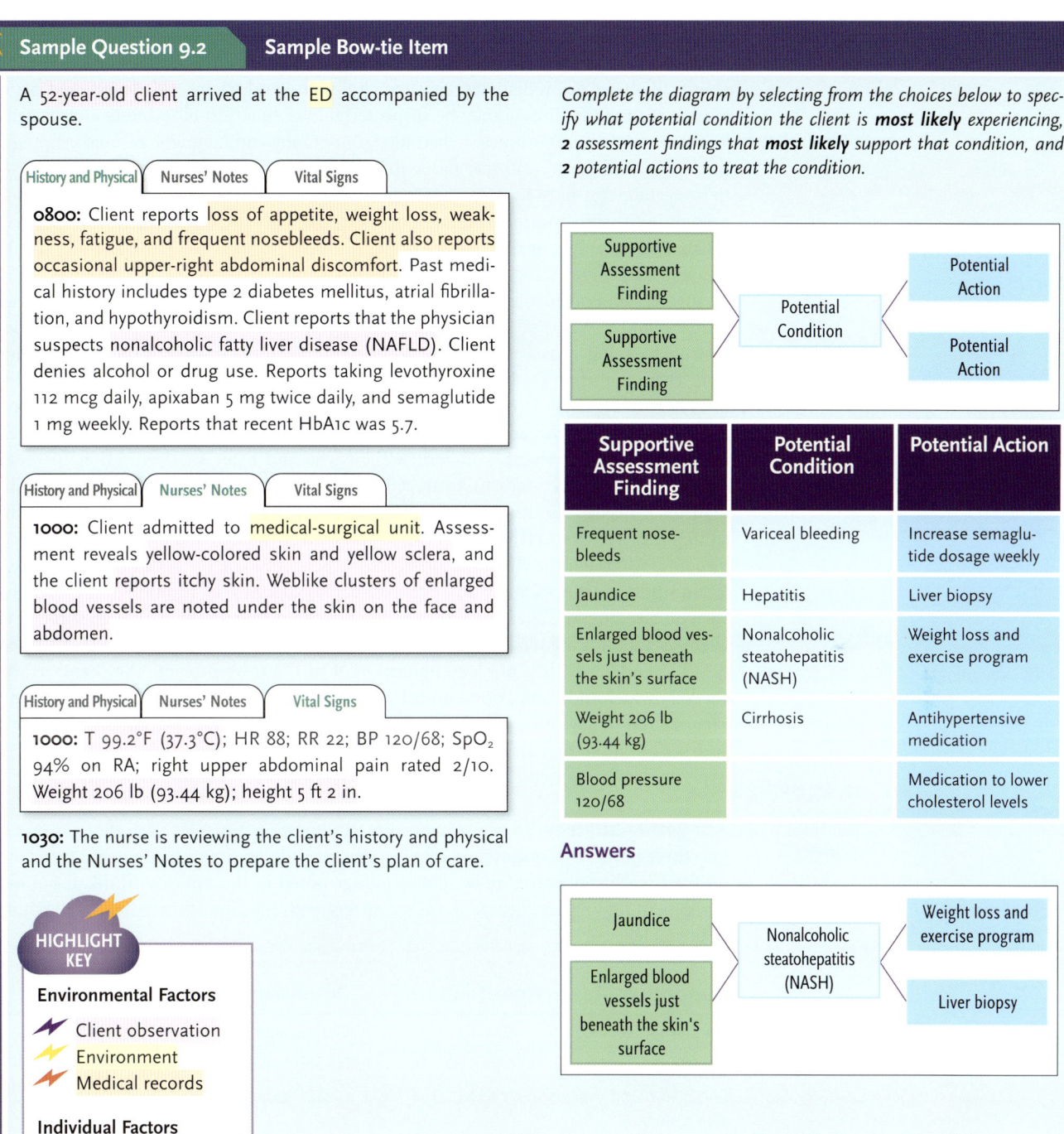

Sample Question 9.2 — Sample Bow-tie Item

A 52-year-old client arrived at the ED accompanied by the spouse.

History and Physical

0800: Client reports loss of appetite, weight loss, weakness, fatigue, and frequent nosebleeds. Client also reports occasional upper-right abdominal discomfort. Past medical history includes type 2 diabetes mellitus, atrial fibrillation, and hypothyroidism. Client reports that the physician suspects nonalcoholic fatty liver disease (NAFLD). Client denies alcohol or drug use. Reports taking levothyroxine 112 mcg daily, apixaban 5 mg twice daily, and semaglutide 1 mg weekly. Reports that recent HbA1c was 5.7.

Nurses' Notes

1000: Client admitted to medical-surgical unit. Assessment reveals yellow-colored skin and yellow sclera, and the client reports itchy skin. Weblike clusters of enlarged blood vessels are noted under the skin on the face and abdomen.

Vital Signs

1000: T 99.2°F (37.3°C); HR 88; RR 22; BP 120/68; SpO$_2$ 94% on RA; right upper abdominal pain rated 2/10. Weight 206 lb (93.44 kg); height 5 ft 2 in.

1030: The nurse is reviewing the client's history and physical and the Nurses' Notes to prepare the client's plan of care.

HIGHLIGHT KEY

Environmental Factors
- Client observation
- Environment
- Medical records

Individual Factors
- Specialty

Complete the diagram by selecting from the choices below to specify what potential condition the client is **most likely** experiencing, 2 assessment findings that **most likely** support that condition, and 2 potential actions to treat the condition.

Supportive Assessment Finding	Potential Condition	Potential Action
Frequent nosebleeds	Variceal bleeding	Increase semaglutide dosage weekly
Jaundice	Hepatitis	Liver biopsy
Enlarged blood vessels just beneath the skin's surface	Nonalcoholic steatohepatitis (NASH)	Weight loss and exercise program
Weight 206 lb (93.44 kg)	Cirrhosis	Antihypertensive medication
Blood pressure 120/68		Medication to lower cholesterol levels

Answers

- Jaundice
- Enlarged blood vessels just beneath the skin's surface
→ Nonalcoholic steatohepatitis (NASH)
→ Weight loss and exercise program
→ Liver biopsy

Rationale: Nonalcoholic fatty liver disease (NAFLD) is a liver condition that affects individuals who drink little to no alcohol. The primary characteristic of the disorder is storage of too much fat in the liver cells. The primary complication of NAFLD is progression to nonalcoholic steatohepatitis (NASH), an aggressive form of fatty liver disease, which is marked by liver inflammation and may progress to advanced scarring (cirrhosis) and liver failure. Symptoms of NASH include severe tiredness, weakness, weight loss, yellowing of the skin or eyes (jaundice), weblike clusters of enlarged blood vessels on the skin, and itching. If NASH results in cirrhosis symptoms, fluid retention, internal bleeding, muscle wasting, and confusion occur. Cirrhosis can lead to liver failure and the need for a liver transplant. Some risk factors for fatty liver disease include obesity, diabetes or prediabetes, elevated cholesterol and triglyceride levels, and hypertension. Fatty liver disease may be suspected if liver function blood tests are abnormal and elevated. Imaging studies such as ultrasonography and magnetic resonance imaging may show fat deposits and scar tissue in the liver. However, liver biopsy is the only way to be certain that fatty liver disease is present. Based on analysis of the biopsy, if fat is present but there is no inflammation or tissue damage, the diagnosis is NAFLD. If fat, inflammation, and liver damage are present, the diagnosis is NASH. If there is scar tissue, known as *fibrosis,* it probably indicates developing cirrhosis. If the client has NASH, no medication is available to reverse the fat buildup in the liver. Although jaundice and visible blood vessels may be seen in cirrhosis, there is no evidence of fluid retention, internal bleeding, muscle wasting, or confusion; therefore cirrhosis is not a likely condition. There is also no evidence to suggest fibrosis. In some cases, the liver damage stops or even reverses itself. However, in others the disease continues to progress. Therefore it is important to control any conditions that may contribute to fatty liver disease. Treatments and lifestyle changes include weight loss and exercise; medication to reduce cholesterol or triglycerides or to treat hypertension if needed; medication to control diabetes if needed; limiting over-the-counter medications; avoiding alcohol; and consulting with a liver specialist. There is no supporting evidence that this client has variceal bleeding. Although the client has nosebleeds, these could be the result of altered coagulation studies or due to many other causes such as allergies. In addition, if the client had variceal bleeding, the client would most likely be vomiting blood. Although some of the client's symptoms are related to hepatitis, the client indicates that the physician suspects NAFLD, and hepatitis is not a complication of this health problem. The client's HbA1c was 5.7, which indicates good control of the diabetes. Therefore there is no reason to increase the semaglutide, which is an antidiabetic medication. The client's blood pressure is normal, so there is no need for antihypertensive therapy. There is no evidence of hyperlipidemia, so medication to lower the cholesterol level is not indicated.

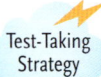

Test-Taking Strategy: To begin answering this question, organize your thought process into three parts. This question is asking you to decide on the potential condition based on the client's supportive assessment findings noted in the options. Think about each assessment finding and decide if it is consistent with the conditions listed, as illustrated in the table.

Supportive Assessment Finding	Potential Condition
Frequent nosebleeds	Coagulopathy
Jaundice	NASH, hepatitis, cirrhosis
Enlarged blood vessels just beneath the skin's surface	NASH, cirrhosis
Weight 206 lb (93.44 kg)	Nonspecific, although it is a risk factor for fatty liver disease
BP 120/68	Normal and therefore not related

The frequent nosebleeds are most likely related to coagulopathy from the client being on anticoagulant therapy. Jaundice could be related to NASH, hepatitis, or cirrhosis.

Enlarged blood vessels beneath the skin surface could be related to NASH or cirrhosis. Weight, although nonspecific, is a risk factor for fatty liver disease. The blood pressure is normal and therefore is not related to any potential condition. Considering that most supportive assessment findings relate to NASH and cirrhosis, you would choose NASH as the potential condition because there is no other evidence of cirrhosis, such as fluid retention, internal bleeding, muscle wasting, or confusion. After you have identified the most likely potential condition based on supportive assessment findings, the next part of your thought process will be to decide on the most appropriate nursing actions for the care of the client with NASH. To decide on the two actions the nurse would perform, think about whether there are data to support performing each action, as illustrated in the table.

Potential Action	Supporting Data
Increase semaglutide dosage weekly	No
Liver biopsy	Yes
Weight loss and exercise program	Yes
Antihypertensive medication	No
Medication to lower cholesterol level	No

In NASH, a liver biopsy is needed to confirm this condition versus NAFLD, therefore there are data to support the need for this test. Thinking about the pathophysiology and the causes of NASH, you would be able to determine that there are data to support the need for a weight loss and exercise program. The client's HbA1c is 5.7, therefore there are no data to support increasing the semaglutide. The client's blood pressure is 120/68, therefore there are data to support the need for antihypertensive medication. There is no evidence of high cholesterol, therefore there are no data to support starting a medication for this.

Content Area: Medical-Surgical Nursing
Priority Concept: Inflammation; Tissue Integrity
Reference(s): Ignatavicius et al., 2024, pp. 1220–1221, 1229

Trend Item

Similar to the Bow-tie for the Stand-Alone test items, the Trend item begins with a client situation that includes assessment data. The client information is presented in the form of a medical record, such as Nurses' Notes, history and physical, physician orders, input and output record, or laboratory and diagnostic tests. The difference between the Bow-tie and the Trend item is that the Trend item *presents data gathered over a period of time* rather than at one point in time. Therefore in the Trend item, the candidate examines trends in data over time to determine changes in the client's condition. The Trend item can measure more than one cognitive skill in the item. In addition, any NGN item type (except a Bow-tie item) will be used in a Trend item. Samples of a Trend item are presented in Sample Question 9.3 and Sample Question 9.4.

THINKING SPACE

Sample Question 9.3 — Sample Trend Item

A 34-year-old G4P4 client delivered a fourth baby 3 hours ago via vaginal delivery and was transferred to the postpartum unit. The postpartum nurse received hand-off report from the labor and delivery nurse.

> **Nurses' Notes**
>
> **1100:** Other children are 7, 5, and 2 years of age. Epidural was used for pain management during labor. Labor was 8 hours, and the obstetrician artificially ruptured the membranes. Oxytocin was administered to induce labor. Stage 2 vaginal laceration, which was repaired after delivery. Rh negative and Group B streptococcus (GBS) negative. Last fundal assessment was firm, dark-red lochia. Plans to breast-feed/chest-feed. Newborn's Apgar scores were 8, 9, and 9. Birth weight was 7 lb 12 oz (3.26 kg). First stool passed. Skin-to-skin care for 1 hour after birth, 3 feedings since birth. Erythromycin eye prophylaxis given, vitamin K injection administered.
>
> **1115:**
> Breast: Soft, no pain to palpation.
> Breath sounds: Clear to auscultation.
> Fundus: Firm, midline, at level of umbilicus.
> Lochia: Lochia rubra, dark red.
> Perineum: Laceration well approximated with sutures in place. Reports mild pain in the area.
> Bladder: No bladder distention.
> Abdomen: Soft, active bowel sounds in all quadrants.
> Lower extremities: Deep tendon reflexes 1+, peripheral edema 1+ nonpitting.
>
> **1130:**
> Breast: Soft, no pain to palpation.
> Breath sounds: Clear to auscultation.
> Fundus: Firm, midline, at level of umbilicus.
> Lochia: Lochia rubra, dark red.
> Perineum: Laceration well approximated with sutures in place. Reports mild pain in the area.
> Bladder: Has not voided, slight bladder distention.
> Abdomen: Soft, active bowel sounds in all quadrants.
> Lower extremities: Deep tendon reflexes 1+, peripheral edema 1+ nonpitting.
>
> **1145:**
> Breast: Soft, no pain to palpation.
> Breath sounds: Clear to auscultation.
> Fundus: Soft, boggy, deviated laterally to the left.
> Lochia: Large clots, large amount of lochia rubra, dark red.
> Perineum: Laceration well approximated with sutures in place. Reports mild pain in the area.
> Bladder: Bladder distention noted on palpation of the abdomen.
> Abdomen: Soft, active bowel sounds in all quadrants.
> Lower extremities: Deep tendon reflexes 1+, peripheral edema 1+ nonpitting.

At the 1145 time point, select which findings would be expected, indicating normal postpartum progression, and which findings would be unexpected, indicating a **need for follow-up**.

Assessment Finding	Expected	Unexpected
Breast	☒	☐
Breath sounds	☒	☐
Fundus	☐	☒
Lochia	☐	☒
Perineum	☒	☐
Bladder	☐	☒
Abdomen	☒	☐
Lower extremities	☒	☐

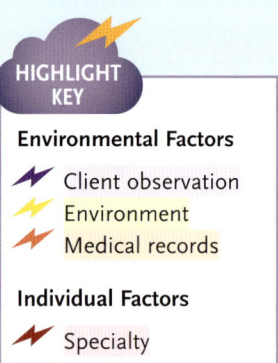

HIGHLIGHT KEY

Environmental Factors
- Client observation
- Environment
- Medical records

Individual Factors
- Specialty

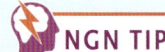 **NGN TIP**

Remember: Any NGN item type (except a Bow-tie item) is used in a Trend item. This sample Trend item provides client data in the form of a medical record presenting Nurses' Notes data over time. The item type for this question is a Matrix Multiple Choice item. In this item type, you need to select one response option for each row.

Rationale: The nurse needs to consider all assessment findings and how they relate to one another to decide what could be happening with the client and to plan care accordingly. In comparing the findings at 1145 with previous assessment findings, the nurse would determine that there are changes, specifically with the fundus, the lochia, and the bladder assessment findings. Breasts are expected to be soft without pain to palpation during the first 1 to 2 days. On days 2 to 3, they are filling, and on days 3 to 5 they are full but soften with breast-feeding/chest-feeding. There should be no firmness, heat, pain, or engorgement of the breasts. Breath sounds should be clear to auscultation; crackles could indicate possible fluid overload, which can occur after oxytocin administration and would require follow-up. The fundus should be firm and midline and should involute approximately 1 cm or 1 finger-breadth per day. If it is soft, boggy, or higher than the expected level, this could indicate uterine atony. The lochia should be dark red, also known as *lochia rubra*, on days 1 to 3. On days 4 to 10 it changes to lochia serosa, which is brownish-red or pink. After 10 days it changes to lochia alba, which is yellowish white. There may be a few clots, and sometimes there is a fleshy odor. Unexpected findings include a large amount of lochia, large clots, or foul odor. Any of these findings could indicate uterine atony or infection. Expected findings for the perineum would include minimal edema, and if a laceration or episiotomy is present, the edges should be approximated and any pain controlled by analgesics and nonpharmacologic interventions. Unexpected findings would be pronounced edema, bruising, hematoma, redness, warmth, or drainage, which could indicate bleeding or infection. The client should be able to void, and there should be no bladder distention noted. An overdistended bladder could cause lateral fundal displacement, uterine atony, and excessive lochia. The abdomen should be soft with active bowel sounds in all quadrants. The client should expect to have a bowel movement by day 2 or 3 after birth. The lower extremities may have peripheral edema from the fluid and medications. Deep tendon reflexes should be 1+ to 2+. There should be no pain, tenderness, redness, or thrombophlebitis. The assessment findings in this scenario that are expected are related to the breast, breath sounds, perineum, abdomen, and lower extremities; the assessment findings that indicate the need for follow-up are related to the fundus, lochia, and bladder.

Test-Taking Strategy: Note that this question is asking you about assessment findings that are expected or unexpected, indicating the need for follow-up in the postpartum period. This question is testing you on whether you can recognize signs of a complication. As illustrated in the table, categorize the assessment findings based on the complication you suspect, if any.

Assessment Finding	Possible Complication
Breast	N/A—expected as milk is being produced
Breath sounds	N/A—normal assessment finding
Fundus	Uterine atony
Lochia	Uterine atony/bleeding
Perineum	N/A—expected after vaginal birth
Bladder	Uterine atony due to bladder distension and lateral fundal displacement
Abdomen	N/A—normal assessment finding
Lower extremities	N/A—expected after oxytocin and fluid administration

N/A, Not applicable.

The assessment findings that are associated with one of the complications would then be those that you select as indicating a need for follow-up, whereas the findings that are not clearly associated with a possible complication would be selected as normal or expected. Note that although an assessment finding could be abnormal, such as with the peripheral edema, it could still be expected. Peripheral edema is expected after oxytocin and fluid administration in the postpartum period and therefore does not require follow-up at this time. This thinking process can be applied to the assessment findings for the breast and perineum as well. The breath sounds and abdomen are normal assessment findings.

Content Area: Obstetric-Newborn Nursing
Priority Concept: Perfusion; Reproduction
Reference(s): Lowdermilk et al., 2024, pp. 426, 728

Sample Question 9.4 — Sample Trend Item

The nurse on the pediatric medical-surgical nursing unit is caring for a 12-year-old child admitted 2 days ago with acute poststreptococcal glomerulonephritis (APSGN). The child is being treated with medications, low-sodium diet, and close monitoring. At 0900, the nurse performs an assessment, reviews the results of the laboratory studies performed early in the day, and then compares the findings with those performed on the day of admission.

Laboratory Tests

Test	Reference Range
Sodium	135–145 mEq/L (135–145 mmol/L)
Potassium	3.5–5.0 mEq/L (3.5–5.0 mmol/L)
Blood urea nitrogen	10–20 mg/dL (3.6–7.1 mmol/L)
Creatinine	0.5–1.2 mg/dL (44–106 μmol/L)
ASO titer	<200; In children younger than 5 years of age, <100

Urinalysis	Reference Range
Specific gravity	1.003–1.030
Bilirubin	Negative
Glucose	Negative
Hemoglobin	Negative
pH	4.0–8.0
Protein	0-trace
Leukocytes	Negative
Nitrites	Negative
Bacteria	Negative

NGN TIP

Remember: Any NGN item type (except a Bow-tie item) can be used in a Trend item. This sample Trend item provides client data in the form of a medical record presenting admission assessment data and current assessment data. This sample measures the cognitive skills *Recognize Cues* and *Evaluate Outcomes*. The item type for this question is Highlight-in-Text. In this item type, you need to select parts of the text based on what the question is asking you to select. For this question, you need to select the findings that indicate improvement in the child's condition.

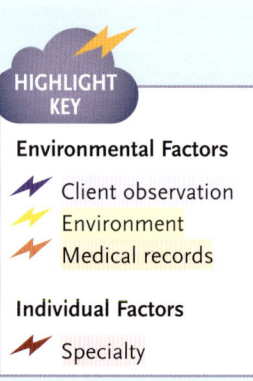

HIGHLIGHT KEY

Environmental Factors
- ⚡ Client observation
- ⚡ Environment
- ⚡ Medical records

Individual Factors
- ⚡ Specialty

At **0900**, highlight the findings that indicate improvement in the child's condition.

	Admission	0900
VS	T: 98.7°F (37°C) HR: 92 RR: 18 BP: 158/88 SpO₂: 99% on RA	T: 98.9°F (37.2°C) HR: 92 RR: 18 **BP: 116/70** SpO₂: 99% on RA
Nurses' Notes	Weight: 100 lb; appears lethargic Periorbital edema present Oropharynx red, erythematous, with positive exudate Neck: Anterior cervical lymphadenopathy Respiratory: Lungs clear to auscultation bilaterally Cardiovascular: 2+ radial and pedal pulses; 3+ pitting edema to bilateral lower extremities GI: Abdomen flat, nondistended; bowel sounds present in all quadrants Renal/urinary: Dark urine noted; urine output 15 mL/h	**Weight: 95 lb; alert, active** **No periorbital edema present** **Oropharynx pink and moist, no exudates** **Neck: No lymphadenopathy** Respiratory: Lungs clear to auscultation bilaterally Cardiovascular: 2+ radial and pedal pulses; **1+ pitting edema to bilateral lower extremities** GI: Abdomen flat, nondistended; bowel sounds present in all quadrants **Renal/urinary: Clear yellow urine noted; urine output 30 mL/h**
Laboratory results	Sodium: 138 mEq/L (138 mmol/L) Potassium: 3.9 mEq/L (3.9 mmol/L) Blood urea nitrogen: 32 mg/dL (11.4 mmol/L) Creatinine: 2.0 mg/dL (176.7 μmol/L) ASO titer: 480 Todd units **Urinalysis:** Specific gravity 1.040 Bilirubin: Negative Glucose: Negative Hemoglobin: Positive pH: 6.0 Protein: 3+ Leukocytes: Negative Nitrites: Negative Bacteria: Negative	Sodium: 138 mEq/L (138 mmol/L) Potassium: 3.9 mEq/L (3.9 mmol/L) **Blood urea nitrogen: 22 mg/dL (7.8 mmol/L)** **Creatinine: 1.6 mg/dL (141.3 μmol/L)** **ASO titer: 140 Todd units** **Urinalysis:** **Specific gravity: 1.030** Bilirubin: Negative Glucose: Negative **Hemoglobin: Negative** pH: 6.0 **Protein: Trace** Leukocytes: Negative Nitrites: Negative Bacteria: Negative

Rationale: Acute glomerulonephritis can occur on its own or secondary to another disorder, and it can range from mild to severe. Common features include oliguria, edema, hypertension, circulatory congestion, hematuria, and proteinuria. A common cause is streptococcal infection, resulting in APSGN. This occurs primarily in school-age children and is uncommon in children younger than 3 years of age. APSGN usually occurs 1 to 2 weeks following a throat infection and 3 to 6 weeks following a skin infection. Often the association with the infection is not recognized because of the latent period between the infection and the nephritis. The infection can sometimes still be present with APSGN. Initial signs include facial puffiness with periorbital edema, anorexia, decreased urine output, and cola-colored urine. The client also exhibits paleness, irritability, lethargy, and an overall unwell appearance. Facial edema is prominent in the morning and then spreads to the extremities, abdomen, and genitalia throughout the day. Blood pressure may be elevated (mildly to severely), and severe symptoms may include hypertensive encephalopathy, pulmonary and circulatory congestion, or hematuria. The initial signs of improvement in the child with APSGN are increased urinary output, decreased body weight, improved appetite, decreased blood pressure, and decreased gross hematuria. During the acute phase, urinalysis reveals hematuria, proteinuria, and increased specific gravity. The urine is discolored, and red blood cells are present along with leukocytes, epithelial cells, and red blood cell casts. Bacteria are not present, and urine cultures are negative. Throat cultures of the pharynx may be positive for streptococci. Electrolyte levels may be normal or may be out of range. Blood urea nitrogen and creatinine levels may be elevated with kidney injury. The antistreptolysin O (ASO) titer will be elevated. The chest x-ray may show cardiac enlargement, pulmonary congestion, and pleural effusion during the acute phase of the disease. Therapeutic management involves rest; improving fluid balance by monitoring vital signs, body weight, and intake and output; and administering diuretics if fluid volume overload is present. Antihypertensives and anticonvulsants may be needed in severe disease. A decreased sodium diet is needed for clients with hypertension and edema. Antibiotic therapy is used for children with confirmed streptococcal infection.

Findings that indicate improvement in the child's condition with treatment include:

- *Vital signs:* All vital signs except the blood pressure were within normal limits at admission and are normal at present. The blood pressure has improved with treatment.
- *Nurses' Notes:* The child has lost weight as the fluid balance has improved. The child's mental status has improved as the child is no longer lethargic and rather is alert and active. The oropharynx is now pink, moist, and without exudates, and the lymphadenopathy is no longer present, indicating that the antibiotics are helping the infection. The edema in the lower extremities is decreasing, indicating that fluid balance is improving. The urine color has normalized, and the urine output is increasing, which indicate improved fluid balance and renal function. All other findings on assessment were normal at admission and are normal at present.
- *Laboratory results:* The electrolytes were normal at admission and remain normal at present. The blood urea nitrogen and creatinine levels were elevated and are improving with treatment. The ASO titer is also decreasing, which indicates improvement. The specific gravity is improving, which indicates improved fluid balance. Hemoglobin is no longer detectable in the urine, and the protein is decreasing as well, which indicate improvement in the condition. Other results on the urinalysis were normal at admission and are normal at present.

Test-Taking Strategy: Note that this question is asking you about assessment findings that indicate improvement in the child's condition. This question is testing you on whether you can recognize abnormalities and then whether you can determine trends and changes in those findings and evaluate improvement, decline, or no change. As illustrated in the table, categorize the assessment findings as improved, declined, or unchanged/unrelated.

Test-Taking Strategy

> **THINKING SPACE**

Assessment Finding	Improved, Declined, Unchanged/Unrelated
T: 98.9°F (37.2°C)	Unchanged/Unrelated
HR: 92	Unchanged/Unrelated
RR: 18	Unchanged/Unrelated
BP: 116/70	Improved
SpO_2: 99% on RA	Unchanged/Unrelated
Weight: 95 lb	Improved
No periorbital edema present	Improved
Oropharynx pink and moist, no exudates	Improved
No lymphadenopathy	Improved
Lungs clear to auscultation bilaterally	Unchanged/Unrelated
2+ radial and pedal pulses	Unchanged/Unrelated
1+ pitting edema to bilateral lower extremities	Improved
Abdomen flat, nondistended	Unchanged/Unrelated
Bowel sounds present in all quadrants	Unchanged/Unrelated
Clear yellow urine	Improved
Urine output: 30 mL/h	Improved
Sodium: 138 mEq/L (138 mmol/L)	Unchanged/Unrelated
Potassium: 3.9 mEq/L (3.9 mmol/L)	Unchanged/Unrelated
Blood urea nitrogen: 22 mg/dL (7.8 mmol/L)	Improved
Creatinine: 1.6 mg/dL (141.3 µmol/L)	Improved
ASO titer: 140 Todd units	Improved
Specific gravity: 1.030	Improved
Bilirubin: Negative	Unchanged/Unrelated
Glucose: Negative	Unchanged/Unrelated
Hemoglobin: Negative	Improved
pH: 6.0	Unchanged/Unrelated
Protein: Trace	Improved
Leukocytes: Negative	Unchanged
Nitrites: Negative	Unchanged/Unrelated
Bacteria: negative	Unchanged/Unrelated

The assessment findings that indicate an improvement would be the ones that you would highlight as the answers to this question. Note that there are no assessment findings that indicate a decline, whereas there are many findings that are unchanged or unrelated. Any findings that are unchanged or unrelated would not be highlighted.

Content Area: Pediatric Nursing
Priority Concept: Fluid and Electrolyte Balance; Infection
Reference(s): Hockenberry et al., 2024, pp. 776–779

What Are Unfolding Case Studies?

The Unfolding Case Study presents the client situation *over time* through several phases of care in the clinical scenario. The time between phases can be minutes, hours, or even days. The client may initially be evaluated in an ED at an acute care hospital, at a clinic, at an urgent care center, at school, or at home. As the scenario changes, or "unfolds," NGN test items require you to use all of the information, including the information in the current phase of the client's care, to answer each question. On the NCLEX®, you will always have access to the case study, including all of the phases as the case emerges and unfolds. There are six NGN items in an Unfolding Case Study. Each of the six items represents one of the CJ cognitive skills.

As described in Chapter 1, the Unfolding Case Study presents a client with initial data describing the clinical situation. These data will typically be part of a client's medical record. The client will either be experiencing an urgent or emergent health problem or will be at risk for experiencing an urgent or emergent health problem. You will need the information in the initial clinical scenario to answer the first NGN test item that will measure the CJ cognitive skill *Recognize Cues*. The second NGN test item will measure your ability to *Analyze Cues,* those cues you recognized as relevant. As the clinical scenario continues, the client's condition will change over time (minutes, hours, days) through several phases of care, and new information will be presented as the case unfolds. Four additional NGN test items will follow and measure the remaining CJ cognitive skills *(Prioritize Hypotheses, Generate Solutions, Take Actions, Evaluate Outcomes)* based on which client data are provided. Sample Questions 9.5, 9.6, 9.7, 9.8, 9.9, and 9.10 accompany an Unfolding Case Study in which a client's condition changes and requires immediate intervention during the home visit by the nurse.

 How Are Stand-Alone Items and Unfolding Case Studies Different?

There are similarities and differences between Stand-Alone items and Unfolding Case Studies. Box 9.2 illustrates these similarities and differences.

BOX 9.2   Stand-Alone Items and Unfolding Case Studies: Similarities and Differences

Stand-Alone Items	Unfolding Case Studies
Present a realistic clinical situation commonly encountered in practice by the new nursing graduate.	Present a realistic clinical situation commonly encountered in practice by the new nursing graduate.
The clinical situation is accompanied by one item, either a Bow-tie or a Trend item.	The case is accompanied by six NGN items.
The Bow-tie item provides a client situation at *one point in time,* and the Trend item presents client information such as VS, Nurses' Notes, and I&O information *over time.*	Presents the client's story *over time* through several phases of care in the clinical situation. The time between phases can be minutes, hours, or even days.
Information will be presented in a medical record format.	Information will be presented in a medical record format.

THINKING SPACE

Sample Question 9.5 — Unfolding Case Study: Question 1: Recognize Cues—Highlight-in-Text

0700: The nurse plans a visit to a client who was discharged from the hospital 1 week ago. The nurse reviews the discharge summary in the history and physical and the Nurses' Notes from the previous home visit that occurred on the day after hospital discharge.

History and Physical | Nurses' Notes | Vital Signs

1 week ago discharge summary: A 32-year-old client sustained a T6 spinal cord injury 3 months ago from a motor vehicle accident that caused paralysis of the lower body. The client was sideswiped by a truck, which caused the car to roll over three times and end up in a ditch off the roadway. The client was pinned in the car, and the front end and side of the car crushed the lower half of their body. The client was hospitalized for 3 months. During hospitalization, emergency treatment was administered, and once stabilized, the client was monitored for complications. The client received rehabilitative therapy including PT and OT, and home care services were initiated for discharge. The client is married, and the client's spouse stays at home caring for their two children, who are 7 and 10 years of age. Prior to the injury, the client was a forklift driver at an industrial manufacturing company. The client has no previous medical history, does not take any medications, does not smoke, and drinks occasionally at social gatherings.

History and Physical | **Nurses' Notes** | Vital Signs

One day post-discharge: Client alert and oriented. Sitting up in wheelchair. Reports using a transfer board with spouse's assistance to get out of bed and transfer to the wheelchair. Reports sitting in the wheelchair all day. Reports fair appetite and is drinking fluids. Reports tiredness and falling asleep in the wheelchair during the day. Reports sweating during the night, which awakens the client; the sweating stops when repositioning to the side, but the client has difficulty falling back to sleep. Reports muscle spasms in the lower body. No complaints of headache. Reports self-catheterizes every 6 hours. Last bowel movement was on the day of hospital discharge. VS: T 98.6°F (37°C); HR 86; RR 18; BP 120/78.

1000: The home health care nurse arrives at the client's home and after introductions performs a focused assessment.

Highlight the findings in the assessment that are **immediate** concern.

History and Physical | Nurses' Notes | **Vital Signs**

VS: T 99.2°F (37.3°C); HR 58; RR 18; BP 150/90.

History and Physical | **Nurses' Notes** | Vital Signs

Alert and oriented. Reports poor appetite over the past few days, and is nauseated. Reports tiredness and continued sweating during the night. Muscle spasms in the lower body worsening and was incontinent once during the night. Reports feeling as though is getting the flu because of nausea, nasal stuffiness, and pounding headache. States last bowel movement was 4 days ago.

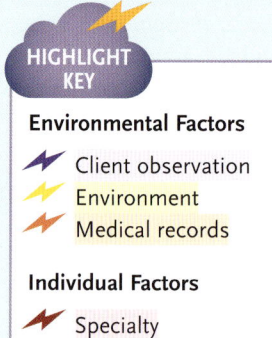

HIGHLIGHT KEY

Environmental Factors
⚡ Client observation
⚡ Environment
⚡ Medical records

Individual Factors
⚡ Specialty

Rationale: Spinal cord injury is caused by trauma to the spinal cord that leads to partial or complete disruption of the nerve tracts and neurons. Spinal cord edema develops following the injury, and necrosis can develop as a result of compromised capillary circulation and venous return. Loss of motor function, sensation, reflex activity, and bowel and bladder function may result. Common causes of spinal cord injury include motor vehicle accidents, falls, sporting and industrial accidents, and gunshot or stab wounds. The client's temperature is slightly elevated at 99.2°F (37.3°C), and the client is at risk for infection, specifically a urinary tract infection. The client had an episode of incontinence and is self-catheterizing, which increases this risk. The client's heart rate is low and is a concern because the baseline is 86. Respirations are unchanged and not a concern. The client's blood pressure is elevated from baseline and would be an immediate concern for the nurse. Other immediate concerns for this client would be the report of nausea, continued sweating, worsening muscle spasms, and incontinence. Other new and concerning findings are the nasal stuffiness, pounding headache, and constipation.

Test-Taking Strategy: Remember to first identify normal/usual or abnormal/expected (not relevant) client findings and abnormal/not expected (relevant) client findings requiring follow-up. The client findings can be categorized as shown in the table.

Client Finding	Normal/Usual or Abnormal/Expected (Not Relevant)	Abnormal/Not Expected (Relevant Requiring Follow-up)
T 99.2°F (37.3°C)	☐	☒
HR 58	☐	☒
RR 18	☒	☐
BP 150/90	☐	☒
Alert and oriented	☒	☐
Reports poor appetite over the past few days and is nauseated	☐	☒
Reports tiredness and continued sweating during the night	☐	☒
Worsening muscle spasms in the lower body	☐	☒
Incontinent once during the night	☐	☒
Nausea, nasal stuffiness, and pounding headache	☐	☒
States last bowel movement was 4 days ago	☐	☒

Thinking about what could be happening to the client will help you determine which findings are expected versus those that are unexpected. Unexpected findings are the parts of the Nurses' Notes that should be highlighted in this question.

Content Area: Medical-Surgical Nursing
Priority Concept: Perfusion; Tissue Integrity
Reference(s): Ignatavicius et al., 2024, pp. 921–929

Sample Question 9.6 — Unfolding Case Study: Question 2: Analyze Cues—Drop-Down Rationale

1020: The nurse analyzes the assessment findings that are of immediate concern to make an interpretation about the client's condition.

Complete the following sentence by choosing from the lists of options provided.

The nurse determines that the client assessment findings would *most likely* be the result of **noxious stimuli** caused by the **constipation**.

Options for 1	Options for 2
Anxiety	Infection
Noxious stimuli	Paralysis
Urinary incontinence	Constipation
Further spinal cord damage	Worsening muscle spasms

THINKING SPACE

Rationale: Autonomic dysreflexia, sometimes referred to as *autonomic hyperreflexia*, is a potentially life-threatening condition in which noxious visceral or cutaneous stimuli cause a sudden massive, uninhibited reflex sympathetic discharge in individuals with high-level spinal cord injury. Symptoms include pounding headache; flushed face and/or red blotches on the skin above the level of the injury; sweating above the level of the injury; nasal stuffiness; nausea; slow heart rate; goose bumps below the level of the injury; and cold, clammy skin below the level of the injury. The causes of autonomic dysreflexia are typically gastrointestinal, gynecologic-urologic, and vascular stimulation. Specific risk factors are bladder distention, urinary tract infection, epididymitis or scrotal compression, bowel distention or impaction from constipation, or irritation from hemorrhoids. Other causes of autonomic dysreflexia are pain; circumferential constriction of the thorax, abdomen, or an extremity (e.g., from tight clothing); contact with hard or sharp objects; and temperature fluctuations. There is no information indicating that the client has anxiety. Further spinal cord damage is unlikely unless another injury occurred; in addition, the client's assessment findings do not indicate that this is the case.

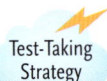

Test-Taking Strategy: Begin answering this question by noting that you need to select the correct option for the first part of the question in order to answer the question correctly. Thinking about the description in the clinical situation and assessment findings, decide whether each option could be a cause of those signs or symptoms.

Option	Possible Explanation of Signs/Symptoms
Anxiety	No
Noxious stimuli	Yes
Urinary incontinence	No
Further spinal cord damage	No

Anxiety and urinary incontinence could occur as a result of autonomic dysreflexia but are not a cause. Bladder distention, however, is a cause. Further spinal cord damage would be caused by additional injury but not by autonomic dysreflexia as a complication of an existing spinal cord injury. Next, you need to use your nursing knowledge to determine which factors precipitate autonomic dysreflexia. Remember *GGUV*—gastrointestinal, gynecologic-urologic, and vascular; thus constipation is a precipitant of this complication.

Content Area: Medical-Surgical Nursing
Priority Concept: Perfusion; Tissue Integrity
Reference(s): Ignatavicius et al., 2024, pp. 921–929

| Sample Question 9.7 | Unfolding Case Study: Question 3: Prioritize Hypotheses—Multiple Response Select N |

1030: The nurse reviews the findings from the focused assessment performed on the client and identifies the potential risk conditions of concern.

Select the **3** conditions the client is at **highest** risk for developing.
- ☒ Infection
- ☐ Malnutrition
- ☐ Spinal shock
- ☐ Hyperthermia
- ☒ Skin breakdown
- ☐ Neurogenic shock
- ☒ Autonomic dysreflexia

Rationale: Based on the client assessment data, the client is exhibiting signs of autonomic dysreflexia, an abrupt, uncontrolled sympathetic response elicited by stimuli below the level of injury. The client is also at risk for skin breakdown because of a report of sitting in the wheelchair all day. In addition, the client is at risk for infection, specifically a urinary tract infection. The client reports an episode of incontinence, and there is a slight increase in the temperature. Catheterization every 6 hours also places the client at risk. Although the client reports nausea and a poor appetite, there is no evidence that malnutrition is a risk. Spinal shock occurs immediately after the injury as the cord's response to the injury. This client's injury occurred 3 months ago. Clients who sustain a spinal cord injury can experience abnormal temperature control as either hypothermia or hyperthermia. Although this client is experiencing some disturbances of sweating, there are no extreme temperature fluctuations occurring; this requires monitoring, but hyperthermia is not a high priority at this time. Neurogenic shock is a type of distributive shock characterized by hypotension, bradycardia, and peripheral vasodilation and attributed to severe central nervous system damage such as head or cervical cord trauma or high thoracic cord injuries. Although the client has a low pulse rate, there are no data indicating that this condition is a risk.

Test-Taking Strategy: Thinking about autonomic dysreflexia as the most likely complication occurring in this clinical scenario, consider each option and how it may or may not be pertinent. Also note that the question asks for the *highest risk,* which means that some or all of the options may be correct, but you need to decide on the three most important options in this situation. Using the thinking process illustrated in the table, first determine whether the option could be a potential problem as it relates to spinal cord injury, and then from there, determine whether there are supporting data for that problem.

Option	Related/Unrelated	Supporting Data
Infection	Related	Yes
Malnutrition	Related	No
Spinal shock	Related	No
Hyperthermia	Related	No
Skin breakdown	Related	Yes
Neurogenic shock	Related	No
Autonomic dysreflexia	Related	Yes

If you determine that the option is related and supporting data are present, it is likely correct. Also, note that this question asks for a specific number of options to choose. As you can see, all options are related in some way, so it is really important to rely on the available data to determine the highest priorities. The only three options with data to support that they are occurring are infection, skin breakdown, and autonomic dysreflexia.

Content Area: Medical-Surgical Nursing
Priority Concept: Perfusion; Tissue Integrity
Reference(s): Ignatavicius et al., 2024, pp. 921–929

Sample Question 9.8 — Unfolding Case Study: Question 4: Generate Solutions—Matrix Multiple Choice

1040: Based on the highest-risk conditions, the nurse quickly prepares a plan of care for the client and potential interventions.

For each potential intervention, select whether the intervention is indicated or not indicated in the care of the client.

Potential Intervention	Indicated	Not Indicated
Assist the client in getting back to bed, and place the client in the supine position.	☐	☒
Check the blood pressure frequently.	☒	☐
Check for bladder distention.	☒	☐
Check for bowel impaction.	☒	☐
Contact the physician.	☒	☐
Place cold packs on the back of the client's neck and in the axilla areas.	☐	☒
Administer sublingual nifedipine.	☐	☒

THINKING SPACE

Rationale: The client is exhibiting symptoms of autonomic dysreflexia including a lower than baseline heart rate of 58, blood pressure of 150/90, sweating during the night, nausea, nasal stuffiness, and pounding headache. The client also reports that the last bowel movement was 4 days ago, so the client could be experiencing bowel impaction, a cause of autonomic dysreflexia. Other risk factors include bladder distention, and the nurse would plan to assess for this occurrence. The nurse would plan to notify the physician and obtain orders for additional interventions if necessary. The nurse would place the client in the upright sitting position because the supine position would exacerbate the hypertension. The nurse would also plan to monitor the blood pressure frequently. If blood pressure elevation does not exceed 150/90, the nurse would continue to observe the client. If the blood pressure exceeds 150/100 and a cause is either not found or found but not likely to be eliminated quickly, pharmacologic treatment should be initiated. If blood pressure elevation is between 150/100 and 180/120, the client may be treated with sublingual nifedipine. Because a likely cause is known for this client and because the blood pressure is 150/90, nifedipine would be contraindicated at this time. Clients who sustain a spinal cord injury can experience abnormal temperature control as either hypothermia or hyperthermia. Cold packs would cause chills and shaking and could lead to unwanted alterations in temperature.

Test-Taking Strategy: Note that this question is asking you to identify potential interventions that are indicated and those that are not indicated. For each action, think about whether that action could improve/would be necessary or could worsen the autonomic dysreflexia. Remember *GGUV*—gastrointestinal, gynecologic-urologic, and vascular—and organize your thought process as illustrated in the table.

Potential Intervention	Improve/Necessary or Worsen
Assist the client in getting back to bed, and place the client in the supine position.	Worsen
Check the blood pressure frequently.	Improve/necessary
Check for bladder distention.	Improve/necessary
Check for bowel impaction.	Improve/necessary
Contact the physician.	Improve/necessary
Place cold packs on the back of the client's neck and in the axilla areas.	Worsen
Administer sublingual nifedipine.	Worsen

Remember that positioning is important for managing blood pressure abnormalities. Recall that temperature changes can worsen the condition. Note that the blood pressure needs to exceed a certain parameter before antihypertensive medications would be indicated.

Content Area: Medical-Surgical Nursing
Priority Concept: Perfusion; Tissue Integrity
Reference(s): Ignatavicius et al., 2024, pp. 921–929

Sample Question 9.9 — Unfolding Case Study: Question 5: Take Actions—Multiple Response Select All That Apply

1040: The nurse quickly considers the plan of care and intervenes to manage the complication the client is experiencing.

Which of the following actions would the nurse perform **immediately**? *Select all that apply*.

- ☒ Catheterize the client.
- ☒ Loosen the client's clothing.
- ☒ Digitally remove impacted stool.
- ☒ Assist the client in getting back to bed, and place the client in the upright position.
- ☐ Send a urine specimen to the lab for culture and sensitivity.
- ☐ Teach the client about measures to prevent autonomic dysreflexia.
- ☐ Call EMS to transport the client to the hospital.

Rationale: Autonomic dysreflexia is a potentially life-threatening condition in which noxious visceral or cutaneous stimuli cause a sudden massive, uninhibited reflex sympathetic discharge in individuals with high-level spinal cord injury. The causes of autonomic dysreflexia are typically gastrointestinal, gynecologic-urologic, and vascular stimulation. Specific risk factors are bladder distention, urinary tract infection, epididymitis or scrotal compression, bowel distention or impaction from constipation, or irritation from hemorrhoids. The nurse would immediately take actions to decrease the client's blood pressure and identify and eliminate the noxious stimuli. The nurse would help the client back to bed in a head-elevated position to prevent further increases in blood pressure. The nurse would loosen clothing because tight clothing causes cutaneous stimulation. The nurse would assess for bladder distention and then catheterize the client and digitally remove the stool. It is not necessary to call EMS unless immediate measures do not resolve the condition and the condition becomes life threatening. There are no orders for culture and sensitivity of the urine, although the physician may prescribe this to rule out a urinary tract infection. The nurse would obtain the urine

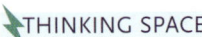

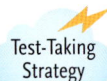

specimen and discuss this intervention with the physician; this, however, would not be an immediate intervention. The nurse would teach the client about measures to prevent autonomic dysreflexia, but this is not an immediate intervention; measures to resolve the complication are the priority.

Test-Taking Strategy: Note the strategic word *immediately*. Knowing that the client is experiencing the complication of autonomic dysreflexia, decide whether each listed intervention would address this complication. Remember *GGUV*—gastrointestinal, gynecologic-urologic, and vascular—and organize your thinking process as noted in the table.

Immediate Nursing Action	GGUV
Catheterize the client.	Gynecologic-urologic
Loosen the client's clothing.	Vascular
Digitally remove the impacted stool.	Gastrointestinal
Assist the client in getting back to bed, and place the client in the upright position.	Vascular
Send a urine specimen to the lab for culture and sensitivity.	N/A
Teach the client about measures to prevent autonomic dysreflexia.	N/A
Call EMS to transport the client to the hospital.	N/A

GGUV, Gastrointestinal, gynecologic-urologic, and vascular; *N/A*, not applicable.

Note that catheterizing the client, loosening the client's clothing, digitally removing impacted stool, and assisting the client to the upright position address GGUV and are the immediate actions. Sending a urine culture, teaching the client about measures to prevent autonomic dysreflexia, and calling EMS do not directly address the cause and therefore would be eliminated.

Content Area: Medical-Surgical Nursing
Priority Concept: Perfusion; Tissue Integrity
Reference(s): Ignatavicius et al., 2024, pp. 921–929

Sample Question 9.10 — Unfolding Case Study: Question 6: Evaluate Outcomes—Matrix Multiple Choice

1050: The nurse has performed the interventions, assesses the client, and makes the following notations in the Nurses' Notes.

Vital Signs

1050: VS: T 99.2°F (37.3°C); HR 78; RR 18; BP 132/78.

Nurses' Notes

1050: Client assisted to bed; sitting upright. Bladder distended, 400 mL urine output via catheterization. Urine obtained for culture and sensitivity pending physician's order. Moderate amount of stool removed digitally.

1100: Client teaching initiated about measures to prevent autonomic dysreflexia. Reports a mild headache and nasal stuffiness.

For each client statement, select whether the statement indicates that the client understood or requires further teaching.

Client Statement	Understood	Requires Further Teaching
"I need to follow the bowel regimen every day."	☒	☐
"A low-fiber diet will help with the abdominal discomfort and muscle spasms."	☐	☒
"It's best to go back to bed during the day and limit the amount of time I spend in the wheelchair to 2 to 3 hours a day."	☐	☒
"I should check my bladder to see if it is distended and make sure that I don't allow it to get too full."	☒	☐
"I will call 911 immediately to take me to the hospital if I experience any of these symptoms again."	☐	☒
"I need to have my spouse help me check my skin to be sure there is no redness or skin breakdown."	☒	☐

Rationale: The nurse needs to teach the client about the causes of autonomic dysreflexia, measures to take to prevent its occurrence, and actions to take if an episode occurs. The causes of autonomic dysreflexia are typically gastrointestinal, gynecologic-urologic, and vascular stimulation. Specific risk factors are bladder distention, urinary tract infection, epididymitis or scrotal compression, bowel distention or impaction from constipation, or irritation from hemorrhoids. The nurse would teach the client about these causes and measures to prevent this occurrence. Measures to prevent autonomic dysreflexia include emptying the bladder so it does not become distended, preventing bladder infections, controlling pain with nonpharmacologic or pharmacologic measures as prescribed, eating a high-fiber diet and achieving adequate fluid intake, and performing bowel care including taking stool softeners to avoid stool impaction. It is best that the client be out of bed rather than in bed because of the complications associated with staying in bed, so it would not be helpful to limit the time spent in the wheelchair. However, the nurse would teach client to shift weight to a different position in the wheelchair to prevent scrotal pressure or skin integrity issues. The client would be instructed on the signs and symptoms of autonomic dysreflexia so it can be detected early and immediate interventions to resolve it can be initiated. Finally, the client would be instructed on measures to take if autonomic dysreflexia occurs. The nurse would also teach the client how to check the blood pressure and to sit up straight if an episode occurs. The client would be taught not to lie down or recline because this can increase the blood pressure even more. The nurse would teach the client to monitor the blood

THINKING SPACE

pressure every 5 minutes during the episode to check for improvement. The nurse would also teach the client how to quickly determine the cause, such as bladder distention, bowel impaction, or skin problems. The client would be instructed to loosen any clothing that is tight, self-catheterize, and quickly do a rectal check for any stool in the rectum. The nurse would notify the physician of the event, even if the symptoms resolve. If the client is unable to resolve the problem, then EMS would be called. The nurse would also instruct the client to carry a medical identification card indicating the risk for autonomic dysreflexia.

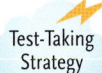

Test-Taking Strategy: Note that the question is asking about evidence to support whether the client teaching has been either understood or not understood, therefore necessitating further teaching. For each option below, decide whether the actions described in the client statement would help prevent autonomic dysreflexia. Organize your thoughts as illustrated in the table.

Client Statement	Helpful/Not Helpful/Not Necessary
"I need to follow the bowel regimen every day."	Helpful
"A low-fiber diet will help with the abdominal discomfort and muscle spasms."	Not Helpful
"It's best to go back to bed during the day and limit the amount of time I spend in the wheelchair to 2 to 3 hours a day."	Not Helpful
"I should check my bladder to see if it is distended and make sure that I don't allow it to get too full."	Helpful
"I will call 911 immediately to take me to the hospital if I experience any of these symptoms again."	Not Necessary
"I need to have my spouse help me check my skin to be sure there is no redness or skin breakdown."	Helpful

Recall that a high-fiber diet, rather than a low-fiber diet, is helpful in preventing constipation. Limiting time in the wheelchair is not an option for this client because of complications associated with staying in bed. It is not necessary to call 911 immediately as this action does not prevent, but rather treats, the problem.

Content Area: Medical-Surgical Nursing
Priority Concept: Perfusion; Tissue Integrity
Reference(s): Ignatavicius et al., 2024, pp. 921–929

CHAPTER 10

NGN Practice Test: Putting It All Together

As described in Chapter 9, complex clinical scenarios provide the foundation for the NGN test items as part of the current NCLEX®. Two types of NGN clinical scenarios are presented: the Unfolding Case Study and the Stand-Alone item. Each Unfolding Case Study includes six test item types that measure the clinical judgment (CJ) cognitive skills identified in the NCLEX-RN® and NCLEX-PN® Test Plans. Two types of Stand-Alone items are also included: the Trend item and the Bow-tie item. Both item types provide client information that requires you to make one or more clinical judgments. Thus these item types can measure more than one CJ cognitive skill.

This chapter allows you the opportunity to practice all of the NGN test item types you will encounter on the NCLEX®, starting with Unfolding Cases Studies and ending with Stand-Alone Trend and Bow-tie items. The answers, rationales, test-taking strategies, CJ cognitive skills, priority concepts, and references for these test item types are presented at the end of the book. To correctly answer the questions related to these practice clinical scenarios, you will need to apply one or more CJ cognitive skills. Chapters 3 to 8 describe these cognitive skills and present test-taking strategies on how to answer test items related to each skill if you need to review them.

Unfolding Case Studies

Unfolding Case Study 1

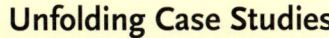 **Unfolding Case Study 1**

The nurse is caring for a 56-year-old client in the ED.

*Highlight the findings that require **immediate** follow-up.*

> **Nurses' Notes**
>
> **2215:** Spouse brought client to ED after finding a suicide note and their gun cabinet unlocked. Reports that client is "not the same person" after being hospitalized 3 months ago with severe COVID-19 and mechanically ventilated for over 2 weeks. Client states that since being discharged from the hospital, has periods of heart palpitations, insomnia, apathy, depressed mood, and anorexia. Reports that drinking alcohol every night helps to relax, but still becomes anxious and depressed at times. Is very worried about getting COVID again because the client's sibling, whom the client recently visited, tested positive yesterday. Has frequent nightmares about the hospital experience because the client nearly died. Lost 35 lb (15.9 kg) during the hospital stay, but states still weighs more than 260 lb (117.9 kg). Was considering suicide this evening because the client was afraid of possibly "being reinfected and dying this time." Recently diagnosed with type 2 DM controlled by diet and metformin.

Practice Question 10.2 — Unfolding Case Study 1

The nurse is caring for a 56-year-old client in the ED.

Nurses' Notes

2215: Spouse brought client to ED after finding a suicide note and their gun cabinet unlocked. Reports that client is "not the same person" after being hospitalized 3 months ago with severe COVID-19 and mechanically ventilated for over 2 weeks. Client states that since being discharged from the hospital, has periods of heart palpitations, insomnia, apathy, depressed mood, and anorexia. Reports that drinking alcohol every night helps to relax, but still becomes anxious and depressed at times. Is very worried about getting COVID again because the client's sibling, whom the client recently visited, tested positive yesterday. Has frequent nightmares about the hospital experience because the client nearly died. Lost 35 lb (15.9 kg) during the hospital stay, but states still weighs more than 260 lb (117.9 kg). Was considering suicide this evening because the client was afraid of possibly "being reinfected and dying this time." Recently diagnosed with type 2 DM controlled by diet and metformin.

For each client finding, select which finding is associated with which client condition. Some findings may be consistent with more than one condition.

Client Findings	Generalized Anxiety Disorder	Major Depressive Disorder	Posttraumatic Stress Disorder (PTSD)
Had recent near-death experience	☐	☐	☐
Anorexia	☐	☐	☐
Depressed mood	☐	☐	☐
Apathy	☐	☐	☐
Nightmares	☐	☐	☐
Potential suicide risk	☐	☐	☐
Excessive worry	☐	☐	☐
Insomnia	☐	☐	☐

Practice Question 10.3 — Unfolding Case Study 1

The nurse is caring for a 56-year-old client in the ED.

Nurses' Notes

2215: Spouse brought client to ED after finding a suicide note and their gun cabinet unlocked. Reports that client is "not the same person" after being hospitalized 3 months ago with severe COVID-19 and mechanically ventilated for over 2 weeks. Client states that since being discharged from the hospital, has periods of heart palpitations, insomnia, apathy, depressed mood, and anorexia. Reports that drinking alcohol every night helps to relax, but still becomes anxious and depressed at times. Is very worried about getting COVID again because the client's sibling, whom the client recently visited, tested positive yesterday. Has frequent nightmares about the hospital experience because the client nearly died. Lost 35 lb (15.9 kg) during the hospital stay, but states still weighs more than 260 lb (117.9 kg). Was considering suicide this evening because the client was afraid of possibly "being reinfected and dying this time." Recently diagnosed with type 2 DM controlled by diet and metformin.

2330: Social worker (SW) interviewed client and administered several screening assessments for selected mental health conditions. Client admitted to flashbacks about hospitalization and feels guilty about putting family through that experience. States was "lazy" and did not wear a mask or social distance at an important corporate meeting. As a result, the client developed a COVID-19 infection, which worsened and led to the hospital stay and mechanical ventilation. Expressed remorse for upsetting spouse and apologized to both the client's spouse and SW.

Complete the following sentence by selecting from the lists of options provided.

The **priority** for the client's care is to **1 [Select]** because the client most likely has **2 [Select]**.

Options for 1	Options for 2
Begin intensive counseling	Paranoid personality disorder
Ensure personal safety	Dissociative identity disorder
Start drug therapy	Posttraumatic stress disorder
Refer the client to a spiritual advisor	Generalized anxiety disorder

Practice Question 10.4 — Unfolding Case Study 1

The nurse is caring for a 56-year-old client in the ED.

Nurses' Notes

2215: Spouse brought client to ED after finding a suicide note and their gun cabinet unlocked. Reports that client is "not the same person" after being hospitalized 3 months ago with severe COVID-19 and mechanically ventilated for over 2 weeks. Client states that since being discharged from the hospital, has periods of heart palpitations, insomnia, apathy, depressed mood, and anorexia. Reports that drinking alcohol every night helps to relax, but still becomes anxious and depressed at times. Is very worried about getting COVID again because the client's sibling, whom the client recently visited, tested positive yesterday. Has frequent nightmares about the hospital experience because the client nearly died. Lost 35 lb (15.9 kg) during the hospital stay, but states still weighs more than 260 lb (117.9 kg). Was considering suicide this evening because the client was afraid of possibly "being reinfected and dying this time." Recently diagnosed with type 2 DM controlled by diet and metformin.

2330: Social worker (SW) interviewed client and administered several screening assessments for selected mental health conditions. Client admitted to flashbacks about hospitalization and feels guilty about putting family through that experience. States was "lazy" and did not wear a mask or social distance at an important corporate meeting. As a result, the client developed a COVID-19 infection, which worsened and led to the hospital stay and mechanical ventilation. Expressed remorse for upsetting spouse and apologized to both the client's spouse and SW.

Which of the following orders would the nurse anticipate for the client at this time? **Select all that apply.**

☐ Begin antidepressant drug therapy.
☐ Admit to the acute psychiatric unit.
☐ Refer to a case manager.
☐ Refer to a spiritual advisor.
☐ Begin intensive psychotherapy.
☐ Place on suicide precautions.
☐ Limit visitors to immediate family.

Practice Question 10.5 — Unfolding Case Study 1

The nurse is caring for a 56-year-old client in the ED.

Nurses' Notes

2215: Spouse brought client to ED after finding a suicide note and their gun cabinet unlocked. Reports that client is "not the same person" after being hospitalized 3 months ago with severe COVID-19 and mechanically ventilated for over 2 weeks. Client states that since being discharged from the hospital, has periods of heart palpitations, insomnia, apathy, depressed mood, and anorexia. Reports that drinking alcohol every night helps to relax, but still becomes anxious and depressed at times. Is very worried about getting COVID again because the client's sibling, whom the client recently visited, tested positive yesterday. Has frequent nightmares about the hospital experience because the client nearly died. Lost 35 lb (15.9 kg) during the hospital stay, but states still weighs more than 260 lb (117.9 kg). Was considering suicide this evening because the client was afraid of possibly "being reinfected and dying this time." Recently diagnosed with type 2 DM controlled by diet and metformin.

2330: Social worker (SW) interviewed client and administered several screening assessments for selected mental health conditions. Client admitted to flashbacks about hospitalization and feels guilty about putting family through that experience. States was "lazy" and did not wear a mask or social distance at an important corporate meeting. As a result, the client developed a COVID-19 infection, which worsened and led to the hospital stay and mechanical ventilation. Expressed remorse for upsetting spouse and apologized to both the client's spouse and SW.

0150: Client admitted to the acute psychiatric unit for one-on-one observation; started on sertraline and psychotherapy.

*The nurse plans health teaching about sertraline before administering the first dose to the client. Select the **5** statements the nurse would include in the health teaching about this medication.*

- ☐ "This drug is one of the most effective ways to treat PTSD and depression."
- ☐ "We will be monitoring you for sedation effects while you are here."
- ☐ "Let me know if you have trouble urinating or having a bowel movement."
- ☐ "Let me know if you have trouble sleeping or feel nervous while on the drug."
- ☐ "We will be monitoring you carefully for changes in your vital signs."
- ☐ "You might experience mild nausea and feel agitated when you start this drug."
- ☐ "Your liver and kidney function will need to be monitored by lab testing."

Practice Question 10.6 — Unfolding Case Study 1

The nurse is interviewing a 56-year-old client at the ambulatory mental health clinic.

Nurses' Notes

2215: Spouse brought client to ED after finding a suicide note and their gun cabinet unlocked. Reports that client is "not the same person" after being hospitalized 3 months ago with severe COVID-19 and mechanically ventilated for over 2 weeks. Client states that since being discharged from the hospital, has periods of heart palpitations, insomnia, apathy, depressed mood, and anorexia. Reports that drinking alcohol every night helps to relax, but still becomes anxious and depressed at times. Is very worried about getting COVID again because the client's sibling, whom the client recently visited, tested positive yesterday. Has frequent nightmares about the hospital experience because the client nearly died. Lost 35 lb (15.9 kg) during the hospital stay, but states still weighs more than 260 lb (117.9 kg). Was considering suicide this evening because the client was afraid of possibly "being reinfected and dying this time." Recently diagnosed with type 2 DM controlled by diet and metformin.

2330: Social worker (SW) interviewed client and administered several screening assessments for selected mental health conditions. Client admitted to flashbacks about hospitalization and feels guilty about putting family through that experience. States was "lazy" and did not wear a mask or social distance at an important corporate meeting. As a result, the client developed a COVID-19 infection, which worsened and led to the hospital stay and mechanical ventilation. Expressed remorse for upsetting spouse, and apologized to both the client's spouse and SW.

0150: Client admitted to the acute psychiatric unit for one-on-one observation; started on sertraline and psychotherapy.

Ambulatory Mental Health Clinic—6 Weeks Later

0900: Has history of PTSD, anxiety, and suicidal risk for which client was admitted for short stay in acute psychiatric unit. Today client reports having a more positive outlook without depressed moods and having a good appetite. Sleeps most nights for 7 to 8 hours, and no longer has heart palpitations. Has not consumed alcohol since hospital discharge. Continues to have flashbacks and nightmares about once a week and usually in the evening. Has been following the treatment plan taking sertraline as prescribed and attending psychotherapy sessions twice a week.

For each current client finding, indicate if the client's condition is improving or not improving.

Client Findings	Improving	Not Improving
Has not consumed any alcohol since hospital discharge	☐	☐
States has a more positive outlook without depressed moods and has a good appetite	☐	☐
Has flashbacks and nightmares about once a week	☐	☐
Sleeps most nights for 7 to 8 hours	☐	☐
States no longer has heart palpitations	☐	☐

Unfolding Case Study 2

Practice Question 10.7 — Unfolding Case Study 2

The nurse is caring for a 68-year-old client in the inpatient surgical suite.

Nurses' Notes | Orders

0645: Admitted to surgical suite preoperative area for right anterior total hip arthroplasty (THA). History of several surgeries including hysterectomy, appendectomy, and cholecystectomy. 52–pack-year smoking history, but quit 2 years ago; BMI of 30.1. History of deep vein thrombosis (DVT) × 2, hypertension controlled by diet and drug therapy, high cholesterol controlled by statins, and gastroesophageal reflux disorder (GERD) controlled by antacid PRN. Bilateral hip osteoarthritis with right hip more painful than left. Lives in a second-floor apartment in a rural town. Has no transportation, and depends on family and friends to obtain food and get to medical appointments. Family and friends are willing to help with postoperative recovery and transportation. Advance directive on file. Prepped for surgery.

Which of the following assessment findings place the client at high risk for postoperative venous thromboembolism (VTE)? **Select all that apply.**

☐ History of hypertension
☐ 52–pack-year smoking history
☐ BMI of 30.1
☐ History of high cholesterol
☐ Having a THA
☐ History of cholecystectomy
☐ History of bilateral hip osteoarthritis
☐ History of DVT × 2

Practice Question 10.8 — Unfolding Case Study 2

The nurse is caring for a 68-year-old client in the acute orthopedic unit.

Nurses' Notes | Orders

0645: Admitted to surgical suite preoperative area for right anterior total hip arthroplasty (THA). History of several surgeries including hysterectomy, appendectomy, and cholecystectomy. 52–pack-year smoking history, but quit 2 years ago; BMI of 30.1. History of deep vein thrombosis (DVT) × 2, hypertension controlled by diet and drug therapy, high cholesterol controlled by statins, and gastroesophageal reflux disorder (GERD) controlled by antacid PRN. Bilateral hip osteoarthritis with right hip more painful than left. Lives in a second-floor apartment in a rural town. Has no transportation, and depends on family and friends to obtain food and get to medical appointments. Family and friends are willing to help with postoperative recovery and transportation. Advance directive on file. Prepped for surgery.

1510: Had a right THA 2 days ago, and recovering on the acute orthopedic unit; client's pain being managed with oral opioids and gabapentin. Possible discharge tomorrow. Client will continue taking apixaban 5 mg orally twice a day and ambulating with assistance at least 4 to 5 times each day with a walker at home. Follow up with outpatient PT.

1935: Client reports was unable to ambulate this evening because of sharp chest pain that worsens when taking a deep breath. States has been "belching" since dinner because of eating onions and peppers on a steak. Restless and anxious about pain, but no acute confusion. T 100°F (37.8°C); HR 104 and irregular; RR 20 with dyspnea; BP 114/62; SpO$_2$ 88% on RA. Right THA incision dry and intact without redness. Right pedal pulses nonpalpable, but detected on Doppler; foot warm and not swollen. Posterior tibial and popliteal pulses +2 bilaterally. Able to flex both feet equally; cap refill <3 seconds.

For each client finding, select which finding is associated with which potential client condition. Some findings may be consistent with more than one condition.

Client Findings	Pulmonary Embolism	GERD	Respiratory Infection
Chest pain	☐	☐	☐
Belching	☐	☐	☐
Restlessness	☐	☐	☐
Anxiety	☐	☐	☐
T 100°F (37.8°C)	☐	☐	☐
HR 104 and irregular	☐	☐	☐
RR 20 with dyspnea	☐	☐	☐
SpO$_2$ 88% on RA	☐	☐	☐

Practice Question 10.9 — Unfolding Case Study 2

The nurse is caring for a 68-year-old client in the acute orthopedic unit.

Nurses' Notes | Orders

0645: Admitted to surgical suite preoperative area for right anterior total hip arthroplasty (THA). History of several surgeries including hysterectomy, appendectomy, and cholecystectomy. 52–pack-year smoking history, but quit 2 years ago; BMI of 30.1. History of deep vein thrombosis (DVT) × 2, hypertension controlled by diet and drug therapy, high cholesterol controlled by statins, and gastroesophageal reflux disorder (GERD) controlled by antacid PRN. Bilateral hip osteoarthritis with right hip more painful than left. Lives in a second-floor apartment in a rural town. Has no transportation, and depends on family and friends to obtain food and get to medical appointments. Family and friends are willing to help with postoperative recovery and transportation. Advance directive on file. Prepped for surgery.

1510: Had a right THA 2 days ago, and recovering on the acute orthopedic unit; client's pain being managed with oral opioids and gabapentin. Possible discharge tomorrow. Client will continue taking apixaban 5 mg orally twice a day and ambulating with assistance at least 4 to 5 times each day with a walker at home. Follow up with outpatient PT.

1935: Client reports was unable to ambulate this evening because of sharp chest pain that worsens when taking a deep breath. States has been "belching" since dinner because of eating onions and peppers on a steak. Restless and anxious about pain, but no acute confusion. T 100°F (37.8°C); HR 104 and irregular; RR 20 with dyspnea; BP 114/62; SpO$_2$ 88% on RA. Right THA incision dry and intact without redness. Right pedal pulses nonpalpable, but detected on Doppler; foot warm and not swollen. Posterior tibial and popliteal pulses +2 bilaterally. Able to flex both feet equally; cap refill <3 seconds.

Complete the following sentence by selecting from the lists of options provided.

The **priority** for the client's care is to **1 [Select]** because the client most likely has **2 [Select]**.

Options for 1	Options for 2
Reduce surgical pain	GERD
Decrease stomach pH	Pneumonia
Promote oxygenation	Right leg neurovascular compromise
Prevent bleeding	Pulmonary embolism

Practice Question 10.10 — Unfolding Case Study 2

The nurse is caring for a 68-year-old client in the acute orthopedic unit.

Nurses' Notes

0645: Admitted to surgical suite preoperative area for right anterior total hip arthroplasty (THA). History of several surgeries including hysterectomy, appendectomy, and cholecystectomy. 52–pack-year smoking history, but quit 2 years ago; BMI of 30.1. History of deep vein thrombosis (DVT) × 2, hypertension controlled by diet and drug therapy, high cholesterol controlled by statins, and gastroesophageal reflux disorder (GERD) controlled by antacid PRN. Bilateral hip osteoarthritis with right hip more painful than left. Lives in a second-floor apartment in a rural town. Has no transportation, and depends on family and friends to obtain food and get to medical appointments. Family and friends are willing to help with postoperative recovery and transportation. Advance directive on file. Prepped for surgery.

1510: Had a right THA 2 days ago, and recovering on the acute orthopedic unit; client's pain being managed with oral opioids and gabapentin. Possible discharge tomorrow. Client will continue taking apixaban 5 mg orally twice a day and ambulating with assistance at least 4 to 5 times each day with a walker at home. Follow up with outpatient PT.

1935: Client reports was unable to ambulate this evening because of sharp chest pain that worsens when taking a deep breath. States has been "belching" since dinner because of eating onions and peppers on a steak. Restless and anxious about pain, but no acute confusion. T 100°F (37.8°C); HR 104 and irregular; RR 20 with dyspnea; BP 114/62; SpO$_2$ 88% on RA. Right THA incision dry and intact without redness. Right pedal pulses nonpalpable, but detected on Doppler; foot warm and not swollen. Posterior tibial and popliteal pulses +2 bilaterally. Able to flex both feet equally; cap refill <3 seconds.

The nurse develops a plan of care to manage the client findings. Select the **6** actions that would be appropriate for the nurse to include in the plan of care at this time.

☐ Obtain peripheral venous access.
☐ Place the client in a flat supine position.
☐ Connect the client to a continuous cardiac monitor.
☐ Prepare the client for computed tomography pulmonary angiography.
☐ Apply oxygen by nasal cannula (NC) or mask.
☐ Increase the client's oral apixaban dosage from 5 mg to 10 mg.
☐ Draw blood for laboratory testing, including complete blood count and coagulation studies.
☐ Place the client on continuous oxygen saturation monitoring.

Practice Question 10.11 — Unfolding Case Study 2

The nurse is caring for a 68-year-old client on the acute orthopedic unit.

Nurses' Notes

0645: Admitted to surgical suite preoperative area for right anterior total hip arthroplasty (THA). History of several surgeries including hysterectomy, appendectomy, and cholecystectomy. 52–pack-year smoking history, but quit 2 years ago; BMI of 30.1. History of deep vein thrombosis (DVT) × 2, hypertension controlled by diet and drug therapy, high cholesterol controlled by statins, and gastroesophageal reflux disorder (GERD) controlled by antacid PRN. Bilateral hip osteoarthritis with right hip more painful than left. Lives in a second-floor apartment in a rural town. Has no transportation, and depends on family and friends to obtain food and get to medical appointments. Family and friends are willing to help with postoperative recovery and transportation. Advance directive on file. Prepped for surgery.

1510: Had a right THA 2 days ago, and recovering on the acute orthopedic unit; client's pain being managed with oral opioids and gabapentin. Possible discharge tomorrow. Client will continue taking apixaban 5 mg orally twice a day and ambulating with assistance at least 4 to 5 times each day with a walker at home. Follow up with outpatient PT.

1935: Client reports was unable to ambulate this evening because of sharp chest pain that worsens when taking a deep breath. States has been "belching" since dinner because of eating onions and peppers on a steak. Restless and anxious about pain, but no acute confusion. T 100°F (37.8°C); HR 104 and irregular; RR 20 with dyspnea; BP 114/62; SpO$_2$ 88% on RA. Right THA incision dry and intact without redness. Right pedal pulses nonpalpable, but detected on Doppler; foot warm and not swollen. Posterior tibial and popliteal pulses +2 bilaterally. Able to flex both feet equally; cap refill <3 seconds.

1955: Reports mild chest pain and occasional dyspnea. Supplemental oxygen started at 4 L/min via NC. Orthopedic surgeon notified.

2100: Computed tomography pulmonary angiography (CTPA) confirmed diagnosis of a submassive PE. Orders received.

Orders

2300:
Discontinue apixaban
Fondaparinux 7.5 mg/day subcutaneously
Warfarin 5 mg/day orally
Supplemental oxygen at 5 L/min via NC
Continuous pulse oximetry monitoring
Continuous cardiac monitoring

The nurse revises the plan of care for the client with a confirmed diagnosis of pulmonary embolism. Select whether the following potential nursing actions are indicated or not indicated for the client at this time.

Potential Nursing Actions	Indicated	Not Indicated
Monitor the client's platelet count.	☐	☐
Monitor the client's activated partial thromboplastin time (aPTT).	☐	☐
Assess the client for bleeding or excessive bruising.	☐	☐
Monitor the client's international normalized ratio (INR).	☐	☐
Monitor the client's hematocrit.	☐	☐
Check for availability of protamine sulfate.	☐	☐
Check for availability of phytonadione (vitamin K).	☐	☐

Practice Question 10.12 — Unfolding Case Study 2

The nurse is assessing a 68-year-old client at the orthopedic surgeon's office.

Nurses' Notes

0645: Admitted to surgical suite preoperative area for right anterior total hip arthroplasty (THA). History of several surgeries including hysterectomy, appendectomy, and cholecystectomy. 52–pack-year smoking history, but quit 2 years ago; BMI of 30.1. History of deep vein thrombosis (DVT) × 2, hypertension controlled by diet and drug therapy, high cholesterol controlled by statins, and gastroesophageal reflux disorder (GERD) controlled by antacid PRN. Bilateral hip osteoarthritis with right hip more painful than left. Lives in a second-floor apartment in a rural town. Has no transportation, and depends on family and friends to obtain food and get to medical appointments. Family and friends are willing to help with postoperative recovery and transportation. Advance directive on file. Prepped for surgery.

1510: Had a right THA 2 days ago, and recovering on the acute orthopedic unit; client's pain being managed with oral opioids and gabapentin. Possible discharge tomorrow. Client will continue taking apixaban 5 mg orally twice a day and ambulating with assistance at least 4 to 5 times each day with a walker at home. Follow up with outpatient PT.

1935: Client reports was unable to ambulate this evening because of sharp chest pain that worsens when taking a deep breath. States has been "belching" since dinner because of eating onions and peppers on a steak. Restless and anxious about pain, but no acute confusion. T 100°F (37.8°C); HR 104 and irregular; RR 20 with dyspnea; BP 114/62; SpO2 88% on RA. Right THA incision dry and intact without redness. Right pedal pulses nonpalpable, but detected on Doppler; foot warm and not swollen. Posterior tibial and popliteal pulses +2 bilaterally. Able to flex both feet equally; cap refill <3 seconds.

1955: Reports mild chest pain and occasional dyspnea. Supplemental oxygen started at 4 L/min via NC. Orthopedic surgeon notified.

2100: Computed tomography pulmonary angiography (CTPA) confirmed the diagnosis of a submassive PE. Orders received.

Surgeon's Office—6 Weeks Later

1015: Walking independently with a cane with full weight bearing; states is able to perform ADLs without assistance. Right hip incision healed with hairline scar and slight distal bruising. Taking warfarin as prescribed, and following up on INR testing, but depends mostly on family and friends for transportation to the lab. Right arm bruised, but reports no other bleeding. T 97.9°F (36.6°C); HR 86; RR 18; BP 126/74; SpO2 95% on RA. No adventitious breath sounds; no new report of shortness of breath or chest pain. States a loss of 27 lb (12.2 kg) since hospitalization as part of a new weight-loss program. Also reports that left nonsurgical hip is increasingly painful.

Based on the nurse's focused assessment, which findings indicate that the client is improving or progressing? **Select all that apply.**

☐ No new report of shortness of breath or chest pain
☐ Hip incision healed with hairline scar
☐ SpO$_2$ of 95% on RA
☐ Right arm badly bruised
☐ Recent weight loss of 27 lb (12.2 kg)
☐ Left hip becoming more painful
☐ Walking independently with a cane
☐ Performing ADLs without assistance

Unfolding Case Study 3

Practice Question 10.13 — Unfolding Case Study 3

A 64-year-old client presents to the ED and reports a 2-week history of fever and chills, nausea and abdominal pain, sore throat, cough, fatigue and lethargy, and muscle aches.

History and Physical | Nurses' Notes | Laboratory Results | Diagnostic Results

1000: History of type 1 diabetes mellitus, hypertension, hyperlipidemia, and hypothyroidism. Denies chest pain or shortness of breath. Nonproductive cough, coarse crackles heard in lower lobes bilaterally. Blood glucose levels have been well controlled, but this morning the client reports a level of 375 mg/dL (20.8 mmol/L), prompting the visit to the ED. States recent glycated hemoglobin (A1c) level performed 2 months ago was 7%. Unable to eat, and reports discontinuing medications 3 days ago because of nausea and abdominal pain. Reports increased urination despite inability to tolerate food or fluids. Reports weakness and muscle aches and being confined to the bed for the past 3 weeks. Fruity breath odor noted. POC glucose 400 mg/dL (22.2 mmol/L). T 100.4°F (38°C); HR 96; RR 24; BP 142/90; SpO$_2$ 91% on RA. Weight 175 lb (79.37 kg), height 5 feet 9 inches (stated). Voided: 250 mL.

Medications:
Levothyroxine 125 mcg/day orally
Lisinopril 2.5 mg/day orally
Simvastatin 20 mg/day orally
Insulin glargine 28 units/day subcutaneously
Semaglutide 1 mg/week subcutaneously

1120: The nurse reviews the recent laboratory and diagnostic results.

History and Physical | Nurses' Notes | **Laboratory Results** | Diagnostic Results

Test and Reference Range	Results
Glucose 74–106 mg/dL (3.9–6.1 mmol/L)	440 mg/dL (24.4 mmol/L)
Ketones <0 mg/dL (0.0–0.27 mmol/L)	86.4 mg/dL (4.8 mmol/L)
White blood cells (WBCs) 5000–10,000/mm^3 (5–10 × 10^9/L)	9900/mm^3 (9 × 10^9/L)
Blood urea nitrogen (BUN) 10–20 mg/dL (2.9–8.2 mmol/L)	22 mg/dL (9.0 mmol/L)
Creatinine 0.6–1.2 mg/dL (53–106 μmol/L)	1.0 mg/dL (88.3 μmol/L)
Potassium 3.5–5.0 mEq/L (3.5–5.0 mmol/L)	5.9 mEq/L (5.9 mmol/L)
Sodium 136–145 mEq/L (136–145 mmol/L)	150 mEq/L (150 mmol/L)
Thyroid-stimulating hormone (TSH) 2–10 mIU/mL (0.4–4.8 mIU/L)	4.0 mIU/mL (4.0 mIU/L)
D-dimer <0.4 mcg/mL (<3 nmol/L)	15 mcg/mL (112.5 nmol/L)
Creatine kinase (CK) 20–200 U/L (20–215 U/L)	140 U/L (150.5 U/L)
C-reactive protein (CRP) <1 mg/dL (<10.0 mg/L)	10.2 mg/dL (102 mg/L)
Troponin I <0.03 ng/mL (<0.35 mcg/L)	0.01 ng/mL (0.17 mcg/L)
Blood culture: no growth	Pending
Urinalysis	
WBCs: 0–4 low-power field	0 (0)
Ketones: none	Positive
Urine culture: no growth	Pending
Arterial Blood Gases (ABGs)	
pH: 7.35–7.45	pH 7.30
PCO$_2$: 35–45 mm Hg	PCO$_2$ 27 mm Hg
HCO$_3$: 21–28 mEq/L	HCO$_3$ 14 mEq/L
PO$_2$: 80–100 mm Hg	PO$_2$ 85 mm Hg
SARS-CoV-2: PCR negative	Positive

Practice Question 10.13 — Unfolding Case Study 3—cont'd

History and Physical	Nurses' Notes	Laboratory Results	Diagnostic Results

Chest x-ray: Bilateral pulmonary infiltrates compatible with COVID-19 pneumonitis
ECG: NSR

*Select the 4 laboratory findings that require **immediate** follow-up.*

☐ A1c
☐ BUN
☐ Sodium
☐ Glucose
☐ D-dimer
☐ Potassium
☐ C-reactive protein
☐ Arterial blood gases

Practice Question 10.14 — Unfolding Case Study 3

A 64-year-old client presents to the ED and reports a 2-week history of fever and chills, nausea and abdominal pain, sore throat, cough, fatigue and lethargy, and muscle aches.

History and Physical

1000: History of type 1 diabetes mellitus, hypertension, hyperlipidemia, and hypothyroidism. Denies chest pain or shortness of breath. Nonproductive cough, coarse crackles heard in lower lobes bilaterally. Blood glucose levels have been well controlled, but this morning the client reports a level of 375 mg/dL (20.8 mmol/L), prompting the visit to the ED. States recent glycated hemoglobin (A1c) level performed 2 months ago was 7%. Unable to eat, and reports discontinuing medications 3 days ago because of nausea and abdominal pain. Reports increased urination despite inability to tolerate food or fluids. Reports weakness and muscle aches and being confined to the bed for the past 3 weeks. Fruity breath odor noted. POC glucose 400 mg/dL (22.2 mmol/L). T 100.4°F (38°C); HR 96; RR 24; BP 142/90; SpO_2 91% on RA.
Weight 175 lb (79.37 kg), height 5 feet 9 inches (stated). Voided: 250 mL.

Medications:
Levothyroxine 125 mcg/day orally
Lisinopril 2.5 mg/day orally
Simvastatin 20 mg/day orally
Insulin glargine 28 units/day subcutaneously
Semaglutide 1 mg/week subcutaneously

1120: The nurse reviews the recent laboratory and diagnostic results.

Laboratory Results

Test and Reference Range	Results
Glucose 74–106 mg/dL (3.9–6.1 mmol/L)	440 mg/dL (24.4 mmol/L)
Ketones <0 mg/dL (0.0–0.27 mmol/L)	86.4 mg/dL (4.8 mmol/L)
White blood cells (WBCs) 5000–10,000/mm³ (5–10 × 10⁹/L)	9900/mm³ (9 × 10⁹/L)
Blood urea nitrogen (BUN) 10–20 mg/dL (2.9–8.2 mmol/L)	22 mg/dL (9.0 mmol/L)
Creatinine 0.6–1.2 mg/dL (53–106 µmol/L)	1.0 mg/dL (88.3 µmol/L)
Potassium 3.5–5.0 mEq/L (3.5–5.0 mmol/L)	5.9 mEq/L (5.9 mmol/L)
Sodium 136–145 mEq/L (136–145 mmol/L)	150 mEq/L (150 mmol/L)
Thyroid-stimulating hormone (TSH) 2–10 mIU/mL (0.4–4.8 mIU/L)	4.0 mIU/mL (4.0 mIU/L)
D-dimer <0.4 mcg/mL (<3 nmol/L)	15 mcg/mL (112.5 nmol/L)
Creatine kinase (CK) 20–200 U/L (20–215 U/L)	140 U/L (150.5 U/L)
C-reactive protein (CRP) <1 mg/dL (<10.0 mg/L)	10.2 mg/dL (102 mg/L)
Troponin I <0.03 ng/mL (<0.35 mcg/L)	0.01 ng/mL (0.17 mcg/L)
Blood culture: no growth	Pending

Urinalysis

WBCs: 0–4 low-power field	0 (0)
Ketones: none	Positive
Urine culture: no growth	Pending

Arterial Blood Gases (ABGs)

pH: 7.35–7.45	pH 7.30
PCO_2: 35–45 mm Hg	PCO_2 27 mm Hg
HCO_3: 21–28 mEq/L	HCO_3 14 mEq/L
PO_2: 80–100 mm Hg	PO_2 85 mm Hg
SARS-CoV-2: PCR negative	Positive

Practice Question 10.14 — Unfolding Case Study 3—cont'd

| History and Physical | Nurses' Notes | Laboratory Results | **Diagnostic Results** |

Chest x-ray: Bilateral pulmonary infiltrates compatible with COVID-19 pneumonitis
ECG: NSR

For each client finding, specify if the finding is consistent with the disease process of DKA or COVID-19. Each finding may support more than one disease process.

Client Findings	DKA	COVID-19
Fever and chills	☐	☐
Nausea	☐	☐
Abdominal pain	☐	☐
Increased urination	☐	☐
Cough	☐	☐
Lung crackles	☐	☐
High C-reactive protein level	☐	☐
High glucose level	☐	☐
ABG results	☐	☐

Practice Question 10.15 — Unfolding Case Study 3

A 64-year-old client presents to the ED and reports a 2-week history of fever and chills, nausea and abdominal pain, sore throat, cough, fatigue and lethargy, and muscle aches.

History and Physical | Nurses' Notes | Laboratory Results | Diagnostic Results

1000: History of type 1 diabetes mellitus, hypertension, hyperlipidemia, and hypothyroidism. Denies chest pain or shortness of breath. Nonproductive cough, coarse crackles heard in lower lobes bilaterally. Blood glucose levels have been well controlled, but this morning the client reports a level of 375 mg/dL (20.8 mmol/L), prompting the visit to the ED. States recent glycated hemoglobin (A1c) level performed 2 months ago was 7%. Unable to eat, and reports discontinuing medications 3 days ago because of nausea and abdominal pain. Reports increased urination despite inability to tolerate food or fluids. Reports weakness and muscle aches and being confined to the bed for the past 3 weeks. Fruity breath odor noted. POC glucose 400 mg/dL (22.2 mmol/L). T 100.4°F (38°C); HR 96; RR 24; BP 142/90; SpO_2 91% on RA. Weight 175 lb (79.37 kg), height 5 feet 9 inches (stated). Voided: 250 mL.

Medications:
Levothyroxine 125 mcg/day orally
Lisinopril 2.5 mg/day orally
Simvastatin 20 mg/day orally
Insulin glargine 28 units/day subcutaneously
Semaglutide 1 mg/week subcutaneously

1120: The nurse reviews the recent laboratory and diagnostic results.

History and Physical | Nurses' Notes | Laboratory Results | Diagnostic Results

Test and Reference Range	Results
Glucose 74–106 mg/dL (3.9–6.1 mmol/L)	440 mg/dL (24.4 mmol/L)
Ketones <0 mg/dL (0.0–0.27 mmol/L)	86.4 mg/dL (4.8 mmol/L)
White blood cells (WBCs) 5000–10,000/mm³ (5–10 × 10⁹/L)	9900/mm³ (9 × 10⁹/L)
Blood urea nitrogen (BUN) 10–20 mg/dL (2.9–8.2 mmol/L)	22 mg/dL (9.0 mmol/L)
Creatinine 0.6–1.2 mg/dL (53–106 μmol/L)	1.0 mg/dL (88.3 μmol/L)
Potassium 3.5–5.0 mEq/L (3.5–5.0 mmol/L)	5.9 mEq/L (5.9 mmol/L)
Sodium 136–145 mEq/L (136–145 mmol/L)	150 mEq/L (150 mmol/L)
Thyroid-stimulating hormone (TSH) 2–10 mIU/mL (0.4–4.8 mIU/L)	4.0 mIU/mL (4.0 mIU/L)
D-dimer <0.4 mcg/mL (<3 nmol/L)	15 mcg/mL (112.5 nmol/L)
Creatine kinase (CK) 20–200 U/L (20–215 U/L)	140 U/L (150.5 U/L)
C-reactive protein (CRP) <1 mg/dL (<10.0 mg/L)	10.2 mg/dL (102 mg/L)
Troponin I <0.03 ng/mL (<0.35 mcg/L)	0.01 ng/mL (0.17 mcg/L)
Blood culture: no growth	Pending
Urinalysis	
WBCs: 0–4 low-power field	0 (0)
Ketones: none	Positive
Urine culture: no growth	Pending
Arterial Blood Gases (ABGs)	
pH: 7.35–7.45	pH 7.30
PCO_2: 35–45 mm Hg	PCO_2 27 mm Hg
HCO_3: 21–28 mEq/L	HCO_3 14 mEq/L
PO_2: 80–100 mm Hg	PO_2 85 mm Hg
SARS-CoV-2: PCR negative	Positive

Practice Question 10.15 — Unfolding Case Study 3—cont'd

| History and Physical | Nurses' Notes | Laboratory Results | **Diagnostic Results** |

Chest x-ray: Bilateral pulmonary infiltrates compatible with COVID-19 pneumonitis
ECG: NSR

Complete the following sentence by selecting from the lists of options provided.

The client is at **highest** risk for developing **1 [Select]**, as evidenced by **2 [Select]** and **3 [Select]**.

Options for 1	Options for 2	Options for 3
Seizures	BUN	Chills
Acute kidney injury	Fever	Creatinine levels
Myxedema coma	D-dimer level	Chest x-ray result
Respiratory failure	Lung crackles	TSH level
Thromboembolism	History of hypothyroidism	Immobility

Practice Question 10.16 — Unfolding Case Study 3

A 64-year-old client presents to the ED and reports a 2-week history of fever and chills, nausea and abdominal pain, sore throat, cough, fatigue and lethargy, and muscle aches.

History and Physical

1000: History of type 1 diabetes mellitus, hypertension, hyperlipidemia, and hypothyroidism. Denies chest pain or shortness of breath. Nonproductive cough, coarse crackles heard in lower lobes bilaterally. Blood glucose levels have been well controlled, but this morning the client reports a level of 375 mg/dL (20.8 mmol/L), prompting the visit to ED. States recent glycated hemoglobin (A1c) level performed 2 months ago was 7%. Unable to eat, and reports discontinuing medications 3 days ago because of nausea and abdominal pain. Reports increased urination despite inability to tolerate food or fluids. Reports weakness and muscle aches and being confined to the bed for the past 3 weeks. Fruity breath odor noted. POC glucose 400 mg/dL (22.2 mmol/L).
VS: T 100.4°F (38°C); HR 96; RR 24; BP 142/90; SpO$_2$ 91% on RA.
Weight 175 lb (79.37 kg), height 5 feet 9 inches (stated). Voided: 250 mL.

Medications:

Levothyroxine 125 mcg/day orally
Lisinopril 2.5 mg/day orally
Simvastatin 20 mg/day orally
Insulin glargine 28 units/day subcutaneously
Semaglutide 1 mg/week subcutaneously

1120: The nurse reviews the recent laboratory and diagnostic results.

Laboratory Results

Test and Reference Range	Results
Glucose 74–106 mg/dL (3.9–6.1 mmol/L)	440 mg/dL (24.4 mmol/L)
Ketones <0 mg/dL (0.0–0.27 mmol/L)	86.4 mg/dL (4.8 mmol/L)
White blood cells (WBCs) 5000–10,000/mm³ (5–10 × 10⁹/L)	9900/mm³ (9 × 10⁹/L)
Blood urea nitrogen (BUN) 10–20 mg/dL (2.9–8.2 mmol/L)	22 mg/dL (9.0 mmol/L)
Creatinine 0.6–1.2 mg/dL (53–106 μmol/L)	1.0 mg/dL (88.3 μmol/L)
Potassium 3.5–5.0 mEq/L (3.5–5.0 mmol/L)	5.9 mEq/L (5.9 mmol/L)
Sodium 136–145 mEq/L (136–145 mmol/L)	150 mEq/L (150 mmol/L)
Thyroid-stimulating hormone (TSH) 2–10 mIU/mL (0.4–4.8 mIU/L)	4.0 mIU/mL (4.0 mIU/L)
D-dimer <0.4 mcg/mL (<3 nmol/L)	15 mcg/mL (112.5 nmol/L)
Creatine kinase (CK) 20–200 U/L (20–215 U/L)	140 U/L (150.5 U/L)
C-reactive protein (CRP) <1 mg/dL (<10.0 mg/L)	10.2 mg/dL (102 mg/L)
Troponin I <0.03 ng/mL (<0.35 mcg/L)	0.01 ng/mL (0.17 mcg/L)
Blood culture: no growth	Pending
Urinalysis	
WBCs: 0–4 low-power field	0 (0)
Ketones: none	Positive
Urine culture: no growth	Pending
Arterial Blood Gases (ABGs)	
pH: 7.35–7.45	pH 7.30
PCO$_2$: 35–45 mm Hg	PCO$_2$ 27 mm Hg
HCO$_3$: 21–28 mEq/L	HCO$_3$ 14 mEq/L
PO$_2$: 80–100 mm Hg	PO$_2$ 85 mm Hg
SARS-CoV-2: PCR negative	Positive

Practice Question 10.16 — Unfolding Case Study 3—cont'd

History and Physical	Nurses' Notes	Laboratory Results	Diagnostic Results

Chest x-ray: Bilateral pulmonary infiltrates compatible with COVID-19 pneumonitis.
ECG: NSR

1145: Hospital admission is planned, and the nurse reassesses the client.

History and Physical	Nurses' Notes	Laboratory Results	Diagnostic Results

1145: VS: T 100.4°F (38°C); HR 98; RR 24; BP 146/92; SpO$_2$ 89% on RA. POC glucose 500 mg/dL (27.7 mmol/L). Client is alert but lethargic, yet arousable. Voiding 200 mL/h. Dry cough. No shortness of breath. Coarse crackles heard in lower lobes bilaterally.

Specify whether the following potential nursing actions are indicated or not indicated for the client at this time.

Potential Nursing Actions	Indicated	Not Indicated
O$_2$ via NC	☐	☐
0.45% NS infusion	☐	☐
Insulin glargine bolus	☐	☐
Continuous infusion of regular insulin diluted in NS	☐	☐
IV potassium	☐	☐
Continuous cardiac monitoring	☐	☐
Enoxaparin subcutaneously daily	☐	☐
Ceftriaxone	☐	☐

Practice Question 10.17 — Unfolding Case Study 3

1345: The ED physician orders are initiated, and the client with DKA and COVID-19 is transferred to the acute care medical unit for hospital admission. The admitting physician prescribes laboratory studies, and the nurse contacts the laboratory for the test results.

History and Physical	**Nurses' Notes**	Laboratory Results	Diagnostic Results

1345: Client is alert and oriented on admission. VS: T 99.4°F (37.4°C); HR 88; RR 20; BP 138/90; SpO$_2$ 90% on RA. Lab contacted for testing.

1415: The laboratory results are reported, and the nurse reviews the results and subsequent orders.

History and Physical	Nurses' Notes	**Laboratory Results**	Diagnostic Results

Test and Reference Range	Results
Glucose 74–106 mg/dL (3.9–6.1 mmol/L)	240 mg/dL (12.6 mmol/L)
Blood urea nitrogen (BUN) 10–20 mg/dL (2.9–8.2 mmol/L)	18 mg/dL (5.22 mmol/L)
Creatinine 0.6–1.2 mg/dL (53–106 µmol/L)	1.2 mg/dL (106 µmol/L)
Potassium 3.5–5.0 mEq/L (3.5–5.0 mmol/L)	4.0 mEq/L (4.0 mmol/L)
Sodium 136–145 mEq/L (136–145 mmol/L)	150 mEq/L (150 mmol/L)

*Based on the client assessment and laboratory findings, select the **3 priority** actions.*

☐ Administer IV potassium.
☐ Offer a sports drink for sipping.
☐ Check hourly urine output amounts.
☐ Teach the client about ways to prevent dehydration.
☐ Administer 5% dextrose in 0.45% NS.

Practice Question 10.18 — Unfolding Case Study 3

0700: The hand-off report from the night nurse to the day nurse has been completed. The night nurse reports that the prescriptions to treat the client's DKA were implemented on the previous evening shift. The night nurse also reports that the client had a comfortable night and that laboratory results and vital signs were checked every 4 hours during the night and remained stable.

0730: The day nurse assesses the client and reviews the most current laboratory results, which were drawn at 0600.

*Tabs: History and Physical | Nurses' Notes | **Laboratory Results** | Diagnostic Results*

Test and Reference Range	Results
Glucose 74–106 mg/dL (3.9–6.1 mmol/L)	240 mg/dL (12.6 mmol/L)
Blood urea nitrogen (BUN) 10–20 mg/dL (2.9–8.2 mmol/L)	18 mg/dL (5.22 mmol/L)
Creatinine 0.6–1.2 mg/dL (53–106 μmol/L)	1.2 mg/dL (106 μmol/L)
Potassium 3.5–5.0 mEq/L (3.5–5.0 mmol/L)	4.0 mEq/L (4.0 mmol/L)
Sodium 136–145 mEq/L (136–145 mmol/L)	150 mEq/L (150 mmol/L)

For each client finding, select whether the finding indicates that the treatment plan is effective or ineffective.

Previous Client Finding	Current Client Finding	Effective	Ineffective
Glucose 240 mg/dL (12.6 mmol/L)	Glucose 190 mg/dL (10.64 mmol/L)	☐	☐
Potassium 4.0 mEq/L (4.0 mmol/L)	Potassium 4.0 mEq/L (4.0 mmol/L)	☐	☐
Urine output 200 mL/h	Urine output 45 mL/h	☐	☐
Sodium 150 mEq/L (150 mmol/L)	Sodium 150 mEq/L (150 mmol/L)	☐	☐

Unfolding Case Study 4

Practice Question 10.19 — Unfolding Case Study 4

A 70-year-old client presents to the ED.

*Highlight the findings that require **immediate** follow-up.*

History and Physical

1200: 70-year-old client admitted to ED reporting chest heaviness and difficulty breathing for 2 days. Symptoms increase with activity and subside with rest after a few minutes. Past medical history of type 2 DM, hypertension, hyperlipidemia, hypothyroidism, and osteoarthritis. Currently smokes 1 pack of cigarettes per day × 20 years. Medications include sliding-scale insulin aspart prior to meals and at bedtime, insulin glargine at bedtime, lisinopril, atorvastatin, levothyroxine, and naproxen.

Nurses' Notes

1200: Appears nontoxic, well nourished, and well hydrated. Skin warm, dry, and intact. Lungs clear to auscultation bilaterally, no adventitious sounds. No use of accessory muscles. HR irregularly irregular. S1 and S2 noted, no S3 or S4; no murmurs, rubs, or gallops. No peripheral edema. Abdomen soft, nontender, and nondistended. Bowel sounds present × 4. Cranial nerves II to XII grossly intact.

Vital Signs

1200: VS: T 97.5°F (36.4°C) oral; HR 130 and irregular; RR 20; BP 108/59; SpO$_2$ 95% on RA. Height: 165 cm (5 feet 5 inches) Weight: 180 lb (81.6 kg) BMI: 30
1200: I: 120 mL water (oral)
1230: O: 140 mL clear, yellow urine

Laboratory and Diagnostic Results

ECG:
Atrial fibrillation with rapid ventricular response, rate 130
Acute anterior and lateral MI
Intraventricular conduction delay
No ST elevation

Test and Reference Range	Results
Sodium 136–145 mEq/L (136–145 mmol/L)	136 mEq/L (136 mmol/L)
Potassium 3.5–5.0 mEq/L (3.5–5.0 mmol/L)	3.8 mEq/L (3.8 mmol/L)
Calcium 9–10.5 mg/dL (2.25–2.62 mmol/L)	9.2 mg/dL (2.4 mmol/L)
Chloride 98–106 mEq/L (98–106 mmol/L)	98 mEq/L (98 mmol/L)
Glucose 74–106 mg/dL (3.9–6.1 mmol/L)	212 mg/dL (11.8 mmol/L)
Blood urea nitrogen (BUN) 10–20 mg/dL (2.9–8.2 mmol/L)	22 mg/dL (7.8 mmol/L)
Creatinine 0.6–1.2 mg/dL (53–106 μmol/L)	1.0 mg/dL (88.3 μmol/L)
Glomerular filtration rate >60 mL/min/1.73 m^2	70 mL/min/1.73 m^2
White blood cells (WBCs) 5000–10,000/mm^3 (5.0–10 × 10^9/L)	6000/mm^3 (6.0 × 10^9/L)
Red blood cells (RBCs) 4.2–6.1 × 10^{12}/L (4.2–6.2 × 10^{12}/L)	4.6 × 10^{12}/L (4.6 × 10^{12}/L)
Hemoglobin (Hgb) 12–18 g/dL (120–180 g/L)	Hgb: 13 g/dL (130 g/L)
Hematocrit (Hct) 37%–52% (0.37–0.54 volume fraction)	38% (0.38 volume fraction)

Cardiac Markers

Troponin T <0.1 ng/mL (0.1 mcg/L)	0.8 ng/mL (0.8 mcg/L)

Practice Question 10.20 — Unfolding Case Study 4

A 70-year-old client presents to the ED.

History and Physical | Nurses' Notes | Vital Signs | Laboratory and Diagnostic Results

1200: 70-year-old client admitted to ED reporting chest heaviness and difficulty breathing for 2 days. Symptoms increase with activity and subside with rest after a few minutes. Past medical history of type 2 DM, hypertension, hyperlipidemia, hypothyroidism, and osteoarthritis. Currently smokes 1 pack cigarettes per day × 20 years. Medications include sliding-scale insulin aspart prior to meals and at bedtime, insulin glargine at bedtime, lisinopril, atorvastatin, levothyroxine, and naproxen.

History and Physical | Nurses' Notes | Vital Signs | Laboratory and Diagnostic Results

1200: Appears nontoxic, well nourished, and well hydrated. Skin warm, dry, and intact. Lungs clear to auscultation bilaterally, no adventitious sounds. No use of accessory muscles. HR irregularly irregular. S1 and S2 noted, no S3 or S4; no murmurs, rubs, or gallops. No peripheral edema. Abdomen soft, nontender, and nondistended. Bowel sounds present × 4. Cranial nerves II to XII grossly intact.

History and Physical | Nurses' Notes | Vital Signs | Laboratory and Diagnostic Results

1200: VS: T 97.5°F (36.4°C) oral; HR 130 and irregular; RR 20; BP 108/59; SpO$_2$ 95% on RA. Height: 165 cm (5 feet 5 inches) Weight: 81.6 kg (180 lb) BMI: 30.
1200: I: 120 mL water (oral)
1230: O: 140 mL clear, yellow urine

History and Physical | Nurses' Notes | Vital Signs | Laboratory and Diagnostic Results

1230:
ECG:
Atrial fibrillation with rapid ventricular response, rate 130
Acute anterior and lateral MI
Intraventricular conduction delay
No ST elevation

Test and Reference Range	Results
Sodium 136–145 mEq/L (136–145 mmol/L)	136 mEq/L (136 mmol/L)
Potassium 3.5–5.0 mEq/L (3.5–5.0 mmol/L)	3.8 mEq/L (3.8 mmol/L)
Calcium 9–10.5 mg/dL (2.25–2.62 mmol/L)	9.2 mg/dL (2.4 mmol/L)
Chloride 98–106 mEq/L (98–106 mmol/L)	98 mEq/L (98 mmol/L)
Glucose 74–106 mg/dL (3.9–6.1 mmol/L)	212 mg/dL (11.8 mmol/L)
Blood urea nitrogen (BUN) 10–20 mg/dL (2.9–8.2 mmol/L)	22 mg/dL (7.8 mmol/L)
Creatinine 0.6–1.2 mg/dL (53–106 μmol/L)	1.0 mg/dL (88.3 μmol/L)
Glomerular filtration rate >60 mL/min/1.73 m^2	70 mL/min/ 1.73 m^2
Complete Blood Count (CBC)	
White blood cells (WBCs) 5000–10,000/mm^3 (5.0–10 × 10^9/L)	6000/mm^3 (6.0 × 10^9/L)
Red blood cells (RBCs) 4.2–6.1 × 10^{12}/L (4.2–6.2 × 10^{12}/L)	4.6 × 10^{12}/L (4.6 × 10^{12}/L)
Hemoglobin (Hgb) 12–18 g/dL (120–180 g/L)	Hgb: 13 g/dL (130 g/L)
Hematocrit (Hct) 37%–52% (0.37–0.54 volume fraction)	38% (0.38 volume fraction)
Cardiac Markers	
Troponin T <0.1 ng/mL (0.1 mcg/L)	0.8 ng/mL (0.8 mcg/L)

The nurse monitors for complications based on the data collection findings. Complete the following sentence by selecting from the lists of options provided.

The client is at **highest** risk for developing **1 [Select]** as evidenced by **2 [Select]**.

Options for 1	Options for 2
Fluid volume overload	I&O
Diminished cardiac output	Respiratory assessment
Decreased renal perfusion	Neurologic assessment
Venous thromboembolism	Cardiovascular assessment

Practice Question 10.21 — Unfolding Case Study 4

A 70-year-old client presents to the ED.

History and Physical

1200: 70-year-old client admitted to the ED reporting chest heaviness and difficulty breathing for 2 days. Symptoms increase with activity and subside with rest after a few minutes. Past medical history of type 2 DM, hypertension, hyperlipidemia, hypothyroidism, and osteoarthritis. Currently smokes 1 pack cigarettes per day × 20 years. Medications include sliding-scale insulin aspart prior to meals and at bedtime, insulin glargine at bedtime, lisinopril, atorvastatin, levothyroxine, and naproxen.

Nurses' Notes

1200: Appears nontoxic, well nourished, and well hydrated. Skin warm, dry, and intact. Lungs clear to auscultation bilaterally, no adventitious sounds. No use of accessory muscles. HR irregularly irregular. S1 and S2 noted, no S3 or S4; no murmurs, rubs, or gallops. No peripheral edema. Abdomen soft, nontender, and nondistended. Bowel sounds present × 4. Cranial nerves II to XII grossly intact.

Vital Signs

1200: VS: T 97.5°F (36.4°C) oral; HR 130 and irregular; RR 20; BP 108/59; SpO$_2$ 95% on RA. Height: 165 cm (5 feet 5 inches) Weight: 81.6 kg (180 lb) BMI: 30
1200: I: 120 mL water (oral)
1230: O: 140 mL clear, yellow urine

Laboratory and Diagnostic Results

1215:
ECG:
Atrial fibrillation with rapid ventricular response, rate 130
Acute anterior and lateral MI
Intraventricular conduction delay
No ST elevation

Test and Reference Range	Results
Sodium 136–145 mEq/L (136–145 mmol/L)	136 mEq/L (136 mmol/L)
Potassium 3.5–5.0 mEq/L (3.5–5.0 mmol/L)	3.8 mEq/L (3.8 mmol/L)
Calcium 9–10.5 mg/dL (2.25–2.62 mmol/L)	9.2 mg/dL (2.4 mmol/L)
Chloride 98–106 mEq/L (98–106 mmol/L)	98 mEq/L (98 mmol/L)
Glucose 74–106 mg/dL (3.9–6.1 mmol/L)	212 mg/dL (11.8 mmol/L)
Blood urea nitrogen (BUN) 10–20 mg/dL (2.9–8.2 mmol/L)	22 mg/dL (7.8 mmol/L)
Creatinine 0.6–1.2 mg/dL (53–106 µmol/L)	1.0 mg/dL (88.3 µmol/L)
Glomerular filtration rate >60 mL/min/1.73 m^2	70 mL/min/1.73 m^2
Complete Blood Count (CBC)	
White blood cells (WBCs) 5000–10,000/mm^3 (5.0–10 × 10^9/L)	6000/mm^3 (6.0 × 10^9/L)
Red blood cells (RBCs) 4.2–6.1 × 10^{12}/L (4.2–6.2 × 10^{12}/L)	4.6 × 10^{12}/L (4.6 × 10^{12}/L)
Hemoglobin (Hgb) 12–18 g/dL (120–180 g/L)	Hgb: 13 g/dL (130 g/L)
Hematocrit (Hct) 37%–52% (0.37–0.54 volume fraction)	38% (0.38 volume fraction)
Cardiac Markers	
Troponin T <0.1 ng/mL (0.1 mcg/L)	0.8 ng/mL (0.8 mcg/L)

The nurse has completed the admission assessment and is initiating the client's plan of care. The nurse notes that the cardiologist has been consulted and has ordered further diagnostic testing.

Based on this clinical scenario, complete the following sentence by selecting from the lists of options provided.

The **priority** and most **specific** diagnostic test would be **1 [Select]** to assess for **2 [Select]**.

Options for 1	Options for 2
D-dimer level	Blood clots
Chest x-ray	Cardiomegaly
Cardiac catheterization	Hyperthyroidism
Trended electrolyte levels	Hypokalemia or hyperkalemia
Thyroid-stimulating hormone	Blockages and narrowed vessels

Practice Question 10.22 — Unfolding Case Study 4

Progress Notes

1400: The consulting cardiologist ordered cardiac catheterization for a 70-year-old client with a suspected MI. Stents were placed, and blood flow was re-established to the affected areas of the heart. The procedure has been completed, and the nurse is monitoring the client on the intermediate care unit. The left femoral vein was used as the insertion site for the procedure.

Which of the following actions would the nurse plan for this client following cardiac catheterization? **Select all that apply.**

☐ Assess for shortness of breath.
☐ Keep both extremities straight.
☐ Encourage activity as tolerated.
☐ Apply a soft knee brace to the left leg.
☐ Position the client in the supine position.
☐ Monitor the client for changes in mental status.
☐ Monitor vital signs every 15 minutes initially.
☐ Assess the insertion site for bloody drainage or hematoma.
☐ Apply sequential compression devices to both lower extremities.
☐ Assess circulation, sensation, and motion of the affected extremity.

Practice Question 10.23 — Unfolding Case Study 4

A 70-year-old client was diagnosed with acute MI and postmyocardial heart failure with an ejection fraction of 30%. The nurse is initiating discharge teaching related to medication therapy.

The nurse is teaching the client about discharge medications. Choose the **most likely** options for the missing information in the table by selecting from the lists of options.

Medication	Dose, Route, Frequency	Drug Class	Indication
1 [Select]	81 mg/day orally	Antiplatelet	MI prevention
Carvedilol	6.25 mg twice daily orally	Beta blocker	4 [Select]
Atorvastatin	20 mg/day orally	3 [Select]	Atherosclerotic cardiovascular disease
Lisinopril	5 mg/day orally	Angiotensin-converting enzyme inhibitor	5 [Select]
Nitroglycerin	2 [Select]	Vasodilator	Acute angina

Options for 1	Options for 2	Options for 3	Options for 4	Options for 5
Aspirin	0.6 mg sublingually every 15 minutes as needed up to 5 times	Fibrate	Acute angina	Hypertension
Ibuprofen	0.4 mg sublingually every 5 minutes as needed up to 3 times	Bile acid sequestrant	Hypertension	Hyperlipidemia
Diclofenac	0.6 mg sublingually × 1 before strenuous activity	HMG-CoA reductase inhibitor	Heart failure with reduced ejection fraction	Heart failure with reduced ejection fraction

Practice Question 10.24 — Unfolding Case Study 4

The nurse is caring for a 70-year-old client who had a cardiac catheterization yesterday to confirm an MI and has completed discharge teaching using the teach-back method. This morning the nurse is reinforcing discharge teaching with the client.

For each client statement, select whether the statement indicates understanding or no understanding of the health teaching provided.

Client Statements	Understanding	No Understanding
"I should walk 1 mile at least once a day in the beginning."	☐	☐
"I will be sure to carry my nitroglycerin with me."	☐	☐
"I will check my pulse before, during, and after I do my exercises."	☐	☐
"I won't exercise if I notice that my pulse is more than 5 BPM higher than what it usually is."	☐	☐
"I will exercise indoors as much as possible."	☐	☐
"I will make sure to walk at least 3 times per week."	☐	☐
"I need to avoid straining, so I won't do push-ups or pull-ups."	☐	☐

Stand-Alone Items

Stand-Alone Item 1: Trend

Practice Question 10.25 — Stand-Alone Item 1: Trend

The nurse is caring for a 56-year-old client admitted 2 days ago from the ED for recurring atrial fibrillation.

History and Physical | Vital Signs | Nurses' Notes | Laboratory Results

History of atrial fibrillation, heart failure, and hypertension. Cardiac status has been well controlled with medications. Reports feeling skipped heartbeats and heart fluttering over the past 24 hours and swelling in the feet.

History and Physical | **Vital Signs** | Nurses' Notes | Laboratory Results

	1100: Day 1	0800: Day 2	0800: Day 3
T	98°F (36.6°C)	97.6°F (36.4°C)	98.2°F (36.7°C)
HR	84 and irregular	86 and regular	88 and regular
RR	20	20	22
BP	148/90	154/92	168/99
SpO₂	96% on 2 L/min O₂ via NC	96% on 2 L/min O₂ via NC	96% on 2 L/min O₂ via NC
Weight	164 lb (74.38 kg)	165 lb (74.84 kg)	168 lb (76.2 kg)
2400: 24-hour urine output	750 mL	535 mL	

History and Physical | Vital Signs | **Nurses' Notes** | Laboratory Results

1100 Day 1: Reports feeling skipped heartbeats and heart fluttering over the past 24 hours. Reports dyspnea on exertion. Lung sounds clear bilaterally. Oxygen administered. ECG shows atrial fibrillation. Labs drawn. IV catheter inserted. Treated with IV diltiazem, converted to NSR. 1+ ankle edema.

0800 Day 2: Denies feeling skipped heartbeats or heart fluttering. Reports feeling better, but still experiencing dyspnea on exertion. Slight crackles heard in right lung base. NSR on heart monitor. 1+ ankle edema.

0800 Day 3: Labs drawn. Denies feeling skipped heartbeats or heart fluttering. Reports ankles feel swollen, and is worried about another episode of heart failure; still experiencing dyspnea on exertion. Bilateral rhonchi heard in lung bases. NSR on heart monitor. 3+ ankle edema.

History and Physical | Vital Signs | Nurses' Notes | **Laboratory Results**

Test and Reference Range	Results Day 1	Results Day 3
Sodium 136–145 mEq/L (136–145 mmol/L)	141 mEq/L (141 mmol/L)	138 mEq/L (138 mmol/L)
Potassium 3.5–5.0 mEq/L (3.5–5.0 mmol/L)	5.0 mEq/L (5.0 mmol/L)	5.5 mEq/L (5.5 mmol/L)
Glucose 70–110 mg/dL (3.9–6.1 mmol/L)	106 mg/dL (6.0 mmol/L)	100 mg/dL (5.5 mmol/L)
Calcium 9.0–10.5 mEq/L (9.0–10.5 mmol/L)	9.0 mEq/L (9.0 mmol/L)	8.6 mEq/L (8.6 mmol/L)
Blood urea nitrogen (BUN) 8.0–23.0 mg/dL (2.9–8.2 mmol/L)	28 mg/dL (10.0 mmol/dL)	38 mg/dL (13.6 mmol/L)
Creatinine 0.6–1.2 mg/dL (53–106 μmol/L)	1.8 mg/dL (157.2 μmol/L)	3.1 mg/dL (274.1 μmol/L)
Hemoglobin (Hgb) 14.0–18.0 g/dL (140–180 g/L)	14.2 g/dL (142 g/L)	14.0 g/dL (140 g/L)
Hematocrit (Hct) 42%–54% (0.42–0.54 volume fraction)	46% (0.46 volume fraction)	44% (0.44 volume fraction)

*Based on the client assessment findings, select the **5** orders the nurse would anticipate.*

☐ Prepare the client for kidney imaging studies.
☐ Prepare the client for an echocardiogram.
☐ Administer a fluid challenge.
☐ Begin diuretic therapy.
☐ Maintain strict I&O, and record output hourly.
☐ Insert an indwelling urinary catheter.
☐ Prepare the client for hemodialysis.

Stand-Alone Item 2: Trend

Practice Question 10.26 — Stand-Alone Item 2: Trend

The nurse in the surgical unit is caring for a 51-year-old who had a thoracotomy for non–small-cell lung cancer.

Nurses' Notes | Vital Signs

1300: Arrived from the PACU. Alert and oriented × 4. Resting comfortably in bed, no restlessness. Closed chest tube drainage system intact. Upper tube is near right front lung apex; occlusive dressing dry and intact. Lower tube is on the right side near the base of the lung; occlusive dressing dry and intact. Drainage chamber 70 mL red fluid. Water seal chamber fluctuation of fluid, no bubbling. Suction control chamber gently bubbling. No subcutaneous emphysema. No shortness of breath or difficulty breathing. Lung sounds clear bilaterally. HOB elevated. Trachea midline. O_2 2 L/min via NC. Having difficulty with coughing and deep-breathing exercises and using an incentive spirometer. Pain rated 4/10.

1400: Alert and oriented × 4. Reports nausea. Restless; reports pain rated 8/10. Closed chest tube drainage system intact. Occlusive dressings dry and intact. Drainage chamber 170 mL red fluid. Water seal chamber fluctuation of fluid with intermittent bubbling. Suction control chamber gently bubbling. No subcutaneous emphysema. States difficulty breathing due to pain. Lung sounds clear bilaterally. HOB elevated. Trachea midline. O_2 2 L/min via NC. Refusing to cough and deep breathe or use incentive spirometer due to pain. Able to tolerate respiratory treatment with assistance of respiratory therapist. Nausea and pain medication administered as prescribed.

1500: Sleepy but arousable. Restless; reports nausea subsided and pain rated 7/10. Closed chest tube drainage system intact. Occlusive dressings dry and intact. Drainage chamber 170 mL red fluid. Water seal chamber continuously bubbling. Suction control chamber gently bubbling. Small amount subcutaneous emphysema around upper tube near right front lung apex. States difficulty breathing. Lung sounds crackles in lower lobes bilaterally. Trachea slight deviation to the left. O_2 2 L/min via NC. Refusing to cough and deep breathe.

Nurses' Notes | Vital Signs

	1300	1400	1500
T	99.6°F (37.5°C)	100.4°F (38°C)	101.6°F (38.6°C)
HR	88	96	110
RR	18	22	26
BP	100/62	128/88	140/90
SpO_2	94% on 2 L/min O_2 via NC	92% on 2 L/min O_2 via NC	90% on 2 L/min O_2 via NC

Select whether the following potential nursing actions are indicated or not indicated for the client at this time.

Nursing Action	Indicated	Not Indicated
Contact the surgeon.	☐	☐
Clamp the chest tube.	☐	☐
Request an order for a stat chest x-ray.	☐	☐
Request an order for additional pain medication.	☐	☐
Flush the chest drainage tube.	☐	☐
Increase the amount of suction in the suction control chamber.	☐	☐

Stand-Alone Item 3: Trend

Practice Question 10.27 — Stand-Alone Item 3: Trend

A 2-year-old child is seen in the ED, where the ED physician diagnoses moderate acute laryngotracheobronchitis.

Nurses' Notes | Vital Signs

1000: Client is alert and responsive. Resting comfortably in bed, no restlessness. Responsive to verbal and tactile stimuli. Chest symmetrical. Suprasternal retractions with nasal flaring. RR 34. Barking cough, labored breathing, use of accessory muscles. Inspiratory wheezes bilaterally. S1 and S2 noted, pulse 110. No murmurs, rubs, or gallops. No cyanosis, edema, clubbing, or pulsations. Radial pulses 2+ bilaterally. Pedal pulses 2+ bilaterally.

Nurses' Notes | **Vital Signs**

	1000	1015	1030
Temperature	99.6°F (37.5°C)	99.4°F (37.4°C)	99.6°F (37.5°C)
Apical pulse	110	112	112
RR	34	36	34
BP	100/62	98/60	98/60
SpO$_2$	94% on RA	92% on RA	90% on RA

Based on the assessment findings, which interventions would the nurse anticipate the ED physician will order? **Select all that apply.**

☐ Oral dexamethasone
☐ Supplemental oxygen
☐ Cool mist via facemask
☐ Intubation with ventilation
☐ Strict NPO status
☐ Nebulized epinephrine every 20 to 30 minutes prn
☐ Limited interaction between the parents and child

Stand-Alone Item 4: Bow-tie

Practice Question 10.28 — Stand-Alone Item 4: Bow-tie

0830: The nurse is assigned to care for a 70-year-old client in the ED for altered mental status.

History and Physical | Nurses' Notes | Vital Signs | Laboratory Results

0830: Client was brought to ED by a family member for altered mental status. Past medical history includes hypertension, overactive bladder, type 2 diabetes mellitus, and hyperlipidemia. According to the family member, the client has been feeling weak and confused since getting up this morning. Client's speech was slurred, and they appeared disoriented to time and place. Associated with decreased appetite and skipped meals. Client has been taking all medications as prescribed. Medications include lisinopril, oxybutynin, semaglutide, and atorvastatin.

History and Physical | **Nurses' Notes** | Vital Signs | Laboratory Results

0830: Client is restless, disoriented × 4, and agitated. Experiencing an altered level of consciousness, fluctuating between lucidity and confusion. Displays a disorganized thought process and speech pattern. Lungs clear to auscultation bilaterally. Regular cardiac rate and rhythm; no murmurs, rubs, or gallops. Visible skin clean, dry, and intact.

History and Physical | Nurses' Notes | **Vital Signs** | Laboratory Results

0830: T 98.6°F (37°C); HR 110; RR 26; BP 152/88; SpO$_2$ 96% on RA.

History and Physical | Nurses' Notes | Vital Signs | **Laboratory Results**

Test and Reference Range	Result
FSBS 70–99 mg/dL (3.9–5.5 mmol/L)	50 mg/dL (2.78 mmol/L)

*Complete the diagram by selecting from the choices below to specify what potential condition the client is likely experiencing, **2** nursing actions that are appropriate to take, and **2** parameters the nurse would monitor to assess the client's progress.*

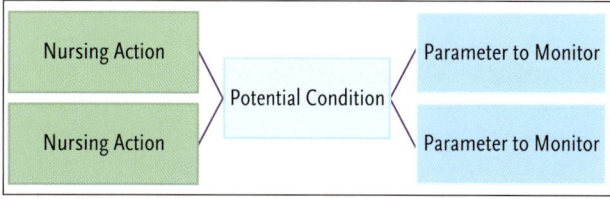

Actions to Take	Potential Condition	Parameters to Monitor
Coordinate neuropsychiatric testing	Anxiety	Suicidal ideation
Administer haloperidol intramuscularly	Delirium	Blood glucose level
Administer lorazepam intramuscularly	Dementia	Cognitive assessment
Administer dextrose 50% (D$_{50}$W) as a bolus injection	Psychosis	Quality-of-life assessment
Administer dextrose 10% (D$_{10}$W) as a continuous intravenous fluid		Extrapyramidal symptoms

Stand-Alone Item 5: Bow-tie

Practice Question 10.29 — Stand-Alone Item 5: Bow-tie

The nurse working in a long-term care facility is caring for a 78-year-old client with Parkinson disease.

History and Physical | Nurses' Notes | Vital Signs

78-year-old client residing in long-term care has been experiencing difficulty with mobility and activities of daily living. Has been experiencing dizziness and weakness upon standing and increased confusion for the past week. Known history of Parkinson disease diagnosed 10 years ago. Symptoms have progressively worsened despite treatment adjustments. Symptoms include bradykinesia, rigidity, resting tremor, and postural instability. Lived alone prior to transitioning to long-term care, and is widowed. Occasional visits from adult children who live out of state.

History and Physical | **Nurses' Notes** | Vital Signs

1000: Skin warm, dry, and intact. Lungs clear to auscultation bilaterally, no adventitious sounds. No use of accessory muscles. S1 and S2 noted, no S3 or S4; no murmurs, rubs, or gallops. No peripheral edema. Abdomen soft, nontender, and nondistended. Bowel sounds present × 4. Urine output: 360 mL in the past 8 hours. Reduced facial expression, infrequent eye blinking.

History and Physical | Nurses' Notes | **Vital Signs**

Lying	Sitting	Standing
HR 86 and regular	HR 98 and regular	HR 110 and regular
BP 154/92	BP 120/80	BP 90/62

Complete the diagram by selecting from the choices below to specify what potential condition the client is likely experiencing, 2 nursing actions that are appropriate to take, and 2 parameters the nurse would monitor to assess the client's progress.

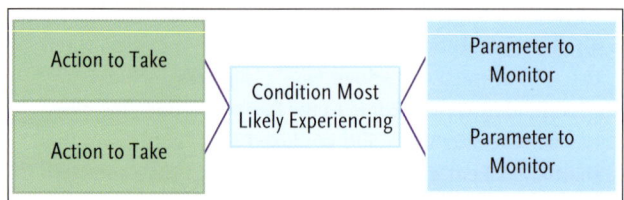

Actions to Take	Potential Condition	Parameters to Monitor
Assist with ambulation	Muscle atrophy	Urine output
Refer to physical therapy	Urinary retention	Gait assessment
Administer midodrine	Orthostatic hypotension	Muscle strength
Provide salt supplementation	Venous thromboembolism	Cognitive assessment
Perform straight catheterization		Positional HR and BP

Stand-Alone Item 6: Bow-tie

Practice Question 10.30 — Stand-Alone Item 6: Bow-tie

The nurse in the birthing suite performs an initial assessment on a newborn and documents the following data in the Nurses' Notes.

> **Nurses' Notes**
>
> **0800:** Newborn of 43 weeks' gestation born via vaginal delivery. Apgar score at 1 minute 3. Newborn limp, skin color bluish, RR 80, grunting during breathing with nasal flaring. Lacks cry with minimal response to gentle slap on soles. Nails and umbilical cord stained a yellow-green color. Blood glucose 40 mg/dL (2.2 mmol/L). Profuse scalp hair. Length 23 inches (58.42 cm), weight 5.5 lb (2500 g). SpO$_2$ 90% on RA.

Complete the diagram by selecting from the choices below to specify what potential condition the client is likely experiencing, **2** nursing actions that are appropriate to take, and **2** parameters the nurse would monitor to assess the client's progress.

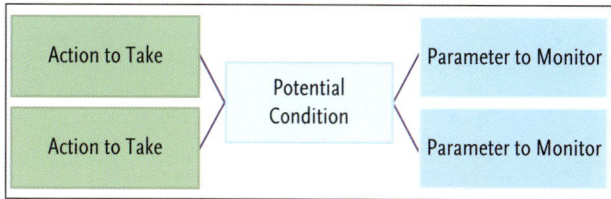

Actions to Take	Potential Condition	Parameters to Monitor
Suctioning	Acrocyanosis	Skin color
Oxygen therapy	Meconium aspiration syndrome	Umbilical cord color
Early feedings with dextrose	Large for gestational age	Blood glucose level
Phototherapy with a biliblanket	Transient tachypnea	Weight
Abdominal decompression with an NG tube		SpO$_2$

CHAPTER 3

Answers to Practice Questions

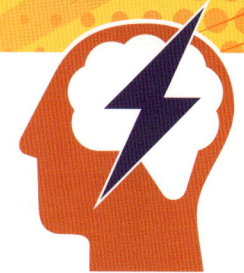

Practice Question 3.1 — Multiple Response Grouping

The nurse is caring for a newborn who was born 10 minutes ago.

Nurses' Notes

1025: 35-week-old baby born via cesarean section. Weight 4.4 lb (2000 g); length 19 in. (48.3 cm). Newborn crying with limp body posture and arms and legs very relaxed. Deep reflexes diminished and skin mottled. Intermittent expiratory grunting with occasional apneic episodes and fine crackles throughout lung fields bilaterally. VS: T 96.7°F (35.9°C) axillary; HR 132 and regular; RR 54; BP 68/40. Systolic murmur heard; changes intensity when newborn moves.

*For each body system listed below, select the newborn findings that require **immediate** follow-up. Each body system may support more than one relevant newborn finding.*

Body Systems	Newborn Findings
Respiratory	☐ RR 54
	☒ Intermittent expiratory grunting
	☐ Fine crackles
	☒ Occasional apneic episodes
Neuromuscular	☒ Arms and legs relaxed
	☐ Crying
	☒ Limp body posture
	☒ Diminished deep reflexes
Cardiovascular/Metabolic	☐ Skin mottled
	☒ Axillary temperature 96.7°F (35.9°C)
	☐ HR 132 and regular
	☐ Presence of systolic murmur

Rationale: For the respiratory system, the relevant client findings that require immediate follow-up are the newborn's expiratory grunting and apneic episodes because they indicate respiratory distress and impaired gas exchange. Fine crackles are common and expected, but coarse crackles would be abnormal and more concerning to the nurse. The normal/usual newborn RR is 30 to 60, so the RR is normal and expected. Mottled skin and crying are also typical for newborns. However, the arms and legs of a newborn are usually in a flexed position rather than a relaxed one. The limp posture and relaxed extremities with diminished deep reflexes could be the result of hypotonia or muscle atrophy, conditions that could result in respiratory compromise. These significant findings require immediate follow-up. The cardiovascular/metabolic findings, including the presence of a systolic murmur, are typical for a newborn with the exception of the body temperature, which is below normal. A subnormal temperature (hypothermia) may lead to systemic complications such as hypoglycemia and acidosis and would therefore be concerning to the nurse and require immediate follow-up. The normal newborn HR is 100 to 160.

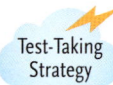

Test-Taking Strategy: Similar to the approach you would take for the sample questions in this chapter, you would identify normal/usual or abnormal and expected (not relevant), and abnormal and not expected (relevant) client findings for the newborn in this clinical scenario to measure *Recognize Cues*. The newborn's findings can be categorized as shown in the table.

Newborn Assessment Findings	Abnormal and Not Expected (Relevant) and Requiring Immediate Follow-up	Normal/Usual or Abnormal but Expected (Not Relevant) and Not Requiring Immediate Follow-up
Respirations: 40–60	☐	☒
Intermittent expiratory grunting	☒	☐
Fine crackles	☐	☒
Occasional apneic episodes	☒	☐
Arms and legs relaxed	☒	☐
Crying	☐	☒
Relaxed body posture	☒	☐
Diminished deep reflexes	☒	☐
Skin mottled	☐	☒
Axillary temperature: 96.7°F (35.9°C)	☒	☐
HR: 132 and regular	☐	☒
Presence of systolic murmur	☐	☒

Recall that a baby born between 34 and 36 weeks is considered to be a late preterm newborn, which may result in abnormal assessment findings. These findings are relevant and require immediate follow-up by the nurse to *Recognize Cues*.

Content Area: Obstetrics-Newborn Nursing
Priority Concepts: Gas Exchange; Perfusion
Reference(s): Lowdermilk et al., 2024, pp. 459–462

Practice Question 3.2   Highlight-in-Text

The nurse is caring for a 20-year-old client in the college campus health care clinic.

*Highlight the findings that require **immediate** follow-up.*

Nurses' Notes

1355: Client came to clinic with report of ==shakiness, unusual sweating, nausea, and vomiting==. Is concerned about getting sick with "stomach flu" or STI during "finals week." Attended a fraternity party 3 nights ago where food and alcohol were consumed. Had "sex" for first time with college football player after the party. Nausea and vomiting started this morning but has worsened with shakiness and diaphoresis. Alert and oriented × 4. Medical history of asthma since early childhood, meningitis last year, and COVID-19 twice in the past 2 years. Most recently was ==diagnosed with diabetes mellitus (DM) type 1==, which has been controlled by insulin and intermittent glucose monitoring. Skin cool and clammy. Breath sounds clear throughout lung fields. S₁ and S₂ present. Abdomen soft and round; BS × 4. Peripheral pulses 2+ and strong. VS: T 97.8°F (36.6°C); HR 92 and regular; RR 18; BP 106/50; SpO₂ 98% on RA; ==FSBG 52 mg/dL (2.9 mmol/L)==. (Reference range 74–106 mg/dL (4.1–5.9 mmol/L).

Rationale: The client presented with acute clinical findings including shakiness, diaphoresis, nausea, and vomiting, which need immediate follow-up to prevent or manage potentially life-threatening fluid and electrolyte imbalances. Cool and clammy skin occurs with diaphoresis and would not require immediate follow-up or be concerning to the nurse. The nurse would want to collect more data about the client's recent onset of diabetes mellitus type 1 because this condition could be related to the acute client findings. Additionally, the client's finger stick blood glucose (FSBG) value is below the reference range of 74 to 106 mg/dL (4.1–5.9 mmol/L), which requires immediate follow-up to ensure adequate major organ function. However, it is not at a critical low value at this point. The other client findings, including vital signs, are within normal limits. The client's history of infections and asthma are likely not significant or related to the client's current findings.

Test-Taking Strategy: Remember to first identify normal/usual or abnormal and expected (not relevant), and abnormal and not expected (relevant) client findings to determine which findings require immediate follow-up by the nurse. The client's findings can be categorized as shown in the table.

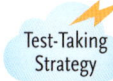
Test-Taking Strategy

Client Findings	Abnormal and Not Expected (Relevant) and Requiring Immediate Follow-Up	Normal/Usual or Abnormal but Expected (Not Relevant) and Not Requiring Immediate Follow-Up
Shakiness	☒	☐
Diaphoresis	☒	☐
Nausea and vomiting	☒	☐
Presence of S_1 and S_2	☐	☒
History of COVID-19	☐	☒
Recent onset DM	☒	☐
T 97.8°F (36.6°C)	☐	☒
BP 106/50	☐	☒
FSBG 52 mg/dL (2.9 mmol/L)	☒	☐

Next, review the findings that are abnormal and not expected for this particular client. These client findings are the significant cues in this clinical scenario and provide the correct responses to this test item measuring *Recognize Cues*.

Content Area: Medical-Surgical Nursing
Priority Concepts: Glucose Regulation; Fluid and Electrolyte Balance
Reference(s): Ignatavicius et al., 2024, pp.1369; Pagana et al., 2022, pp. 240–241

Practice Question 3.3 — Drag-and-Drop Cloze

The nurse is caring for a 78-year-old client who was hospitalized for evacuation of a subdural hematoma.

Nurses' Notes

0730: Very drowsy this morning but can be aroused with gentle shaking. Remains oriented × 4. Does not readily respond when spoken to, but eventually answers in 1 to 2 words. Immediately after surgery a week ago, the client was alert and oriented, communicative, and continent of bowel and bladder. No adventitious or diminished breath sounds. S_1 and S_2 present; no additional heart sounds. BS hyperactive × 4 and abdomen slightly distended. Had 2 incontinent diarrheal stools during the night. Able to move all extremities, but right arm continues to be weak. Skin intact; no reddened areas noted. Plan to send to PT and OT this morning. Temperature increased from 98°F (36.7°C) last evening to 100.2°F (37.9°C) currently.

Complete the following sentence by selecting from the word choices below.

The nurse determines that the client findings that require *immediate* follow-up are **drowsiness**, **incontinent diarrheal stools**, **speech difficulty**, and **elevated temperature**.

Word Choices

Drowsiness
No adventitious or diminished breath sounds
Right arm weakness
Hyperactive BS × 4
Incontinent diarrheal stools
Speech difficulty
Elevated temperature

Rationale: Immediately after surgery, the client was alert and oriented, communicative, and continent of bowel and bladder. The client's LOC changed from alert and oriented to drowsy and oriented. A decrease in LOC suggests that the client is likely clinically deteriorating, and this change would therefore be of immediate concern to the nurse and require follow-up. The client is less communicative and incontinent, which are also significant changes that would concern the nurse. The elevated temperature is not expected and could indicate a serious or life-threatening condition requiring immediate follow-up. The client's arm weakness was present after surgery, so this finding is expected and not concerning. Bowel sounds are hyperactive and expected when a client has diarrhea. Having no adventitious breath sounds is a desirable finding indicating that breath sounds are normal.

Test-Taking Strategy: To answer this test item correctly, you need to first compare the client's current assessment data with the previous data. Then categorize the client's findings as you would do for the other test items that measure *Recognize Cues*.

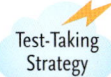

Client Findings	Abnormal and Not Expected (Relevant) Requiring Immediate Follow-up	Normal/Usual or Abnormal and Expected (Not Relevant) Not Requiring Immediate Follow-up
Drowsiness	☒	☐
No adventitious or diminished breath sounds	☐	☒
Elevated temperature	☒	☐
Right arm weakness	☐	☒
Hyperactive BS × 4	☐	☒
Incontinent diarrheal stools	☒	☐
Speech difficulty	☒	☐

To *Recognize Cues,* select the client findings that you determined to be abnormal and not expected (not relevant) because these findings require immediate follow-up to prevent potentially life-threatening conditions.

Content Area: Medical-Surgical Nursing
Priority Concepts: Cognition; Elimination
Reference(s): Ignatavicius et al., 2024, pp. 560–561

Practice Question 3.4 — Multiple Response Select All That Apply

The nurse is caring for a 43-year-old client in the inpatient psychiatric unit.

Nurses' Notes

1100: Admitted to unit for observation and treatment related to a suicide attempt. Attempted to cut both wrists, which are currently bandaged. Client was in a severe motor vehicle accident 5 months ago, resulting in tetraplegia. Has been living in a group home with full-time caregiver for assistance with ADLs since discharge from rehabilitation. Has no family living in the area. Has stage 3 sacral pressure injury covered with gauze dressing. Recently completed a course of antibiotics for infected sacral wound. Wears an external condom catheter and follows bowel regimen, but has frequent problems with urine leakage and bowel incontinence. Is able to transfer with supervision from bed to wheelchair using sliding board. Lost 20 lb (9.1 kg) since the accident, and describes appetite as "fair." Does not want to be here because the client is "sick of being in hospitals."

Which of the following findings require **immediate** follow-up related to risk factors for additional or worsening pressure injuries? **Select all that apply.**

- ☐ Attempted suicide
- ☒ Tetraplegia
- ☒ Current stage 3 sacral wound
- ☐ ADL dependent
- ☒ Sliding board for transfers
- ☒ Urinary and bowel incontinence
- ☐ 43 years of age
- ☐ Weight loss of 20 lb (9.1 kg)
- ☐ Fair appetite

Rationale: The nurse recognizes that the client is at high risk for additional or worsening pressure injury due to a number of factors. First, the client already has a stage 3 pressure injury, which resulted in full-thickness skin loss and infection. A local infection can lead to systemic infection and possibly sepsis, a potentially life-threatening health problem. The existence of a pressure injury suggests that the client is vulnerable to skin breakdown. As a result of the client's accident, the client has impaired mobility and is unable to walk. Impaired mobility is a major risk factor for skin breakdown and would be a concern for the nurse. Using a sliding board for transfers can lead to skin friction and shearing, especially due to decreased skin sensation. To add to impaired mobility, the client's skin is frequently soiled by urine and feces. Excessive skin moisture is a major risk factor and would therefore alert the nurse that the client is at high risk for skin and tissue breakdown. The client is not an older adult, meaning that skin should not be thinning to make the client vulnerable for skin integrity issues. Weight loss and fair appetite are likely not of concern at the moment because the client's original weight is not known, and those with tetraplegia have better mobility at a lower weight. The client's ADL dependence is expected and would not cause skin integrity problems. Attempted suicide is a relevant cue of immediate concern to the nurse and health care team; however, it is not a risk factor for the development of pressure injuries.

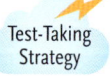

Test-Taking Strategy: To answer this question that assesses your ability to *Recognize Cues*, you need to think about what client findings could lead to additional problems with skin and tissue integrity as categorized in the table.

Client Findings	Abnormal or Expected, but Is a Risk Factor for Pressure Injury	Normal/Usual, Abnormal or Expected, but Not a Risk Factor for Pressure Injury
Attempted suicide	☐	☒
Tetraplegia	☒	☐
Current stage 3 sacral wound	☒	☐
ADL dependent	☐	☒
Uses sliding board for transfers	☒	☐
Urinary and bowel incontinence	☒	☐
43 years of age	☐	☒
Weight loss of 20 lb (9.1 kg)	☐	☒

As you probably realize, this client is at high risk for worsening pressure injury or new pressure injury due to the presence of many risk factors. To *Recognize Cues,* select the client findings that you determined to be abnormal and not expected (relevant) because these findings require immediate follow-up to prevent worsening pressure injury or new pressure injury.

Content Area: Foundations of Nursing
Priority Concepts: Tissue Integrity; Stress and Coping
Reference(s): Ignatavicius et al., 2024, pp. 445–446; Potter et al., 2023, pp. 1319–1321

Practice Question 3.5 — Matrix Multiple Choice

The nurse is caring for an 85-year-old client in the ED.

Nurses' Notes

1640: Client transported to ED via ambulance from skilled nursing facility. Family present and very concerned about client's condition. Client alert and oriented × 1 (person). Has difficulty talking due to shortness of breath. Reports feeling very "winded." Placed in sitting position; supplemental oxygen in place at 3 L/min. Skin warm and dry. Crackles present in both lungs; S_3 present. Abdomen slightly distended; BS present and distant × 4. Able to move all extremities. Peripheral pulses present and bounding. Cap refill >3 sec. Pitting 3+ edema in both feet. VS: T 97°F (36.1°C); HR 100 and irregular; RR 28; BP 138/76; SpO_2 92% on oxygen.

Complete the following table by selecting whether each client finding requires **immediate** *follow-up or does not require immediate follow-up.*

Client Findings	Requires Immediate Follow-Up	Does Not Require Immediate Follow-Up
Shortness of breath	☒	☐
Alert and oriented × 1	☐	☒
Crackles in both lungs	☒	☐
Bounding peripheral pulses	☒	☐
RR 28	☒	☐
BP 138/76	☐	☒
HR 100 and irregular	☐	☒
Cap refill >3 sec	☐	☒
Pitting 3+ edema both feet	☒	☐

Rationale: The client likely has excess body fluid or fluid overload as evidenced by pitting 3+ edema in both feet, bilateral crackles, and bounding peripheral pulses. Fluid overload in a client of advanced age can cause pulmonary edema (fluid in the lungs), which is a life-threatening condition. Therefore these findings require immediate follow-up. The client is already experiencing shortness of breath and tachypnea, which are likely contributing to the client's lack of orientation from hypoxia. Adequate oxygenation is needed to ensure proper functioning of body tissues, especially major organs like the heart, brain, and kidneys. Therefore being short of breath and tachypneic require immediate follow up. A capillary refill of more than 3 seconds is expected in older clients who typically have less elastic blood vessels and atherosclerosis. The client's blood pressure is somewhat elevated but would also be expected in clients who have excess fluid volume, or hypervolemia. A heart rate of 100 is within the normal range for adults.

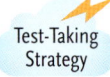

Test-Taking Strategy: Remember to first identify normal/usual or abnormal and expected (not relevant), and abnormal and not expected (relevant) client findings to determine which findings require immediate follow-up by the nurse. The client's findings can be categorized as shown in the table.

Client Findings	Abnormal and Not Expected (Relevant) and Requiring Immediate Follow-Up	Normal/Usual or Abnormal but Expected (Not Relevant) and Not Requiring Immediate Follow-Up
Shortness of breath	X	☐
Alert and oriented × 1	☐	X
Crackles in both lungs	X	☐
Bounding peripheral pulses	X	☐
RR 28	X	☐
BP 138/76	☐	X
HR 100 and irregular	☐	X
Cap refill >3 sec	☐	X
Pitting 3+ edema both feet	X	☐

To *Recognize Cues,* select the client findings that you determined to be abnormal and not expected (not relevant) because these findings require immediate follow-up to prevent potentially life-threatening conditions.

Content Area: Medical-Surgical Nursing
Priority Concepts: Perfusion; Gas Exchange
Reference(s): Ignatavicius et al., 2024, pp. 560–561

Practice Question 3.6 — Multiple Response Select N

The nurse is caring for a 13-year-old client in the Urgent Care Center.

Nurses' Notes

0850: Newcomer parent brought child for urgent care. Reports being in the country for only 2 weeks; speaks English fluently. Reports that child started having new GI symptoms 2 days ago, which could have been "caused by something eaten at the shelter." Child started with lack of appetite and nausea but progressed to fever and vomiting with occasional diarrhea. Last night, the child went to bed earlier than usual and showed no interest in playing games or watching TV. This morning parent noted dark urine in the toilet. Child's current temperature is 103.2°F (39.6°C). States feeling very tired and wants to go to bed.

*Select the **4** findings that require **immediate** follow-up.*

- ☒ Anorexia
- ☐ Occasional diarrhea
- ☒ Nausea and vomiting
- ☒ Elevated temperature
- ☐ Fatigue
- ☐ Wants to sleep
- ☒ Dark urine

Rationale: The child experienced new GI symptoms 2 days ago that included anorexia, nausea/vomiting, and elevated temperature (fever). These findings are significant and of immediate concern to the nurse because the child could become dehydrated and have electrolyte imbalances. These imbalances of fluids and electrolytes are potentially life-threatening and require immediate follow-up. Having dark urine is also of concern because this finding could be due to increased bilirubin caused by liver inflammation or dysfunction or by biliary obstruction. The liver is a vital organ needed for many body functions. The child's diarrhea is *not* concerning at this time because it is only occasional and commonly occurs in children with GI distress. Fatigue and desire to sleep are expected because of the client's GI symptoms and would not be of concern for the nurse at this time. Hypovolemia caused by fluid loss through vomiting (combined perhaps with occasional diarrhea) can also cause these symptoms.

Test-Taking Strategy: For this test item, you need to categorize the client findings as those that are within normal/usual limits or abnormal but expected (not relevant), or abnormal and not expected (relevant), as shown in the table, to *Recognize Cues*. Then you will be able to easily select the correct options.

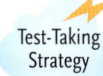
Test-Taking Strategy

Client Findings	Abnormal and Not Expected (Relevant) Requiring Immediate Follow-up	Normal/Usual or Abnormal and Expected (Not Relevant) Not Requiring Immediate Follow-up
Anorexia	X	☐
Occasional diarrhea	☐	X
Nausea and vomiting	X	☐
Fever	X	☐
Fatigue	☐	X
Wants to sleep	☐	X
Dark urine	X	☐

To *Recognize Cues,* select the client findings that you determined to be abnormal and not expected (not relevant) because these findings require immediate follow-up to prevent potentially life-threatening conditions.

Content Area: Pediatric Nursing
Priority Concepts: Elimination; Fluid and Electrolyte Balance
Reference(s): Hockenberry et al., 2024, pp. 815

CHAPTER 4

Answers to Practice Questions

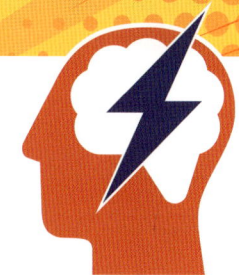

Practice Question 4.1 — Drop-Down Rationale

A 45-year-old client diagnosed with CKD requires dialysis. As a candidate for both hemodialysis and peritoneal dialysis, the client decides that peritoneal dialysis is the better option for their lifestyle. The client is hospitalized and undergoes insertion of the peritoneal dialysis catheter, and the first dialysis procedure is ordered. The nurse documents predialysis assessment data and reviews laboratory results.

Vital Signs | Laboratory Results

1100: T 98.2°F (36.8°C); apical HR 90 and regular; BP 146/98; RR 16; breath sounds clear bilaterally. Weight 160 lb (72.57 kg)

Vital Signs | **Laboratory Results**

Test and Reference Range	Result
Blood urea nitrogen (BUN) 10–20 mg/dL (3.6–7.1 mmol/L)	30 mg/dL (10.8 mmol/L)
Creatinine 0.5–1.2 mg/dL (44–106 µmol/L)	6.0 mg/dL (528 µmol/L)
Glucose 70–99 mg/dL (3.9–5.5 mmol/L)	110 mg/dL (6.1 mmol/L)
Sodium 135–145 mEq/L (135–145 mmol/L)	150 mEq/L (150 mmol/L)
Potassium 3.5–5.0 mEq/L (3.5–5.0 mmol/L)	5.5 mEq/L (5.5 mmol/L)

During dialysis infusion, the nurse notes a slow inflow of the dialysate, and the client complains of pain. On assessment of the catheter, the nurse notes some fibrin clot formation in the dialysis tubing. **Complete the following sentence by choosing from the lists of options provided.**

The nurse recognizes that the slow inflow, presence of fibrin clots, and complaints of pain are *most likely* the result of the <u>initial dialysis treatment</u> due to the <u>surgical procedure</u>.

Options for 1	Options for 2
Peritonitis	Catheter slippage
Initial dialysis treatment	Surgical procedure
Bowel perforation	Lack of aseptic technique
Abdominal pressure	Elevated BP and laboratory results

Rationale: Pain during the inflow of dialysate is common when a client is initially started on peritoneal dialysis therapy following the surgical procedure and catheter placement. Usually, this pain no longer occurs 1 to 2 weeks after receiving these treatments. Warming the dialysate bags before instillation by using a heating pad to wrap the bag or by using the warming chamber of the automated cycling machine will assist in preventing pain. Slow inflow of the dialysate is not uncommon initially but should always be assessed because it could be due to a kink in the tubing or fibrin clots. Fibrin clot formation is not uncommon after catheter placement, although it is also important to know that it can occur with peritonitis. In this client situation, fibrin clot formation is most likely an expected finding because the client recently had the catheter placed and because there are no associated findings of peritonitis, such as fever. In addition, it is not likely that signs of peritonitis would show just after catheter placement. Milking the tubing may dislodge the fibrin clot and improve flow. Bowel perforation would be exhibited by a brown-colored outflow. Abdominal pressure may occur on inflow and may cause minimal discomfort, but this is an unlikely occurrence in this client situation; also, fibrin clots are not associated with abdominal pressure.

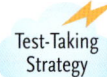

Test-Taking Strategy: The first thing you would do is look at the client data and use knowledge about the peritoneal dialysis procedure and expected and unexpected findings. Think about what the findings presented mean and what could be happening to the client. The elevated BP and laboratory findings are expected in a client with CKD predialysis, indicating the need for dialysis. If the catheter slips and is malpositioned, fluid will not drain in or out. Also, note that this scenario presents a client receiving the first dialysis treatment after insertion of the dialysis catheter. Next, look at the options presented, and think about what you would expect to note in each of these conditions. Construct a table to help organize your thoughts to answer correctly. In a Drop-Down Rationale item, it is important to select the correct answer for the first option so you can correctly pair the information with the second option choices.

Condition	Expected Findings
Peritonitis	Fever, which is not likely to be present initially after insertion, even if there was a lack of aseptic technique
Initial dialysis treatment	Pain, slow inflow, and fibrin clots initially due to a new catheter
Bowel perforation	A complication, but the most likely finding is brown outflow
Abdominal pressure	May be present on inflow, but pain would be minimal and expected; this is unrelated to fibrin clots

Content Area: Medical-Surgical Nursing
Priority Concept: Elimination, Tissue Integrity
Reference(s): Ignatavicius et al., 2024, pp. 1482–1487

Practice Question 4.2 — Drop-Down Rationale

An 80-year-old client who had a cholecystectomy 2 weeks ago was admitted 2 hours ago to the medical-surgical unit from the ED with acute pain located in the left upper abdomen. The client had laboratory testing and a contrast-enhanced CT scan of the abdomen. The nurse conducts an admission assessment and reviews the laboratory and diagnostic results.

Vital Signs | Laboratory Results | Diagnostic Results

1100: T 100.8°F (38.2°C); HR 90; BP 168/88; RR 24; SpO$_2$ 89% on RA; lung sounds clear but diminished to auscultation bilaterally, and breathing is nonlabored.

Vital Signs | **Laboratory Results** | Diagnostic Results

Test and Reference Range	Result
White blood cells (WBCs) 5000–10,000/mm³ (5–10 × 10⁹/L)	16,000/mm³ (16 × 10⁹/L)
Hemoglobin (Hgb) 12–18 g/dL (120–180 g/L)	16 g/dL (160 g/L)
Hematocrit (Hct) 37%–52% (0.37–0.52)	44% (0.44)
Blood urea nitrogen (BUN) 10–20 mg/dL (3.6–7.1 mmol/L)	18 mg/dL (6.48 mmol/L)
Creatinine 0.5–1.2 mg/dL (44–106 μmol/L)	0.8 mg/dL (70.6 μmol/L)
Glucose 70–99 mg/dL (3.9–5.5 mmol/L)	110 mg/dL (6.1 mmol/L)
Alanine aminotransferase (ALT) 4–36 U/L (4–36 U/L)	80 U/L (80 U/L)
Aspartate aminotransferase (AST) 0–35 U/L (0–35 U/L)	88 U/L (88 U/L)
Activated partial thromboplastin time (aPTT) 30–40 sec (30–40 sec)	32 sec (32 sec)
Prothrombin time (PT) 11–12.5 sec (11–12.5 sec)	11.4 sec (11.4 sec)
International normalized ratio (INR) 0.81–1.2 (0.81–1.2)	1.0 (1.0)
Amylase 60–120 U/L (60–120 U/L)	800 U/L (800 U/L)
Lipase 0–160 U/L (0–160 U/L)	320 U/L (320 U/L)

Vital Signs | Laboratory Results | **Diagnostic Results**

CT abdomen with contrast impression: Edema of the uncinate process of the pancreatic head, with peripancreatic fat, consistent with acute interstitial pancreatitis

Based on the assessment findings, complete the following sentence by choosing from the lists of options provided.

As a complication of acute pancreatitis, the client is at **highest** risk for developing **atelectasis** as evidenced by **SpO₂ level**.

Options for 1	Options for 2
Atelectasis	SpO₂ level
Bile duct calculi	PT/INR results
Pulmonary edema	CT abdomen results
Coagulation defects	BUN and creatinine levels

Rationale: Acute pancreatitis is an acute inflammation of the pancreas, and complications associated with acute pancreatitis can sometimes be life-threatening. Atelectasis, bile duct calculi, pulmonary edema, and coagulation defects are all potential complications of acute pancreatitis. Older adults are at risk for developing atelectasis and resultant pneumonia as a complication of acute pancreatitis. The overall clinical presentation, including leukocytosis, hyperglycemia, elevated liver enzymes and pancreatic enzymes, and the CT results, is consistent with acute pancreatitis. The elevation in BP is likely due to pain. Other clinical manifestations include the elevated temperature, RR 24, SpO_2 89% on RA, and diminished lung sounds bilaterally. These findings point to atelectasis as the most likely complication of this condition.

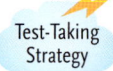

Test-Taking Strategy: You need to interpret the assessment findings to determine what is happening to the client. Note that some findings are expected in acute pancreatitis. Also note that the question is asking about a complication of acute pancreatitis in which the client is at highest risk. Remember to first think about client conditions consistent with the assessment findings or cues. Ask yourself if there are any findings or cues that support or oppose any client conditions. Decide which cues are of concern and which are expected, and establish the significance of the findings within the context of the larger clinical picture. In a Drop-Down Rationale item type, you have to understand both, or all aspects of the concepts being tested in order to receive credit. To answer this question correctly, use the "Supports" strategy as illustrated in the table below.

Assessment Finding	Supports Atelectasis	Supports Bile Duct Calculi	Supports Pulmonary Edema	Supports Coagulation Defects
SpO_2 89% on RA	☒	☐	☒	☐
Age	☒	☐	☐	☐
Elevated WBCs	☒	☐	☐	☐
Diminished lung sounds	☒	☐	☐	☐
RR 24	☒	☐	☐	☐
aPPT, PT, INR	☐	☐	☐	☒

Categorizing the findings of each complication listed in the options is a strategy that will help you analyze cues and determine which client findings support the possible complications. The complication with the most supportive findings is most likely the correct answer for the first option. The low SpO_2 level, the elevated RR, and diminished lung sounds bilaterally support atelectasis. In pulmonary edema, there would be a low SpO_2 level, labored breathing, sputum production, and adventitious lung sounds such as rhonchi or crackles. The coagulation study findings would be normal in atelectasis, whereas these results would be abnormal in coagulation defects. The CT results support acute pancreatitis and differentiate bile duct calculi, as calculi would be noted in the CT results if this complication were present. The BUN and Cr levels are normal and therefore are not related.

Content Area: Medical-Surgical Nursing
Priority Concept: Gas Exchange, Inflammation
Reference(s): Ignatavicius et al., 2024, pp. 1247–1248

Practice Question 4.3 — Drag-and-Drop Cloze

A 7-year-old child is brought to the ED by a parent who reports that the child has had no energy these past few weeks and was very sleepy this morning and difficult to arouse. The nurse assesses the child, gathers data from the parent, and documents the following findings.

Nurses' Notes | Vital Signs

Child sleepy, responds to verbal stimuli and repeated commands slowly
Parent reports that the child has had no sick contacts and has been attending full days of school until today, and the child told the parent about being really tired and had a headache.
Parent reports that the child has been thirsty lately and urinating very frequently, even during the night. Parent reports thinking that the increased urination had to do with the increased fluid intake but became concerned this morning about the child because of the tiredness and feeling weak.
Child cheeks are flushed, skin dry, mucous membranes dry and crusty
Fruity, acetone-like breath odor
Reflexes diminished, muscle strength poor
Denies neck stiffness; no swelling of the neck or lymph nodes
Denies cough or difficulty breathing; lung sounds clear
Immunizations up-to-date
Allergies: No known allergies

Nurses' Notes | **Vital Signs**

Weight: 55 lb (59th percentile), parent reports that child has lost some weight over the past few weeks
Height: 49.25 inches (55th percentile)
BMI: 15.94 (58th percentile)
T: 97.9°F (36.6°C) temporal
HR: 70, pulse weak
RR: 24 deep
BP: 108/70

Complete the following sentence by choosing from the lists of options below.

Based on the assessment findings, the nurse would **most likely** suspect **hyperglycemia** because of **fruity, acetone-like breath odor** and **thirst and increased urination**.

Options for 1	Options for 2	Options for 3
Hyperglycemia	Flushed cheeks	Thirst and increased urination
Influenza	Fruity, acetone-like breath odor	Dry and crusty mucous membranes
Hypoglycemia	Poor muscle strength	Subnormal temperature reading
Hypothyroidism	Sleepiness	Weak pulse

Rationale: Diabetes is a chronic disorder of metabolism characterized by hyperglycemia and insulin resistance. Manifestations include polyphagia, polyuria, polydipsia, weight loss, nocturia, irritability, shortened attention span, fatigue, dry skin, blurred vision, flushed skin, and poor wound healing. Hypoglycemia and hyperglycemia are acute complications associated with diabetes. In hypoglycemia the blood glucose is low, and manifestations include irritability, nervousness, tremors, difficulty concentrating, hunger, headaches, dizziness, pallor and sweating, shallow respirations, and tachycardia. In hyperglycemia the blood glucose is elevated, and manifestations include lethargy, dulled sensorium and confusion, thirst, weakness, nausea and vomiting, abdominal pain, flushed skin and signs of dehydration, dry and crusty mucous membranes, deep and rapid (Kussmaul) respirations, weak pulse, diminished reflexes, paresthesia, and fruity, acetone-like breath odor.

Influenza is a viral infection. Manifestations may be subclinical, mild, moderate, or severe. It is usually characterized by a dry cough, hoarseness, sudden onset of fever and chills, flushed face, photophobia, myalgia, sore throat, headache, and malaise. It is sometimes accompanied by vomiting and diarrhea.

Clinical manifestations of hypothyroidism depend on the extent of dysfunction and the child's age at onset. Manifestations can include impaired growth and development, skin changes (dry skin, puffiness around the eyes, sparse hair), constipation, lethargy, and mental decline.

Test-Taking Strategy: Remember to first think about client conditions consistent with the findings or cues. Ask yourself if there are any findings or cues that support or oppose any client conditions. Decide which cues are of concern, and establish the significance of the findings within the context of the larger clinical picture to determine what the findings mean and what is happening to the child. In a Drag-and-Drop Cloze question, partial credit is given if correct and incorrect answers are chosen. Choosing correctly as you begin answering the question will help you choose the greatest number of correct answers. In this question, thinking about the assessment findings noted and what the parent reports will help you answer the question correctly. Categorize the findings as noted in the table to assist in answering correctly.

Assessment Findings	Hyperglycemia	Influenza	Hypothyroidism	Hypoglycemia
Flushed cheeks	☒	☒	☐	☐
Fruity, acetone-like breath odor	☒	☐	☐	☐
Poor muscle strength	☒	☒	☐	☐
Sleepiness	☒	☐	☒	☐
Thirst and increased urination	☒	☐	☐	☐
Dry crusty mucous membranes	☒	☐	☐	☐
Subnormal temperature reading	☐	☐	☒	☐
Weak pulse	☒	☐	☐	☐

Categorizing the findings of each possible problem using this table is another strategy that will help you analyze cues and determine which condition is most likely occurring. Some findings are related to more than one problem. The condition with the most findings is most likely the correct answer. You need to rely to some extent on your knowledge base of the differences in clinical manifestations for these conditions. Note that most of the manifestations relate to hyperglycemia. Also note that there are no manifestations associated with hypoglycemia, which also cues you to think that the opposite condition (hyperglycemia) is likely the problem.

Content Area: Pediatric Nursing
Priority Concept: Fluid and Electrolyte Balance; Glucose Regulation
Reference(s): Hockenberry et al., 2024, pp. 844–845; 1181–1182; 1193–1208

Practice Question 4.4 — Drop-Down Cloze

A single parent arrives at the homeless mobile medical unit and asks to speak to a nurse about feelings being experienced. The parent is holding their infant and reports that the infant was born 2 months ago. The nurse performs an assessment on the parent and documents vital signs and Nurses' Notes in the medical record.

Vital Signs

T: 98°F (36.6°C)
HR: 68
RR: 18
BP: 188/72
SpO_2: 98% on RA

Nurses' Notes

Parent holding infant; infant still and sleeping
Reports feeling a loss of interest in everything that started a few weeks before the birth of the baby and feels that symptoms are worsening
Feels as though the infant is demanding and does not feel pleasure with caring for the infant; feeling inept as a parent
Expresses fear, worthlessness, guilt, and a lack of ability to care for self and the infant because of being a single parent and unhoused
Has no appetite and has lost weight; difficulty sleeping
Breast-feeding the infant, but does not think that the infant is getting enough milk

Complete the following sentence by choosing from the list of options provided.

Based on the assessment findings, the nurse determines that the parent is **most likely** experiencing **peripartum depression**.

Options

Bipolar disorder
Postpartum psychosis
Postpartum obsessive-compulsive disorder
Peripartum depression

Rationale: *Peripartum depression* is a term used to describe the onset of a depressive disorder during pregnancy or postpartum. The health problem is designated as peripartum because the first episodes of depression occurred during the antepartum period. Manifestations include a depressed mood with loss of interest in usual activities and a loss of usual emotional response to family. Although the person cares for the infant, the parent is unable to feel love or caring, sees the infant as demanding, and sees self as inept. Changes in appetite, sleep patterns, feelings of worthlessness or guilt, and difficulty concentrating and making decisions occur. Most of the symptoms are intensely and consistently present for at least a 2-week period and tend to become worse over time.

Those with bipolar disorder experience periods of irritability, hyperactivity, euphoria, and grandiosity. They exhibit little need for sleep and are not aware they have a problem. Their poor judgment and confusion make self-care and infant care impossible, which can be life-threatening. The depressions of bipolar disorder are characterized by tearfulness, preoccupation with guilt and feelings of worthlessness, and sleep and appetite alterations. Delusions and hallucinations may also be present.

Postpartum psychosis is a state in which the person's ability to recognize reality, communicate, and relate to others is impaired. Manifestations include agitation, irritability, rapidly shifting moods, disorientation, and disorganized behavior.

Postpartum obsessive-compulsive disorder is a health problem in which the parent has consuming thoughts about harming the baby and fear of being alone with the baby. Anxiety and depression occur, and the parent may perform compulsive behaviors to avoid acting on thoughts.

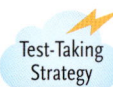

Test-Taking Strategy: Remember to first think about client conditions consistent with the findings or cues. Ask yourself if there are any findings or cues that support or oppose any client conditions. Decide which cues are of concern and unexpected, and establish the significance of the findings within the context of the overall clinical picture. For this question, use knowledge about the manifestations associated with each health problem in the options. It may be helpful to organize the information by creating a table listing the assessment findings and each condition presented in the options and then determining which findings are associated with the condition.

Assessment Findings	Bipolar Disorder Yes/Not Associated/ Possibly	Postpartum Psychosis Yes/Not Associated/ Possibly	Postpartum Obsessive-Compulsive Disorder Yes/Not Associated/ Possibly	Peripartum Depression Yes/Not Associated/ Possibly
Feeling a loss of interest in everything that started before the birth of the baby	Not Associated	Not Associated	Not Associated	Yes
Does not feel pleasure with caring for the infant	Not Associated	Not Associated	Not Associated	Yes
Feeling inept as a parent	Not Associated	Not Associated	Not Associated	Yes
Expressing fear, worthlessness, and guilt	Yes	Not Associated	Not Associated	Yes
Lacks ability to care for self and the infant	Yes	Possibly	Possibly	Yes
Has no appetite and has lost weight	Yes	Possibly	Possibly	Yes
Not able to sleep	Yes	Possibly	Possibly	Yes

Categorizing the assessment findings for each health problem as illustrated in the table and using knowledge of the manifestations of each disorder is a strategy that will help you *Analyze Cues*. Then, connecting this knowledge and analysis of each manifestation with the health problem will help you select the correct option.

Content Area: Maternal-Newborn Nursing
Priority Concept: Reproduction; Stress and Coping
Reference(s): Lowdermilk et al., 2024, pp. 666, 675

Practice Question 4.5 — Multiple Choice Select All That Apply

A 45-year-old client is admitted to the ED because of frequent episodes of chest pain unrelieved by sublingual nitroglycerin. The ECG shows ST segment elevation. Troponin levels are elevated. While awaiting results of diagnostic studies and transfer to the cardiac unit, the nurse monitors the client and checks vital signs.

Vital Signs

- **1200:** HR 88; RR 22; BP 142/86
- **1215:** HR 92; RR 24; BP 120/82
- **1230:** HR 106 and weak; RR 28; BP 100/62
- **1245:** HR 120 and weak; RR 32; BP 90/58

The nurse determines that these vital sign findings **most likely** indicate which complication(s)? **Select all that apply.**

- ☐ Dysrhythmias
- ☐ Pulmonary edema
- ☒ Cardiogenic shock
- ☐ Cardiac tamponade
- ☐ Pulmonary embolism
- ☐ Dissecting aortic aneurysm

Rationale: Cardiogenic shock occurs with severe damage (more than 40%) to the left ventricle. Classic signs include hypotension; a rapid heart rate that becomes weaker; decreased urine output; and cool, clammy skin. The respiratory rate increases as the body develops metabolic acidosis from shock. Dysrhythmias would be detected by changes in the rate and rhythm of the pulse and would be evidenced on the cardiac monitor and ECG. Although ST segment elevation is noted, there is no evidence of dysrhythmias as a complication. Pulmonary edema is evidenced by severe dyspnea and breathlessness with adventitious breath sounds. Cardiac tamponade is accompanied by distant, muffled heart sounds and prominent neck vessels. Pulmonary embolism presents suddenly with severe dyspnea accompanying the chest pain. Dissecting aortic aneurysms usually are accompanied by back pain.

Test-Taking Strategy: Focus on the words *most likely* in the question. Begin answering this question by analyzing each of the options and thinking about the manifestations of the condition and the most likely effect of each condition on the vital signs. Keeping in mind the pathophysiology associated with each condition will help you determine the most likely effect. As illustrated in the table, cardiogenic shock, cardiac tamponade, pulmonary embolism, and dissecting aortic aneurysm are conditions likely to cause the changes in vital signs noted in this clinical scenario.

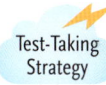

Client Condition	Most Common Vital Signs Effect: Increase, Decrease, or Both Increase or Decrease
Dysrhythmias	P: both, R: both, BP: both (depending on dysrhythmia)
Pulmonary edema	P: increase, R: increase, BP: increase
Cardiogenic shock	P: increase, R: increase, BP: decrease
Cardiac tamponade	P: increase, R: increase, BP: decrease
Pulmonary embolism	P: increase, R: increase, BP: decrease
Dissecting aortic aneurysm	P: increase, R: increase, BP: decrease

Next, you need to consider the other client data presented including the ECG finding (ST segment elevation) and elevated troponin levels. Next, make the connection between these abnormal findings and the most likely client condition—cardiogenic shock. Although the vital signs findings in this clinical scenario are also consistent with cardiac tamponade and pulmonary embolism, the other client data are not usually found in these conditions. This will direct you to cardiogenic shock as the correct answer.

Content Area: Medical-Surgical Nursing
Priority Concept: Gas Exchange, Perfusion
Reference(s): Ignatavicius et al., 2024, pp. 564, 598–603, 667–673, 702–703, 746–747, 761–763, 773, 795–799, 1473

Practice Question 4.6 — Matrix Multiple Response

At 1300 hours, an 86-year-old client with altered mental status who is accompanied by their neighbor is admitted to the medical-surgical unit, and the nurse is performing an assessment. The client has an IV solution of a 1000-mL bag of 0.9% sodium chloride hung at 1200 in the ED that is infusing at 100 mL/h. At 1400 hours, 1 hour after admission, the client's neighbor calls the nurse and reports that the client has a pounding headache, is having trouble breathing, and seems scared. The nurse assesses the client, reviews the laboratory results, and documents in the Nurses' Notes.

Nurses' Notes

1300: Client is weak and reports has not been able to eat or drink in the past 3 days because of anorexia.
Skin is very dry, dry mucous membranes, sleepy.
Client reports a history of heart failure, hypertension, and hyperlipidemia.
Breath sounds clear bilaterally.
Medications include lisinopril, carvedilol, and digoxin.
1400: Client is dyspneic and complaining of chest tightness, coughing, and is pale; neck vein distention is seen. Breath sounds wheezing and congestion bilaterally; 500 mL remaining in the IV bag.

Vital Signs

1300: T 100.2°F (36.8°C); apical HR 72 and regular; BP 100/68; RR 24; SpO₂ 90% on RA
1400: T 100.2°F (36.8°C); apical HR 110 and regular; BP 152/98; RR 28; SpO₂ 89% on RA

Laboratory Results

Test and Reference Range	Result
Blood urea nitrogen (BUN) 10–20 mg/dL (3.6–7.1 mmol/L)	24 mg/dL (8.64 mmol/L)
Creatinine 0.5–1.2 mg/dL (44–106 µmol/L)	1.8 mg/dL (159.4 µmol/L)
Digoxin 0.5–2.0 ng/mL (0.64–2.56 nmol/L)	2.2 ng/mL (2.8 nmol/L)
Sodium 135–145 mEq/L (135–145 mmol/L)	148 mEq/L (148 mmol/L)
Potassium 3.5–5.0 mEq/L (3.5–5.0 mmol/L)	5.2 mEq/L (5.2 mmol/L)

For each assessment finding below, click to specify if the finding is **most likely** *consistent with dehydration, circulatory overload, or digoxin toxicity. Check one response only for each row.*

Assessment Finding	Dehydration	Circulatory Overload	Digoxin Toxicity
Anorexia	☐	☐	☒
Dry mucous membranes	☒	☐	☐
BUN and creatinine levels	☒	☐	☐
Sodium and potassium levels	☒	☐	☐
Digoxin level	☐	☐	☒
Elevation in BP and RR	☐	☒	☐
Wheezing and congestion bilaterally in lungs	☐	☒	☐
Neck vein distention	☐	☒	☐

Rationale: Dehydration is a condition in which the body has a lower than needed amount of body fluid. At admission, this client showed signs of dehydration and reported weakness. The client's skin and mucous membranes were very dry, and the client was sleepy. In addition, the BUN, creatinine, sodium, and potassium are elevated, also noted in dehydration and due to the loss of fluid affecting cellular regulation. The dehydration is likely a result of the client not being able to eat or drink for the past 3 days.

Circulatory overload occurs when the volume of fluid in the body is greater than the body needs, and fluid accumulates faster than the circulatory system can compensate for the large volume of fluid. Fluid exists in greater amounts than needed in the extracellular compartments. An older client is at risk because of changes in the circulatory system due to the aging process. In addition, those with compromised cardiac function, such as a client with heart failure, are at greatest risk. In this client, 400 mL of fluid is infused during a 1-hour period (inadvertently, because the prescribed rate was 100 mL/h), and this is the likely cause of the circulatory overload. Some of the signs and symptoms of circulatory overload include headache, dyspnea, orthopnea, wheezing, tightness in the chest, cough, cyanosis, tachypnea, rapid increase in BP, and distended neck veins.

A client taking digoxin is at risk for digoxin toxicity. The therapeutic digoxin level ranges from 0.5 ng/mL (0.66 nmol/L) to 2.0 ng/mL (2.6 nmol/L). A digoxin level of 2.2 ng/mL (2.8 nmol/L) is above the therapeutic level. Early signs of digoxin toxicity are mental status changes and GI alterations that include anorexia, nausea, vomiting, and diarrhea. Bradycardia or tachycardia can occur, and the client develops visual disturbances such as blurred vision and changes in colors.

Test-Taking Strategy: Begin answering this question by analyzing the data provided in the Nurses' Notes, Laboratory Results, and Vital Signs tabs of the medical record. Note the words *most likely* in the question. For each of the findings, thinking about whether the finding is associated with the client condition and why or why not it is associated will assist in answering the question correctly. Drawing from your nursing knowledge, try to recall the signs and symptoms of the conditions in the question, list the findings from the medical record, and then determine whether they are related or not related. Some findings are the opposite of what you would see; this makes sense because the client is being treated for dehydration with rehydration measures. Therefore thinking about the complications of the treatment, it is possible for opposite findings to be noted depending on outcomes of the treatment. Organize your thinking process as illustrated in the table, listing the most likely findings in the first row and then noting in each row if the listed finding is related or not related.

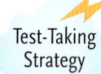
Test-Taking Strategy

Assessment Finding	Dehydration	Circulatory Overload	Digoxin Toxicity
Most likely findings	Dry mucous membranes, mental status changes, weakness, low-grade fever, decreased and concentrated urine, hemoconcentration, elevated BUN and creatinine levels, hypotension	Headache, shortness of breath, cough, elevated BP, puffiness around the eyes, dependent edema, neck vein distention, congestion in the lungs	Anorexia, blurred vision, mental status changes, dysrhythmias, nausea, vomiting, and diarrhea
Anorexia	Not related	Not related	Related
Dry mucous membranes	Related	Not related (opposite)	Not related
BUN and creatinine levels	Related	Not related	Not related
Sodium and potassium levels	Related	Not related	Not related (potassium opposite)
Digoxin level	Not related	Not related	Related
Elevated BP and RR	Not related (opposite)	Related	Not related
Wheezing and congestion bilaterally in lungs	Not related	Related	Not related
Neck vein distention	Not related (opposite)	Related	Not related

This thinking process demonstrates how to consider the findings in the question and analyze and interpret them, fitting them into the clinical picture. Using visual aids is a very helpful way to ensure that you are considering everything you need to and drawing on all available knowledge to direct you to the correct options.

Content Area: Medical-Surgical Nursing
Priority Concept: Fluid and Electrolyte Balance, Perfusion
Reference(s): Ignatavicius et al., 2024, pp. 256–260, 673–674, 699–700, 707

CHAPTER 5

Answers to Practice Questions

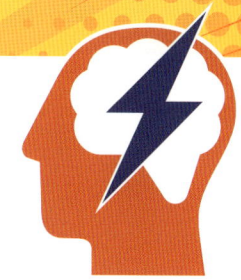

Practice Question 5.1 — Multiple Response Grouping

A 12-year-old client visits the health care clinic for a follow-up visit after laboratory and other testing.

Health History | Nurses' Notes | Diagnostic Tests | Laboratory Results

0900: Parent states that client was diagnosed at 3 years of age with cystic fibrosis (CF).

Health History | Nurses' Notes | Diagnostic Tests | Laboratory Results

0900: VS: T 98.2°F (36.6°C); HR 78; RR 16; BP 118/70; SpO$_2$ 96% on RA; denies pain.
Skin: Warm, dry, intact.
Respiratory: Dry cough. Reports sputum expectoration of thick, white mucus following respiratory treatments. Lung sounds clear to auscultation in all lung fields.
GI: Increased appetite. Reports taking pancreatic enzymes with all meals and snacks. Bowel sounds active × 4 quadrants. Regular bowel movements that are brown and fatty.
GU: Urinating more frequently than usual.
Weight: 91.5 lb (41.5 kg)
Height: 59 inches (149.8 cm)

Health History | Nurses' Notes | Diagnostic Tests | Laboratory Results

0930: Chest x-ray: Mild lung hyperinflation; no chest infiltrates, atelectasis, or bronchiectasis

Health History | Nurses' Notes | Diagnostic Tests | Laboratory Results

Test and Reference Range	Results
0930: Oral glucose tolerance test (OGTT) 2 hours: < 140 mg/dL (7.8 mmol/L)	240 mg/dL (13.37 mmol/L)

For each body system, select the **priority** client need to prevent a complication of the client's health problem. Each body system supports one priority client need.

Body System	Priority Client Need
Respiratory	☒ Oscillatory positive expiratory therapy (PEP)
	☐ Oxygen administration
GI	☒ Pancreatic enzyme therapy
	☐ Low-fat diet
Immune	☐ Prophylactic antibiotic therapy
	☒ Contact precautions with separation from others with CF by at least 6 feet
Endocrine	☒ Insulin administration
	☐ Recombinant human growth hormone administration
Integumentary	☒ High-sodium foods
	☐ Oatmeal baths

199

Rationale: CF is a condition characterized by exocrine (mucus-producing) gland dysfunction and leads to multisystem involvement. CF is inherited as an autosomal recessive trait. CF leads to decreased pancreatic secretion of bicarbonate and chloride and an increase of sodium and chloride in both sweat and saliva. The primary factor responsible for many manifestations of the health problem is mechanical obstruction caused by the increased viscosity of mucous gland secretions. The mucous glands produce a thick, heavy mucoprotein that accumulates and dilates them. Then small passages in organs become obstructed as secretions precipitate or coagulate to form concretions in glands and ducts. Because of the increased viscosity of bronchial mucus, there is a greater resistance to ciliary action, a slower flow rate of mucus, and incomplete expectoration. The retained secretions serve as an excellent medium for bacterial growth. Pulmonary symptoms are produced by the stagnation of mucus with eventual bacterial colonization leading to destruction of lung tissue. The thick mucus also obstructs the bronchi and bronchioles, leading to bronchiectasis, atelectasis, and hyperinflation. Airway clearance therapy (ACT) is a primary need for these clients to assist with the removal of secretions and prevention of pulmonary infection. Chest physiotherapy, percussion and postural drainage, PEP, oscillatory PEP, high-frequency chest compressions, and exercise are among some of the treatments. Oxygen administration may be used for children with acute episodes and exacerbations but must be used cautiously because many children with CF have chronic carbon dioxide retention, and oxygen can be harmful. The extent of GI involvement varies. In many clients, the thick secretions block the pancreatic ducts, leading to cystic dilations and then degeneration and progressive diffuse fibrosis. Essential pancreatic enzymes are unable to reach the duodenum, causing impairment in the digestion and absorption of nutrients, particularly fats and proteins. Excessive stool fat (steatorrhea) and foul-smelling stools are characteristic. Biliary obstruction and fibrosis occur in the liver, and extensive liver involvement with fatty infiltration occurs despite adequate nutrition. Pancreatic enzyme therapy is necessary to treat pancreatic insufficiency and is administered with meals and snacks to ensure that digestive enzymes are mixed with food in the duodenum. In addition, because the uptake of fat-soluble vitamins is decreased, water-miscible forms of these vitamins (A, D, E, and K) along with multivitamins are also needed. The client with CF also requires a well-balanced, high-protein, high-calorie diet with unrestricted fat because of the impaired intestinal absorption.

Prevention of infection is critical in the client with CF. Staff, people with CF, and their families need regular and ongoing education to remind them that all persons with CF have some colonization of secretions in the respiratory tract. Therefore clients with CF should separate from others with CF by at least 6 feet to reduce the chance of cross-infection. In addition, contact precautions are needed for all clients regardless of the pathogens present. The client with CF is also advised to wear a mask in common areas of health care facilities. Antibiotics are not administered to the client with CF as a prophylactic measure. If this were done, then resistance to the antibiotic would develop, and it would not be effective when needed to treat an infection. If an infection is confirmed, such as a respiratory infection, then the client is aggressively treated with antibiotics and possible antifungal medications.

The incidence of cystic fibrosis–related diabetes (CFRD) is a concern because the islets of Langerhans decrease in number as the pancreatic fibrosis develops and progresses. CFRD is diagnosed with an oral glucose tolerance test (OGTT). The result of the OGTT 2 hours after administration of the glucose liquid shows a glucose level of 240 mg/dL (13.37 mmol/L), indicating diabetes. Children with CFRD require close monitoring of blood glucose, administration of insulin injections, management of diet and exercise, and monitoring of glycosylated hemoglobin. The administration of recombinant human growth hormone is being used to achieve optimum growth in children with CF who have growth delay. There is no indication that this child has growth delay.

The abnormally high sodium and chloride concentrations in the sweat are a unique characteristic of CF. Parents will often describe their children as tasting "salty" when they kiss the child. Because of the abnormal salt loss, dehydration and hypochloremic and hyponatremic alkalosis during hyperthermic conditions are concerns. Therefore salt replacement therapy is necessary for the client with CF. The recommended dose of salt replacement for clients with CF is based on the client's symptoms, dietary intake, climate conditions, and exercise or activity level. The easiest and best way for clients with CF to get extra salt is by adding salt to foods and eating foods that are naturally high in salt. Although salt crystals may deposit on the skin, and oatmeal or other types of baths may be helpful, baths are not the priority need.

Test-Taking Strategy: Note that this question is asking for the *priority client needs,* and the options are organized by body system. You are presented with two possible priority needs within each body system, and you are asked to select one option for each system. Also note that you are asked to choose the priority need to prevent complications associated with CF. Remember that when you are asked to prioritize, some or all of the options presented to you are good choices; however, you need to rank the options in order of priority based on what the question is asking about. In this clinical scenario, certain options prevent complications of CF (what the question is asking you), some options manage complications, and other options are not helpful in preventing or managing complications. Organize your thinking process in this way, as illustrated in the table.

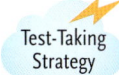
Test-Taking Strategy

Client Need	Prevents Complications	Manages Complications	Not Helpful in Preventing or Managing Complications
Oscillatory PEP	☒	☐	☐
Oxygen administration	☐	☒	☐
Pancreatic enzyme therapy	☒	☐	☐
Low-fat diet	☐	☐	☒
Prophylactic antibiotic therapy	☐	☐	☒
Contact precautions with separation from others with CF by at least 6 feet	☒	☐	☐
Insulin administration	☒	☐	☐
Recombinant human growth hormone administration	☐	☒	☐
High-sodium foods	☒	☐	☐
Oatmeal baths	☐	☒	☐

Choose options that prevent complications as the correct answers for each body system, as this most directly relates to the subject of the question, or what the question is asking about. Options that are used to manage complications or are not related to preventing or managing complications of CF are of lesser priority.

Content Area: Pediatric Nursing
Priority Concepts: Gas Exchange; Glucose Regulation
Reference(s): Hockenberry et al., 2024, pp. 934–943

Practice Question 5.2 — Multiple Response Select N

A 68-year-old client complaining of chest pain is admitted to the medical-surgical nursing unit for acute coronary syndrome.

Nurses' Notes | Laboratory Results | Medication Administration Record

1230: The cardiologist prescribes a continuous IV heparin infusion per protocol. The client weighs 165 lb (74.8 kg), and baseline partial thromboplastin time (PTT) is drawn. A heparin bolus is administered as prescribed, and a continuous infusion is initiated based on the protocol noted in the Medication Administration Record.

Nurses' Notes | Laboratory Results | **Medication Administration Record**

Baseline PTT and every 6 or 12 hours after start of continuous infusion based on protocol.

Heparin 80 units/kg IV bolus prior to start of continuous infusion.

Start heparin 25,000 units in 250 mL D_5W (concentration 100 units/mL) continuous infusion 18 units/kg/h.
Adjust continuous infusion based on the following:
- PTT less than 35 seconds: IV bolus 80 units/kg, increase rate by 4 units/kg/h, PTT in 6 hours
- PTT 35–45 seconds: IV bolus 40 units/kg, increase rate by 2 units/kg/h, PTT in 6 hours
- PTT 46–70 seconds (goal): No bolus, no rate change, PTT in 12 hours
- PTT 71–90 seconds: No bolus, decrease rate by 2 units/kg/h, PTT in 12 hours
- PTT above 90 seconds: No bolus, stop infusion

0700: The next day, the oncoming nurse assigned to monitor the client assesses the client and checks laboratory results drawn 1 hour ago.

Nurses' Notes | Laboratory Results | Medication Administration Record

Client states, "I feel okay; I just have a hard time sleeping since I've been in the hospital. My chest pain is better. I had a nosebleed this morning, but it stopped. I'm ready for breakfast; it should be here soon." The heparin infusion is running at 13.5 mL/h.

Nurses' Notes | **Laboratory Results** | Medication Administration Record

Test and Reference Range	Results
0600: PTT 30–40 seconds	92 seconds

*Select the **3 priority** needs that are of **immediate** concern.*

- ☐ Appetite
- ☐ Chest pain
- ☒ Nosebleed
- ☒ PTT results
- ☒ Heparin infusion
- ☐ Difficulty sleeping

Rationale: The major adverse effects of heparin therapy include heparin-induced thrombocytopenia (HIT) and/or hemorrhage. Other adverse effects include hypersensitivity, local irritation and hematoma, and allergic responses. The priority needs in this scenario that are of immediate concern are the client report of a nosebleed, the PTT results, and the heparin infusion. Nosebleeds can be associated with an adverse effect of HIT or hemorrhage. The PTT results are above the therapeutic range and could also lead to bleeding. The heparin infusion is still running and therefore is of immediate concern. The cardiologist needs to be notified of the nosebleed and supratherapeutic PTT level, and the heparin infusion needs to be stopped. The client is reporting looking forward to having breakfast; this is not a concerning finding related to appetite. The client reports that the chest pain has improved, therefore this is not of immediate concern. The client's difficulty sleeping since being in the hospital is most likely due to the disruption in routine and is not specifically related to the treatment, therefore this is not of immediate concern.

Test-Taking Strategy: Focus on the strategic words *priority* and *immediate,* and note that this question is asking you to prioritize three findings out of a total of six that are of immediate concern to the nurse. Use all of the information provided in the clinical scenario to help you decide on the three most important findings. In addition, thinking about whether these client needs require immediate follow-up to ensure safe client care may help direct you to the correct options. This thinking process is illustrated in the table.

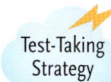
Test-Taking Strategy

Client Finding	Requires Immediate Follow-up	Does Not Require Immediate Follow-up
Appetite	☐	☒
Chest pain	☐	☒
Nosebleed	☒	☐
PTT results	☒	☐
Heparin infusion	☒	☐
Difficulty sleeping	☐	☒

The client is reporting an appetite, which is normal and does not require follow-up; therefore this option can be eliminated. The client's chest pain is improved and therefore does not require follow-up either, so this option can also be eliminated. Although the client is reporting difficulty sleeping, consider the environment as contributing to this. The nurse would want to take measures to address this to promote sleep, but it is not an immediate client need. This leaves you with the three remaining options of nosebleed, PTT results, and the heparin infusion as the correct answer to this question.

Content Area: Pharmacology
Priority Concepts: Clotting; Perfusion
Reference(s): Lilley et al., 2023, pp. 403, 413–414, 423; Ignatavicius et al., 2024, pp. 790, 791–792

Practice Question 5.3 — Drag-and-Drop Rationale

A 70-year-old client had an exploratory laparotomy with colectomy due to small bowel obstruction and was transferred to the postoperative medical-surgical nursing unit 8 hours ago. The oncoming nurse receives report and assesses the client.

Nurses' Notes | Vital Signs

1900: Client received general anesthesia and has a PCA pump with hydromorphone for pain control. Client has been using the PCA pump every 10 minutes for the past 8 hours.

Skin: Warm, dry, intact.

Respiratory: RR 18, unlabored. SpO$_2$ 96% on 2 L/min O$_2$ via NC. Dry cough, no sputum. Lung sounds clear to auscultation in all lung fields.

Cardiovascular: Apical pulse rate 80. Heart sounds: regular rate and rhythm.

GI: Bowel sounds absent × 4 quadrants. Abdomen firm to palpation. Dressing over midline abdominal incision intact with scant amount of serosanguineous drainage noted. Dressing changed per surgeon's order, wound cleansed with normal saline, and dressing reapplied. Incision is well approximated; no redness, swelling, or tenderness at incision site. Pain at incision site rated 2 (on a 0 to 10 pain intensity scale).

Genitourinary: Unable to urinate since arrival to unit 8 hours ago.

Neurologic: Alert and oriented × 3.

Nurses' Notes | **Vital Signs**

T 98.2°F (36.7°C); HR 80; RR 18; BP 138/78; SpO$_2$ 96% on 2 L/min O$_2$ via NC; pain rated 2 (on a 0 to 10 pain intensity scale)

Based on the client findings, complete the following sentence by choosing from the lists of options below.

The client is at **highest** risk for developing __urinary retention__ as evidenced by __urine output__.

Options for 1	Options for 2
Infection	Urine output
Atelectasis	Temperature
Hemorrhage	BP
Urinary retention	RR
Wound dehiscence	Drainage on dressing

Rationale: The client in the postoperative period is at risk for certain complications related to having surgery. In this scenario, the client is at highest risk for developing urinary retention due to the effects of anesthesia and opioid analgesics as well as the type of surgery the client had because of manipulation of the tissues surrounding the bladder. Certain positions can also impair voiding reflexes, and a normal voiding position should be assumed whenever possible.

The client's lack of urine output in at least the past 8 hours is evidence that urinary retention may be a complication that is occurring; the client should void a minimum of 30 mL of urine per hour on average and should be able to initiate the urinary stream without difficulty.

In addition, the GI assessment, which revealed a firm abdomen, is suggestive of urinary retention. Sometimes, straight catheterization following surgery is necessary until the voiding routine is re-established.

Infection can occur after surgery and most often occurs in the wound or at the incision site. It can be caused by poor aseptic technique or contamination of the site. Signs and symptoms include warm, red, and tender skin around the wound or incision site; fever; chills; and purulent drainage. Because the client's temperature is normal and the drainage is serosanguineous, which is normal in the early stage of healing, this complication would not be a concern.

Atelectasis can occur because of the effects of anesthesia, analgesia, and immobilization; signs and symptoms include elevated respiratory rate, dyspnea, fever, crackles, and productive cough. Because this client's respiratory rate is normal, there is no fever, lung sounds are clear, and the cough is dry, atelectasis is most likely not a problem.

Hemorrhage or bleeding can occur after surgery from slipping of a suture or a dislodged clot at an incision site. The client may experience hypotension, weak and rapid pulse, cool and clammy skin, increased respiratory rate, restlessness, and, in the later stages, reduced urine output. The client's lack of urine output is a concern; however, in the absence of these other signs and symptoms, hemorrhage is most likely not a complication occurring currently.

Wound dehiscence occurs when there is separation of wound edges at the suture line. Contributing factors include malnutrition, obesity, radiation to the site, older age, poor circulation, and strain on the suture line. Signs and symptoms include an appearance of underlying tissues at the incision site. The client's incision is well approximated, so this is not a complication that is occurring.

Other complications that can occur after surgery include pneumonia; hypoxemia; PE; hypovolemia; thrombophlebitis; embolus to the brain, heart, or mesentery; deconditioning; paralytic ileus; abdominal distention; nausea and vomiting; UTI; wound evisceration; skin breakdown; intractable pain; and malignant hyperthermia. There are no data indicating that any of these complications are a concern.

Test-Taking Strategy: Focus on what the question is asking about: postoperative complications. Think about what happens during surgery, including the use of anesthesia, manipulation of tissues, medication administration, and immobility. Because the client had surgery, the client is at risk for all of these complications, so you need to look for the data or evidence that a complication is actually happening. Look at each complication listed in the first column, and use your knowledge of pathophysiology to think about the evidence that is needed to support the presence of this complication. Relate this knowledge back to the data provided in the clinical scenario, as illustrated in the table.

Complication	Supporting Evidence
Infection	None—Temperature is normal; incision site without signs of infection
Atelectasis	None—Lung sounds are clear, SpO_2 is normal, RR and work of breathing are normal, cough is dry
Hemorrhage	BP is normal, pulse is normal, RR and work of breathing are normal, alert and oriented × 3 Urine output is inadequate; however, without other signs of bleeding, this likely is not related to this complication
Urinary retention	Inadequate urine output, firm abdomen
Wound dehiscence	Incision is well approximated Serosanguineous drainage can be a sign of future dehiscence but is also a normal part of the healing process; because the incision is not separated, it is not a complication now

As you can see, some of the findings in the clinical scenario can relate to more than one potential complication; however, the highest risk would be for an actual complication that is confirmed based on the available data. Urinary retention can be confirmed based on inadequate urine output, a firm abdomen, and the fact that the client has not urinated for the past 8 hours. Note that there are no data to support infection or atelectasis. The only supporting evidence for hemorrhage is inadequate urine output; recall, however, that hemorrhage would be a later sign, and in the absence of other signs and symptoms this would not be the priority concern. Although serosanguineous drainage is present, it does not confirm wound dehiscence, and there is no evidence to support that this complication is occurring as the incision is well approximated; therefore this is not the priority concern at this time. Remember to consider all data presented in the clinical scenario and organize your thinking process in a way that will allow you to make connections; this will make it much easier to decide on the priority client needs.

Content Area: Foundations of Nursing
Priority Concepts: Elimination; Tissue Integrity
Reference(s): Potter et al., 2023, pp. 1441–1445

Practice Question 5.4 — Multiple Response Select All That Apply

The nurse working at a psychiatric outpatient clinic is performing an intake assessment on a 28-year-old client accompanied by their parent.

Health History | Nurses' Notes

1400: Parent reports that the client has been increasingly withdrawn, spending most of the time in their bedroom for the past 6 months. Parent noticed that the client seems preoccupied and is often talking to oneself. Parent reports that the client has difficulty maintaining employment due to the symptoms. Client admits to hearing voices that tell them they are worthless and others are plotting against them. Client has also been neglecting personal hygiene and refusing to eat meals with the family. Client denies substance use or history of head injury. There is no significant past medical history, and the client has never been hospitalized for psychiatric reasons. There is no known family history of psychiatric disorders. Client lives with parents and a younger sibling. Client has limited social interactions outside of the family and has no close friends.

Health History | Nurses' Notes

1400: Mental status examination:

Appearance: Disheveled and has poor hygiene.

Behavior: Appears withdrawn, avoids eye contact. Observed talking to oneself.

Speech: Tangential and disorganized.

Mood/Affect: Appears anxious and states suspicion of clinical staff. Blunted affect.

Thought Process/Content: Exhibits paranoid delusions with auditory hallucinations that are persecutory in nature.

Cognition: Demonstrates impaired concentration and memory.

Insight/Judgment: Lacks insight into condition as evidenced by denying the need for treatment.

Based on the client's clinical presentation, which of the following are the priority concerns? **Select all that apply.**

- ☒ The client is exhibiting signs of schizophrenia.
- ☐ The client likely has generalized anxiety disorder.
- ☐ The client will require long-term inpatient hospitalization.
- ☐ The client is primarily experiencing delusions of reference.
- ☐ The client's problem-solving abilities and daily functioning are intact.
- ☒ The client is experiencing positive, negative, and cognitive symptoms.

Rationale: Schizophrenia is a complex mental health problem associated with a range of symptoms that affect thoughts, emotions, perceptions, and behaviors. Symptoms are categorized into positive, negative, and cognitive symptoms. The client in this scenario is exhibiting signs of schizophrenia and is experiencing all three categories of symptoms associated with this mental health problem. Positive symptoms include being preoccupied; talking to oneself; hearing voices; tangential speech; and paranoid delusions with auditory hallucinations. Negative symptoms include being increasingly withdrawn; blunted affect; difficulty maintaining employment; and avolition or a decrease in motivation or initiative. Cognitive symptoms include impaired attention, concentration, and memory as well as lack of executive function as evidenced by lacking insight into the condition. The client is not demonstrating symptoms of generalized anxiety disorder. Although the client likely has schizophrenia and treatment is required, long-term inpatient hospitalization is not necessary unless the client poses harm to self or others.

The client is not experiencing delusions of reference (the belief that neutral events or objects have special significance); rather, they are experiencing persecutory delusions, or the belief that they are being targeted or persecuted. Therefore the client's problem-solving abilities are not intact, and they will need a support system to assist with management of the schizophrenia.

Test-Taking Strategy: Note the strategic word *priority*. Recall that schizophrenia is a complex mental health problem typically characterized by positive, negative, and cognitive symptoms. Look at the information provided in the Health History and Nurses' Notes, and decide whether the options are linked to the assessment findings noted.

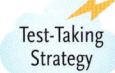
Test-Taking Strategy

Option	Assessment Finding
The client is exhibiting signs of schizophrenia.	Increasingly withdrawn; preoccupied; talking to oneself; difficulty maintaining employment; hearing voices; neglecting personal hygiene; limited social interactions
The client likely has generalized anxiety disorder.	None
The client will require long-term inpatient hospitalization.	None
The client is primarily experiencing delusions of reference.	None; exhibiting paranoid delusions with auditory hallucinations that are persecutory in nature
The client's problem-solving abilities and daily functioning are intact.	None; not intact
The client is experiencing positive, negative, and cognitive symptoms.	Positive: being preoccupied; talking to oneself; hearing voices; tangential speech; paranoid delusions with auditory hallucinations Negative: being increasingly withdrawn; blunted affect; difficulty maintaining employment; avolition/decrease in motivation/initiative Cognitive: impaired attention, concentration, and memory; lack of executive function; lacking insight into condition

There are no findings specific to generalized anxiety disorder, therefore this option can be eliminated. Next, you can eliminate the option about required long-term hospitalization by recalling that schizophrenia can often be safely managed on an outpatient basis with a support system. Note that the client is exhibiting paranoid delusions with auditory hallucinations that are persecutory in nature. You can then eliminate the option stating that the client's problem-solving abilities and daily functioning are intact, noting the assessment findings suggesting otherwise.

Content Area: Mental Health Nursing
Priority Concepts: Mood and Affect; Stress and Coping
Reference(s): Halter, 2022, pp. 191–218

Practice Question 5.5 — Drop-Down in Table

A 59-year-old postmenopausal client with stage IV bilateral breast cancer had a double mastectomy. One month later, the client visits the clinic for a follow-up.

> **Nurses' Notes**
>
> **1500:** Reports experiencing some unusual symptoms.
>
> Reports pelvic pain, vaginal discharge, burning on urination.
>
> Having hot flashes, dizziness; states that left leg feels warm and tender.
>
> Feeling weak, and experiencing bone pain and joint stiffness.
>
> Has been constipated; having stomach cramps, nausea, and vomiting.
>
> Biopsy showed a hormone receptor–positive tumor, and the client is taking tamoxifen.

*For each body system, select the 1 **priority** concern specific to a complication of tamoxifen therapy.*

Body System	Priority Concern
Genitourinary	☒ Pelvic pain
	☐ Vaginal discharge
	☐ Burning on urination
Cardiovascular	☐ Hot flashes
	☐ Dizziness
	☒ Tenderness and warmth to left leg
Musculoskeletal	☐ Weakness
	☒ Bone pain
	☐ Joint stiffness
GI	☐ Constipation
	☐ Stomach cramps
	☒ Nausea and vomiting

Rationale: Tamoxifen is an estrogen modulator that blocks the effects of estrogen in breast tissue. It is used to treat breast cancer and for prevention of breast cancer in those who are at high risk for developing it. This medication works by blocking estrogen receptors, which helps inhibit growth and proliferation of cancer cells. Endometrial cancer is a complication because tamoxifen acts as an estrogen agonist at receptors in the uterus, which can cause proliferation of endometrial tissue, eventually leading to endometrial cancer. In postmenopausal clients, endometrial cancer is often characterized by abnormal menstrual bleeding, so it is an obvious abnormality after menopause. A hysterectomy may be performed as a preventive measure. Another sign of endometrial cancer is pelvic pain. Vaginal discharge may be normal or abnormal and can occur as a side effect of tamoxifen therapy, and it should be addressed, but this is not the highest priority. Burning on urination may be a sign of UTI and needs follow-up, but it is not specifically related to tamoxifen. Vasomotor symptoms such as hot flashes can occur as a side effect of tamoxifen, but this is not the highest priority and can be addressed routinely. Dizziness may also be associated with tamoxifen therapy but is not the highest priority. Tenderness and warmth in the left leg may be a sign of a thromboembolic event, such as DVT, PE, or stroke; therefore this finding is a priority concern. Tamoxifen can cause transient hypercalcemia and subsequent bone pain in clients with bone metastasis, so bone pain is a priority concern and could be an indication of metastasis. In addition, the risk for pathologic fractures with bone metastasis is high. Weakness and joint stiffness are not specifically associated with tamoxifen therapy. Nausea and vomiting commonly occur with tamoxifen therapy; this is a priority concern because of the associated risk of malnutrition, dehydration, and fluid and electrolyte imbalance. Constipation and stomach cramps are not adverse effects that indicate a complication of tamoxifen therapy.

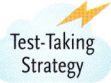

Test-Taking Strategy: Note the strategic word *priority*. The first step in answering this question correctly is to determine which of the concerns listed in the question are adverse effects indicating a complication specifically related to tamoxifen therapy. As shown in the table, think about the effects of tamoxifen on the body. First, use your nursing knowledge of this medication, and recall that it blocks the effects of estrogen by blocking estrogen receptors. Next, think about whether or not the effect is a priority concern. Recalling the effects of this hormone will help you narrow down which options may be related to complications associated with tamoxifen therapy.

Effects	Specifically Related to Tamoxifen Therapy/A Priority Concern-Yes or No
Pelvic pain	☒ /Yes
Vaginal discharge	☒ /No
Burning on urination	☐
Hot flashes	☒ /No
Dizziness	☒ /No
Tenderness and warmth to left leg	☒ /Yes
Weakness	☐
Bone pain	☒ /Yes
Joint stiffness	☐
Constipation	☐
Stomach cramps	☐
Nausea and vomiting	☒ /Yes

From here, you need to prioritize for each body system which of these findings would be of priority concern related to a complication of tamoxifen therapy. Recall that pelvic pain could be a manifestation of endometrial cancer and should be prioritized above vaginal discharge and burning on urination. Tenderness and warmth in the leg are signs of a thrombus and would be the priority over hot flashes and dizziness. Recalling that this medication can cause hypercalcemia in the presence of bone metastasis will assist you in prioritizing bone pain. Remembering that malnutrition, dehydration, and fluid and electrolyte imbalance can occur with nausea and vomiting will assist you in selecting this as the priority.

Content Area: Pharmacology
Priority Concepts: Clotting; Immunity
Reference(s): Lilley et al., 2023, pp. 732–736

Practice Question 5.6 — Multiple Response Select N

The nurse is caring for a 29-year-old gravida 3, para 2 (G3P2) pregnant client who came to the labor and delivery unit experiencing a precipitous labor.

Health History | Nurses' Notes | Vital Signs

1500: 29-year-old G3P2 client at 38 weeks' gestation presented to the labor and delivery unit in active labor. Reports experiencing sudden and intense contractions that started 1 hour ago. Over that time, contractions quickly increased in frequency and intensity. Reports associated pressure in lower back and pelvis, rectal pressure, and spontaneous rupture of membranes shortly after contractions started. Previously had 2 uncomplicated vaginal deliveries at 39 weeks and 38 weeks, both with active labor lasting approximately 6 to 8 hours. Reports no significant medical history and has been taking prenatal vitamins and attending prenatal appointments. Married and has 2 children; reports good social support at home.

Health History | Nurses' Notes | Vital Signs

1500: Fundal height consistent with gestational age. Uterus firm. Contractions regular. Cervix fully dilated, 2+ station. Reassuring fetal heart rate pattern.

Health History | Nurses' Notes | Vital Signs

1500: T 98.2°F (36.7°C); HR 96; RR 18; BP 112/78; SpO₂ 98% on RA

Based on this clinical scenario, select the **5** potential complications that would be of **highest priority** to the nurse.

☐ Placental abruption
☒ Fetal shoulder dystocia
☒ Fetal intracranial trauma
☒ Excessive uterine bleeding
☒ Inadequate fetal oxygenation
☒ Birthing parent perineal trauma

Rationale: Precipitous labor is defined as labor that lasts less than 3 hours from the onset of contractions to the time of delivery. Although it is usually not considered a complication in and of itself, there can be complications that occur after precipitous labor. Postpartum hemorrhage can occur as a result of the increased likelihood of uterine atony, a condition in which the uterus fails to adequately contract after delivery. This leads to excessive uterine bleeding. The rapid labor progression with frequent and intense contractions may lead to inadequate fetal oxygenation. Neonatal trauma can result due to difficulty maneuvering the baby through the birth canal, and complications like fetal shoulder dystocia and intracranial trauma can result. Perineal trauma for the birthing parent, including lacerations in the vaginal walls, perineum, or cervix, may occur from the rapid labor progression. Placental abruption occurs when the placenta partially or completely separates from the uterine wall before delivery. Placental abruption is associated with premature rupture of the membranes.

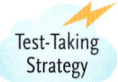

Test-Taking Strategy: Note the strategic words *highest priority*, and note that the question is asking about complications of precipitous labor. Recall that the words *highest priority* indicate the need to prioritize. Some or all of the options may be relevant to the scenario. Also note that the question instructions tell you to choose 5 of the 6 options. Using knowledge, thinking about the pathophysiology, and visualizing the possible complications that can occur with precipitous labor during pregnancy will help direct you to the correct options. Remember that complications are related to the frequent and intense contractions and the quick transport of the fetus through the birth canal.

Complication	Related to Frequent/ Intense Contractions	Related to Quick Transport of Fetus Through Birth Canal
Placental abruption	☐	☐
Fetal shoulder dystocia	☐	☒
Fetal intracranial trauma	☒	☒
Excessive uterine bleeding	☒	☒
Inadequate fetal oxygenation	☒	☐
Birthing parent perineal trauma	☐	☒

Placental abruption is concerning but is not the highest priority in this case because it is not directly related to precipitous labor. Fetal shoulder dystocia, fetal intracranial trauma, excessive uterine bleeding, inadequate fetal oxygenation, and birthing parent perineal trauma are all related to precipitous labor and therefore are the answers to this question.

Content Area: Obstetric-Newborn Nursing
Priority Concepts: Oxygenation; Perfusion
Reference(s): Lowdermilk et al., 2024, pp. 699–700

CHAPTER 6

Answers to Practice Questions

Practice Question 6.1 — Multiple Response Grouping

A 58-year-old client is recovering on the medical-surgical nursing unit from an L4–L5 spinal fusion completed 3 hours ago.

Medication Administration Record

Hydromorphone via PCA, 0.2 mg every 10 minutes, with a 4-mg lock-out dose in 4 hours.

For each body system, specify the potential intervention that would be appropriate for the initial plan of care to monitor for or prevent adverse effects of hydromorphone. **Each body system may support more than one potential nursing intervention.**

Body System	Potential Nursing Intervention
Renal	☒ Assess renal function.
	☒ Monitor I&O.
	☐ Maintain fluid restriction.
Respiratory	☒ Assess RR frequently.
	☒ Ensure that naloxone is available.
	☐ Place the PCA on hold if RR is less than 18.
Cardiovascular	☐ Encourage brisk walking.
	☒ Instruct the client to change positions slowly.
	☒ Assess BP and HR frequently.
Gastrointestinal	☐ Administer methylnaltrexone.
	☒ Administer ondansetron as indicated.
	☒ Ensure adequate intake of fluids and fiber.
Urinary	☒ Assess the bladder frequently.
	☒ Prompt the client to void every 4 hours.
	☐ Perform straight catheterization every 4 hours.

Rationale: Hydromorphone is an opioid analgesic used to manage pain. Adverse effects include increased intracranial pressure (ICP), neurotoxicity, respiratory depression, orthostatic hypotension, constipation, vomiting, and urinary retention. Other adverse effects include cough suppression, biliary colic, euphoria and dysphoria, sedation, and miosis. Hydromorphone can cause birth defects if taken by a pregnant person. Increased ICP can result from hydromorphone owing to retained carbon dioxide from respiratory depression. In addition, opioid-induced neurotoxicity can occur, causing delirium, agitation, myoclonus, and hyperalgesia. Renal impairment, cognitive impairment, and prolonged use are risk factors for increased ICP and neurotoxicity as adverse effects of this medication. Because renal impairment is a risk factor for increased ICP in a client receiving hydromorphone, assessing renal function, monitoring urinary output, maintaining hydration, and reducing the dose in clients with renal impairment are important measures. Respiratory depression is the most serious adverse effect. The RR needs to be assessed frequently for a client on PCA receiving hydromorphone. The PCA will lock out and would need to be placed on hold if the RR is less than 12, or as otherwise prescribed. Naloxone, the antidote to opioid analgesics, needs to be available if respiratory depression occurs. Opioid analgesics lower the BP by blunting the baroreceptor reflex and causing dilation to the peripheral vasculature. The nurse needs to teach the client about symptoms of hypotension such as light-headedness and dizziness and instruct the client to sit or lie down if these symptoms are noticed. Changing positions slowly, while maintaining proper positioning as prescribed by the surgeon, and asking for assistance with activity are important safety measures to prevent hypotension from occurring or to prevent injury if hypotension does occur. Regularly assessing the BP and HR will alert the nurse to this problem. Constipation is an adverse effect associated with opioid analgesics and occurs because of suppression of peristalsis. Fecal impaction, tearing, hemorrhoids, and bowel perforation can result. Initially the nurse would promote motility by ensuring adequate fluid and fiber intake, encouraging activity, and administering prophylactic stimulants such as senna and stool softeners such as docusate. Lactulose or sodium phosphate, stronger osmotic laxatives, may be needed if these measures do not work. Methylnaltrexone, a medication that blocks mu receptors in the intestine, may be given as a last resort for opioid-induced constipation but is not an appropriate intervention initially. Vomiting can occur through stimulation of the chemoreceptor trigger zone in the brain. Remaining still and taking an antiemetic, such as ondansetron, help with this effect if it occurs. Hydromorphone can cause urinary retention by increasing tone in the bladder sphincter, increasing tone in the detrusor muscle, and interfering with voiding by suppressing awareness of bladder stimuli. Clients need to be prompted to void every 4 hours. The nurse needs to assess for urinary retention by monitoring I&O and palpating for bladder distention every 4 to 6 hours. Intermittent straight catheterization may be needed if this complication occurs but is not performed unless clients cannot void on their own.

Test-Taking Strategy: Note that this question is asking for the *appropriate potential nursing interventions* for the *initial* plan of care and that the options are organized by body system. You are presented with three possible interventions within each body system, and you are asked to select one or more option for each system. When answering questions about medications, think about how safety is addressed with each of the options presented and whether the option monitors for or prevents an adverse effect of the medication. Organize your thinking process in this way, as illustrated in the table.

Potential Intervention	Monitors for or Prevents a Potential Adverse Effect	Does Not Address a Potential Adverse Effect
Assess renal function.	X	☐
Monitor I&O.	X	☐
Maintain fluid restriction.	☐	X
Assess RR frequently.	X	☐
Ensure that naloxone is available.	X	☐
Place the PCA on hold if RR is less than 18.	☐	X
Encourage brisk walking.	☐	X
Instruct the client to change positions slowly.	X	☐
Assess BP and HR frequently.	X	☐
Administer methylnaltrexone.	☐	X
Administer ondansetron as indicated.	X	☐
Ensure adequate intake of fluids and fiber.	X	☐
Assess the bladder frequently.	X	☐
Prompt the client to void every 4 hours.	X	☐
Perform straight catheterization every 4 hours.	☐	X

Choose options that address adverse effects as the correct answers for each body system because this most directly relates to the subject of the question, or what the question is asking about. Options that are unrelated to monitoring for or managing adverse effects can be eliminated.

Content Area: Pharmacology
Priority Concepts: Gas Exchange; Tissue Integrity
Reference(s): Lilley et al., 2023, p. 149

Practice Question 6.2 — Multiple Response Select N

An unhoused 72-year-old client is brought to the ED by EMS. The client was found sleeping on a park bench by a jogger who reported that the client had a foul smell and an excessive amount of wetness on a pant leg.

History and Physical | Nurses' Notes | Physician's Orders

0600: Client reports history of peripheral vascular disease and has not received follow-up care.
Has an arterial leg ulcer that is open and draining copious amounts of drainage.
Physician in to see client.

History and Physical | **Nurses' Notes** | Physician's Orders

1600: Client requiring multiple dressing changes through the day owing to the excessive drainage.
1630: Seen by the wound care team.

History and Physical | Nurses' Notes | **Physician's Orders**

0630: Admit to medical-surgical unit for wound care management.
Wound culture.
Pack the wound with sterile, saline-moistened gauze, and then cover with a dry, sterile dressing, with daily dressing changes and as needed.
1700: Begin negative-pressure wound therapy (NPWT).

Which **5** interventions would the nurse include in the plan of care for the client to maintain and ensure a good seal during NPWT?

- ☒ Identify air leaks using a stethoscope.
- ☐ Shave the hair on the skin around the wound.
- ☒ Make sure the periwound skin surface area is dry.
- ☒ Avoid wrinkles when applying the transparent film.
- ☒ Fill uneven skin surfaces with a skin barrier product.
- ☒ Frame the periwound area with a hydrocolloid dressing.
- ☐ Cut the transparent film to extend ½ inch beyond the wound perimeter.
- ☐ Use as many additional dressing layers as needed for identified air leaks.

Rationale: NPWT treats acute and chronic wounds and is a helpful treatment for clients with wounds with copious amounts of drainage. Maintaining an airtight seal is important for NPWT to be effective. To avoid loss of suction, or negative pressure, the wound and dressing must stay sealed. Interventions to assist in maintaining an airtight seal include identifying air leaks using a stethoscope and repairing them with a transparent dressing; filling uneven skin surfaces with a skin barrier product; making sure the periwound skin surface is dry; avoiding wrinkles when applying the transparent film; and framing the periwound area with a hydrocolloid dressing. Rather than shaving, the hair on the skin around the wound needs to be clipped per agency policy. Only one or two additional dressing layers should be used for air leaks because multiple layers reduce moisture vapor transmission and cause maceration of the wound. The transparent film should be cut to extend 1 to 2 inches beyond the wound perimeter.

Test-Taking Strategy: Note that this question is asking you to identify 5 interventions out of a total of 8 listed interventions that the nurse would plan in the care of a client receiving NPWT. Use knowledge about this treatment and the information provided in the clinical scenario to help you decide on the 5 appropriate interventions. Note that the question focuses on maintaining a good seal for NPWT. Thinking about the interventions that would help in this scenario and the interventions that either would not help or pose a safety risk will assist you in answering the question correctly. This thinking process is illustrated in the table.

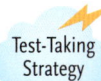
Test-Taking Strategy

Intervention	Helps Maintain/Ensure a Seal	Does Not Help Maintain/Ensure a Seal or Poses a Safety Risk
Identify air leaks using a stethoscope.	X	
Shave the hair on the skin around the wound.		X
Make sure the periwound skin surface area is dry.	X	
Avoid wrinkles when applying the transparent film.	X	
Fill uneven skin surfaces with a skin barrier product.	X	
Frame the periwound area with a hydrocolloid dressing.	X	
Cut the transparent film to extend ½ inch beyond the wound perimeter.		X
Use as many additional dressing layers as needed for identified air leaks.		X

Shaving hair poses a safety risk because of the possibility of injury and therefore can be eliminated. From here, use your nursing knowledge to eliminate the option that states to cut the transparent film ½ inch beyond the wound perimeter and the option that states to use as many additional dressing layers as needed for air leaks, noting that these interventions would not help maintain or ensure a good seal.

Content Area: Foundations of Nursing
Priority Concepts: Perfusion; Tissue Integrity
Reference(s): Potter et al., 2023, pp. 1350–1351, 1375–1378

Practice Question 6.3 — Drag-and-Drop Rationale

A 44-year-old postoperative client returned to the nursing unit from the PACU following a bilateral mastectomy.

Nurses' Notes | Vital Signs | Physician's Orders

1300:
Alert and oriented. Reports incisional pain rated 2/10 (on a 0–10 pain scale).
Bilateral incisions on the chest covered with a dry, sterile dressing; clean, dry, and intact.
Lung sounds clear to auscultation bilaterally. S1S2, no S3S4. +2 peripheral pulses, no edema.
4 Jackson-Pratt drains from the incisional areas: #1 with 5 mL of sanguineous drainage, #2 with 10 mL of sanguineous drainage, #3 with 5 mL of sanguineous drainage, #4 with 10 mL of sanguineous drainage, compressed for suction.

Nurses' Notes | **Vital Signs** | Physician's Orders

1300: T 98.2°F (36.8°C); HR 70; RR 20; BP 146/72; SpO$_2$ 97% at 3 L/min O$_2$ via NC; Pain rated 2/10.

Nurses' Notes | Vital Signs | **Physician's Orders**

1300:
Monitor VS per agency protocol
Titrate oxygen to maintain SpO$_2$ greater than 92%
Monitor incision site for signs of bleeding
Monitor and maintain surgical drains
Enoxaparin 40 mg subcutaneously daily
Apply sequential compression devices (SCDs) below the knee bilaterally for venous thrombosis prevention
Pain management via PCA pump
Clear liquids advance to regular as tolerated
Incentive spirometry per unit protocol
Ondansetron 4 mg IV every 4 hours as needed for nausea

Based on the client findings, complete the following sentence by choosing from the lists of options below.

To ensure client safety, the nurse plans to **first administer enoxaparin** to address **thrombus risk**.

Options for 1	Options for 2
Administer enoxaparin	Pain
Administer pain medication	Infection
Increase supplemental oxygen	Hypoxemia
Empty and compress surgical drains	Thrombus risk

Rationale: Taking into consideration all client data in this clinical scenario, the major concern would be the potential for thrombus formation as a postoperative complication. Enoxaparin, classified as an anticoagulant or low–molecular-weight heparin, is given to postoperative clients as a preventive measure for thrombus formation. To ensure client safety, the nurse would plan to first administer the enoxaparin to address thrombus risk. The other options may be needed but are not the priority at this time. Pain is expected after surgery and needs to be well managed to promote healing. The client's pain is currently rated 2/10, and because the client has a PCA pump as noted in the Physician's Orders, it would not be a priority for the nurse to administer pain medication. Hypoxemia can occur after surgery, related to the effects of anesthesia and immobility in the postoperative period. The client's SpO$_2$ is 97% at 3 L/min O$_2$ via NC, and there is no evidence of hypoxemia; therefore the nurse would not need to increase the oxygen flow rate. Maintaining the surgical drains is an important measure so body fluids are adequately drained and do not build up in the affected area, leading to infection. Because there is only 5 to 10 mL of drainage in each drain, it is not the priority to empty and compress the surgical drains at this time. In addition, the Nurses' Notes indicate that the drains were already compressed for suction.

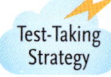

Test-Taking Strategy: Note that this question is asking about nursing interventions to ensure client safety and the rationale behind them. Note the strategic word *first*. This word may indicate that some or all options are correct, and you need to decide which intervention should be planned first. Once you have determined the intervention, then consider the rationale for that intervention. Think about the potential complications of surgery. Because the client had surgery, the client is at risk for pain, infection, hypoxemia, and thrombus, so you need to decide which intervention needs to be planned *first* for client safety considerations. Using this knowledge and the data provided in the clinical scenario, organize your thinking process as illustrated in the table. There needs to be supporting evidence for options for the option to be correct.

Intervention	Supporting Evidence Indicating Priority Intervention
Administer enoxaparin	Recent surgery—prevents thrombus
Administer pain medication	Not needed—pain 2/10, using PCA
Increase supplemental oxygen	Not needed—97% 3 L per NC
Empty and compress surgical drains	Not needed—not full yet; already compressed

The client's pain assessment, SpO_2, and surgical drain assessments do not indicate the need for intervention at this time and therefore do not need to be addressed first. Because administering enoxaparin is a preventive measure to reduce the risk of thrombus following surgery, this intervention should be performed first. Note that the second part of the question requires you to demonstrate that you know the reason for choosing the first option. Use your nursing knowledge to recall that enoxaparin is an anticoagulant commonly used after surgery to prevent formation of a thrombus as a result of the surgery.

Content Area: Medical-Surgical Nursing
Priority Concept: Clotting; Tissue Integrity
Reference(s): Lilley et al., 2023, pp. 408, 412–413; Potter et al., 2023, p. 1335

Practice Question 6.4 — Multiple Response Select All That Apply

A 22-year-old client presents to the outpatient mental health clinic.

History and Physical | Nurses' Notes

1000: Reports no previous history of mental health problems or a family history

History and Physical | Nurses' Notes

1000: Reports feeling "down" and having difficulty maintaining responsibilities with school. States experiencing a hard time finding friends, that peers in class don't think the client is smart, and that they make fun of the client behind the client's back. Reports not speaking to parents and that the only support system is the client's partner. States "putting myself through school." Describes not being able to meet assignment deadlines and thinks about considering quitting school. Counseling at the psychological center and group therapy discussed with the client.

Based on this scenario, which of the following interventions would the mental health nurse plan for the client? **Select all that apply.**

- ☒ Set realistic goals for behavior modification.
- ☒ Reward the client for practicing new behaviors.
- ☐ Provide positive regard for adaptive behaviors only.
- ☒ Encourage the client to practice behavior modification.
- ☐ Help the client identify negative qualities and experiences.
- ☒ Help the client identify their own behaviors needing change.
- ☒ Reinforce self-worth with time and attention by giving one-on-one time.

Rationale: This client is experiencing decreased self-esteem, which could be related to perceived lack of belonging, perceived lack of respect from others, lack of success in role functioning, a disturbed relationship with parents or caregivers, and feeling targeted by peers. Although not reported, a psychiatric disorder could also be a factor for this client. The nurse would help the client describe self in positive ways, fulfill personally significant roles, and engage in meaningful interaction with others. Interventions that would be planned for this client include setting realistic goals for behavior modification; rewarding the client for practicing new behaviors; encouraging the client to practice behavior modification; helping the client identify their own behaviors needing change; and reinforcing self-worth with time and attention by giving one-on-one time. Rather than providing positive regard for adaptive behaviors only, the nurse needs to give unconditional positive regard and avoid acknowledgment or reinforcement of negative behaviors. Instead of helping the client identify negative qualities and experiences, the nurse would help the client identify positive qualities and accomplishments.

Test-Taking Strategy: Note that this question is asking you choose interventions that the nurse would plan for this client based on the information described in the clinical scenario. To decide on the appropriate interventions for the plan of care, first you need to determine based on the information in the scenario that the client is experiencing problems with self-esteem. Next, for each intervention listed, determine whether the intervention would improve or not improve self-esteem. Organize your thinking process as illustrated in the table.

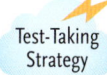

Intervention	Improves Self-Esteem	Does Not Improve Self-Esteem
Set realistic goals for behavior modification.	X	
Reward the client for practicing new behaviors.	X	
Provide positive regard for adaptive behaviors only.		X
Encourage the client to practice behavior modification.	X	
Help the client identify negative qualities and experiences.		X
Help the client identify their own behaviors needing change.	X	
Reinforce self-worth with time and attention by giving one-on-one time.	X	

If you focus on the outcome of improving self-esteem, then you will be able to determine which interventions are appropriate in the plan of care for this client. Options that describe new behaviors, realistic goals, self-worth, and changing behaviors are actions that would improve self-esteem. Options that are limited in scope or that focus on negative adaptations are actions that would not improve self-esteem and therefore should be eliminated.

Content Area: Mental Health Nursing
Priority Concept: Mood and Affect; Stress and Coping
Reference(s): Halter, 2022, p. 250

Practice Question 6.5 — Matrix Multiple Choice

A 32-year-old client is hospitalized in the neurologic unit after sustaining a head injury after falling from a ladder while working in the garage.

Nurses' Notes

0800: Client unresponsive and unable to take in food or fluids. Prepared for central line insertion and total parenteral nutrition (TPN) as prescribed for nutritional support.

Select whether the following potential interventions are indicated or not indicated for the client at this time.

Potential Intervention	Indicated	Not Indicated
Administer insulin.	X	
Assess for diaphoresis.	X	
Monitor the IV site.	X	
Follow Droplet Precautions.		X
Monitor blood glucose level every 6 hours.	X	
Discontinue the infusion if the bag is empty while waiting for the next TPN bag to become available.		X

Rationale: TPN, also called parenteral nutrition (PN), involves IV administration of a complex and highly concentrated solution that contains nutrients and electrolytes. It is formulated to meet the client's nutritional needs. This nutritional support is provided for clients who are unable to digest or absorb nutrition orally or enterally. Clients who are in highly stressed physiologic states that occur with sepsis, head injury, or burns are candidates for TPN. TPN needs to be administered through a central venous catheter (CVC). Safe administration of TPN requires management of the CVC and insertion site to prevent infection as well as ongoing and careful monitoring to prevent metabolic complications. Hypoglycemia and hyperglycemia are potential complications of TPN therapy. The nurse needs to monitor for diaphoresis and needs to assess the blood glucose level every 6 hours to monitor for these complications. For clients receiving TPN who are conscious, other signs and symptoms of these potential complications include shakiness, confusion, loss of consciousness, thirst, headache, lethargy, and increased urination. In addition, to prevent hypoglycemia, the TPN should not be abruptly discontinued, but rather tapered down. If an infusion bag of TPN completes, and it is necessary to wait for the preparation of the next TPN infusion bag, the nurse would infuse a solution of 10% glucose until the TPN infusion bag is available. IV 50% dextrose or glucagon needs to be available to treat hypoglycemia if it occurs. TPN also should not be suddenly increased but instead should be tapered up to prevent hyperglycemia. Insulin may be required during therapy, especially if the client has DM. The client is at risk for infection because of the CVC and because the client is receiving TPN. The nurse needs to monitor the IV site for signs of infection and intervene accordingly to prevent infection and to address it if it is suspected. For TPN therapy, the nurse does not need to follow Droplet Precautions but instead would follow Standard Precautions, unless the client is on Transmission-Based Precautions for another transmissible disease.

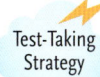

Test-Taking Strategy: Note that the question is asking about actions or interventions that are either indicated or not indicated. An action that is indicated is one that would be appropriate or necessary, whereas, as noted in this question, an action that is not indicated would be one that is unnecessary or could be harmful. The first step in answering this question correctly is to determine which of the potential interventions listed in the options are helpful or not helpful or unnecessary or potentially harmful as they relate to the care necessary for a client receiving TPN. As shown in the table, think about the effects of TPN on the body. Use your nursing knowledge of the indications and effects of TPN.

Potential Intervention	Indicated (Appropriate or Necessary)/Not Indicated (Unnecessary or Harmful)
Administer insulin.	Helpful
Assess for diaphoresis.	Helpful
Monitor the IV site.	Helpful
Follow Droplet Precautions.	Unnecessary
Monitor blood glucose level every 6 hours.	Helpful
Discontinue the infusion if the bag is empty while waiting for the next TPN bag to become available.	Harmful

From here, you can determine that any helpful intervention is a correct option, but any intervention that is not necessary or is harmful is an incorrect option. Recall that blood glucose changes can occur with TPN, therefore any option related to monitoring for complications or managing blood glucose levels would be helpful. Droplet Precautions are not needed for TPN therapy and therefore are unnecessary. Discontinuing the infusion before the next bag is available could be harmful because it could cause a decrease in blood glucose levels and therefore is incorrect.

Content Area: Pharmacology
Priority Concept: Fluid and Electrolyte Balance: Tissue Integrity
Reference(s): Lilley et al., 2023, pp. 862–863; Potter et al., 2023, pp. 1064, 1196

Practice Question 6.6 — Multiple Response Select N

A 46-year-old client is visited by a home health nurse following discharge from the hospital with a diagnosis of new-onset diabetes mellitus.

Nurses' Notes

1000: Discharged from the hospital with a diagnosis of new-onset diabetes mellitus (DM). Admitted to the hospital after reporting increased thirst, increased hunger, and increased urination for 7 days. Client's blood glucose level was significantly elevated on admission, and the client was treated for DKA. After being stabilized, the client was discharged to home with a diagnosis of new-onset DM. Teaching started on self-management and measures to prevent hospitalization. Client reports often feeling hungry, irritable, shaky, and weak as well as having a headache.

Based on the client's reported symptoms, which **5** measures would the home care nurse plan to teach this client to implement when these symptoms occur?

- ☒ Eat 6 saltine crackers.
- ☒ Eat 3 graham crackers.
- ☒ Drink 120 mL of fruit juice.
- ☒ Drink 240 mL of skim milk.
- ☒ Consume 6 to 10 hard candies.
- ☐ Consume 4 tablespoons of honey.
- ☐ Drink 120 mL of a diet soft drink.
- ☐ Decrease carbohydrate intake.
- ☐ Administer insulin based on a sliding scale.

Rationale: Clients with DM need to be taught how to manage hypoglycemia at home. The client's symptoms (hunger, irritability, shakiness, weakness, headache) are indicative of possible hypoglycemia. To manage or treat hypoglycemia at home if the client is conscious, they should be taught to do one of the following: eat 6 saltine crackers, eat 3 graham crackers, or drink 120 mL of fruit juice, 240 mL of skim milk, or 120 mL of nondiet or regular soft drink. The client can also consume 6 to 10 hard candies or 1 tablespoon of honey or syrup. The client would not be instructed to administer insulin based on a sliding scale or to decrease carbohydrate intake as this would worsen the hypoglycemia; these measures would be used to manage *hyperglycemia*.

Test-Taking Strategy: Note that this clinical scenario describes symptoms consistent with hypoglycemia. Thinking about the pathophysiology and recalling the measures that are necessary to manage hypoglycemia will help direct you to the correct options. Remember that the food item given needs to be the correct item and in the correct amount in order to adequately raise the blood glucose while also not raising the blood glucose too high. Using a thinking process as illustrated in the table may be helpful to you.

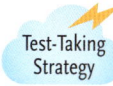

Food Item	Correct Item	Correct Amount
6 saltine crackers	Yes	Yes
3 graham crackers	Yes	Yes
120 mL of fruit juice	Yes	Yes
240 mL of skim milk	Yes	Yes
6 to 10 hard candies	Yes	Yes
4 tablespoons of honey	Yes	No
120 mL of diet soft drink	No	No

Food items that are correct items and are also correct in amount should be chosen as interventions for this scenario. Note that only 1 tablespoon of honey should be given to avoid raising the blood glucose too high. Also note that 120 mL of nondiet (rather than diet) soft drink can be given in the event of hypoglycemia. The last two options should be eliminated, noting that decreasing the intake of carbohydrates and administering insulin based on the sliding scale would further worsen the hypoglycemia. This leaves you with the five correct options: the saltine crackers, graham crackers, fruit juice, skim milk, and hard candies.

Content Area: Medical-Surgical Nursing
Priority Concept: Glucose Regulation; Tissue Integrity
Reference(s): Ignatavicius et al., 2024, pp. 1368–1370

CHAPTER 7

Answers to Practice Questions

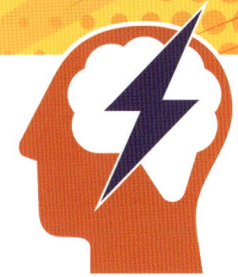

Practice Question 7.1 — Multiple Response Select All That Apply

An occupational nurse employed at a toy factory is called for emergency assistance to a 42-year-old victim of an accident.

Nurses' Notes | Vital Signs

1400: Victim is sitting on the floor leaning against a wall. Victim's index and middle finger were completely severed by a machine saw. The fingers are seen on the floor 2 feet away from the victim.

Nurses' Notes | **Vital Signs**

1400: T 98.2°F (36.7°C); HR 120; RR 22; BP 132/84; SpO$_2$ 95% on RA

Which of the following actions would the nurse take? **Select all that apply.**

- ☒ Call 911 (EMS).
- ☒ Elevate the affected hand above the victim's heart level.
- ☒ Place the fingers in a waterproof, sealed plastic bag.
- ☒ Check the victim for airway or breathing problems.
- ☐ Place the waterproof, sealed bag containing the fingers on ice.
- ☒ Apply direct pressure to the amputation sites with layers of dry gauze.
- ☐ Remove the dry gauze after 10 minutes to check the status of the bleeding.
- ☒ Ensure that the amputated fingers are transported to the hospital with the victim.

Rationale: The nurse needs to call 911 in the event of a traumatic amputation. Emergency care is necessary while waiting for transport of the victim to the hospital. The nurse would assess the victim for airway or breathing problems, examine the amputation sites, and apply direct pressure with layers of dry gauze. The hand is elevated above the victim's heart level to decrease the bleeding. Once the dressing has been applied, it is not removed to prevent dislodging of the clot that may form. The nurse would wrap the completely severed fingers in dry, sterile gauze and place them in a waterproof, sealed plastic bag. The bag is placed in ice water, never directly on ice, as 1 part ice and 3 parts water. The nurse would ensure that the amputated parts are transported to the hospital with the victim. While waiting for EMS to arrive, the nurse would stay with the client and monitor the victim's status including vital signs.

Test-Taking Strategy: Think about the goals of care for a victim of a traumatic amputation. Bleeding needs to be stopped, and adequate peripheral perfusion to the residual part needs to be maintained. The goal for the amputated part is to preserve perfusion for possible reattachment. With these goals in mind, read each option and think about how the action will achieve this goal. This will assist in answering correctly. Using a simple "Yes/No, Why or Why Not" approach with some thinking processes as to the rationale for each option will help you organize the information in a way that will help you answer correctly, as noted in the table.

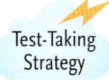
Test-Taking Strategy

Nursing Actions	Yes	No	Why or Why Not
Call 911 (EMS).	☒	☐	Emergency care needed for traumatic event
Elevate the affected hand above the victim's heart level.	☒	☐	To decrease bleeding and swelling
Place the fingers in a waterproof, sealed plastic bag.	☒	☐	To preserve the fingers for reattachment
Check the victim for airway or breathing problems.	☒	☐	To ensure cardiopulmonary stability
Place the waterproof, sealed bag containing the fingers on ice.	☐	☒	Not directly on ice—rather, in ice water; direct ice could damage tissue
Apply direct pressure to the amputation site with layers of dry gauze.	☒	☐	To decrease bleeding
Remove the dry gauze after 10 minutes to check the status of the bleeding.	☐	☒	Removal may dislodge any formed clots
Ensure that the amputated fingers are transported to the hospital with the victim.	☒	☐	For possible reattachment

Remember that test-taking strategies are useful ways to organize information to answer a test question. With Multiple Response Select All That Apply questions, the "Yes/No, Why or Why Not" approach is a helpful way to think through each option.

Content Area: Medical-Surgical Nursing
Priority Concept: Perfusion, Tissue Integrity
Reference(s): Ignatavicius et al., 2024, pp. 1098–1101

Practice Question 7.2 — Drop-Down Rationale

A client who is 4 weeks postpartum presents to the clinic with excessive vaginal bleeding.

Nurses' Notes / Vital Signs

1000: Client is 4 weeks postpartum and reports excessive vaginal bleeding with occasional spurts of excessive blood. Reports pelvic pain and feelings of pelvic heaviness, backache, fatigue, and persistent malaise.

Nurses' Notes / Vital Signs

1000: T 98.9°F (37.1°C); HR 100; RR 20; BP 110/70; SpO₂ 95% on RA

Complete the following sentence by selecting from the lists of options provided.

The nurse would **contact the obstetrician** because the client is *most* likely experiencing **subinvolution of the uterus**.

Options for 1	Options for 2
Contact the obstetrician.	Infection
Instruct the client to apply a heating pad on a low setting to the abdomen.	Septic shock
Teach the client about the warning signs of postpartum complications.	Subinvolution of the uterus

Rationale: Subinvolution refers to a slower than expected return of the uterus to its normal or nonpregnant size after childbirth. The most common causes of subinvolution are retained placental fragments and pelvic infection. Signs include prolonged discharge of lochia, irregular or excessive uterine bleeding, and sometimes profuse hemorrhage. Pelvic pain or feelings of pelvic heaviness, backache, fatigue, or persistent malaise are reported. On bimanual examination, the uterus feels larger and softer than normal. Although infection is a cause of subinvolution of the uterus, the client's temperature is normal; other client findings such as pelvic pain and pressure are not specific to infection when considering the larger picture of the client's health problem. Septic shock is a life-threatening condition caused by a severe localized or systemic infection that requires immediate intervention. Manifestations include signs of shock such as low blood pressure, pale and cool extremities, fever, difficulty breathing, and decreased urine output. The client exhibits no signs of septic shock. If the nurse suspects subinvolution of the uterus, the obstetrician is notified because therapeutic management includes oral administration of methylergonovine, which will promote long and sustained contractions of the uterus. Teaching the client about the warning signs of postpartum complications needs to be done before the client is discharged from the postpartum unit. Heat is not applied to the abdomen because it could cause increased bleeding; additionally, in this situation, an obstetrician order would need to be obtained for the use of heat.

Test-Taking Strategy: Begin to answer this question by determining which health condition the client is experiencing. Focus on the data in the question and medical record. Then use knowledge related to the manifestations associated with infection, septic shock, and subinvolution of the uterus to answer correctly. Create a table as shown to help you organize your thinking in determining the client's health problem.

Assessment Finding	Associated With Infection	Associated With Septic Shock	Associated With Subinvolution
Excessive vaginal bleeding	No	No	Yes
Occasional spurts of excessive blood	No	No	Yes
Pelvic pain	Yes	No	Yes
Pelvic heaviness	Yes	No	Yes
Backache	Yes	No	Yes
Fatigue	Yes	Yes	Yes
Persistent malaise	Yes	Yes	Yes
T 98.9°F (37.1°C); HR 100; RR 20; BP 110/70; SpO$_2$ 95% on RA	No	No	No

Setting up a table will help you determine what is occurring in the client. Noting that the vital signs are within normal range helps you determine that they are unrelated to any of the health problems presented in the question. Although some of the assessment findings relate to all health problems presented, all are associated with subinvolution.

Once you have determined the health problem, think about the pathophysiology of the problem to determine the action that the nurse would take. Time pressure is a consideration with client teaching. Create a table to help you visualize each action, how it may be helpful or not helpful or even worsen the situation, and the rationale.

Nursing Actions	Helpful/Rationale	Not Helpful/Worsen the Situation/Rationale
Contact the obstetrician.	Yes. Therapeutic management to promote contractions of the uterus can be initiated.	
Instruct the client to apply a heating pad on a low setting to the abdomen.		No. This could worsen the situation. Heat dilates the vessels and could lead to increased bleeding. An obstetrician's order for use of heat needs to be obtained.
Teach the client about the warning signs of postpartum complications.		No. Teaching about postpartum complications would have been done before discharge from the hospital.

Content Area: Obstetrics/Newborn Nursing
Priority Concept: Perfusion, Reproduction
Reference(s): Lowdermilk et al., 2024, pp. 419, 730, 777–778

Practice Question 7.3 — Matrix Multiple Response

A 65-year-old client was hospitalized and treated for symptoms of heart palpitations and extreme shortness of breath. On admission, diagnostic studies were performed.

Diagnostic Studies
ECG: atrial fibrillation
CT of the lungs: negative for embolism
Chest x-ray: enlarged left ventricle

The nurse is preparing the client for discharge and provides teaching about prescribed medications. For each medication listed, select the teaching point the nurse would provide to the client. Each teaching point may support more than one medication.

Teaching Point	Amiodarone	Metoprolol	Warfarin
Routine laboratory monitoring	☐	☐	☒
Monitor and report signs of bleeding	☐	☐	☒
Monitor and report shortness of breath	☒	☒	☐
Monitor BP and HR	☒	☒	☐
Consume consistent amounts of green, leafy vegetables	☐	☐	☒

Rationale: Amiodarone is an antidysrhythmic used to treat atrial fibrillation. It causes blood vessels to dilate and can lead to dizziness and hypotension. The client is taught how to check the heart rate and blood pressure. An adverse effect of amiodarone is pulmonary toxicity, and if the client experiences shortness of breath, it could be an indication that this effect is occurring, warranting prescriber notification. Metoprolol is a beta-adrenergic blocker and causes the heart rate and blood pressure to decrease, so the client needs to make sure the heart rate and blood pressure are within prescribed parameters before taking this medication so they do not drop too low. Metoprolol can also cause shortness of breath, coughing, and wheezing; if these occur, the nurse would notify the prescriber. The client taking amiodarone or metoprolol is taught safety measures such as moving slowly from a sitting or lying to a standing position and to immediately sit or lie down if dizziness or light-headedness occurs. The nurse would also instruct the client to contact the prescriber if these symptoms persist. Warfarin is an anticoagulant that requires routine laboratory monitoring for coagulation studies, specifically the international normalized ratio (INR), and dose adjustments are made based on the INR. Because warfarin slows clotting, an adverse effect is bleeding, and the client needs to monitor and report signs of bleeding. Green, leafy vegetables contain vitamin K, which is the antidote for warfarin. The client needs to consume consistent amounts of green, leafy vegetables so the vitamin K from these foods remains at a consistent level in the body and does not inhibit the effects of the warfarin.

Test-Taking Strategy: An important nursing action is to provide teaching to a client. Begin to answer this question by thinking about the medication classifications. Sometimes you will be easily able to recognize medication names and their classifications, and other times you will need to rely solely on knowledge. For example, metoprolol has a common suffix *(-lol),* which helps you determine that this medication belongs to the beta-adrenergic blocker classification. From here, you may need to use your knowledge and determine the other medication classifications. Rather than trying to learn every medication and everything about them, learn medications by associating them with a specific classification. The indications, side effects and adverse effects, and primary nursing considerations and teaching points for a classification will be similar, so if you can associate a medication with a classification, this will really help you in answering pharmacology questions. Organizing information in the format shown in the table when answering pharmacology questions will be a helpful strategy in answering these questions correctly. In this question, recalling the medication classifications and associated side effects and adverse effects as well as the primary nursing considerations will help you determine the teaching points specific to each medication.

Medication Classification	Indications	Side Effects / Adverse Effects	Primary Nursing Considerations/ Teaching Points
Warfarin (anticoagulant)	Long-term prophylaxis of thrombosis	Bleeding	Multiple drug-drug and drug-food interactions Review medications and client's diet to identify any interactions Monitor for bleeding: bruising, urine, stool Safety measures
Amiodarone (antidysrhythmic)	Management of atrial and ventricular dysrhythmias	Pulmonary, cardiac, liver, and thyroid toxicity Ophthalmic effects Photosensitivity	Monitor for signs and symptoms of toxicity Measure HR and BP Report episodes of light-headedness or dizziness
Metoprolol (beta-adrenergic blocker)	Treatment of hypertension, angina, heart failure, and myocardial infarction	Bradycardia, reduced cardiac output, heart block, rebound cardiac excitation	Measure HR and BP Monitor for and report adverse effects such as light-headedness or dizziness, coughing, wheezing

Content Area: Pharmacology
Priority Concept: Clotting, Perfusion
Reference(s): Lilley et al., 2023, pp. 390, 414

Practice Question 7.4 — Matrix Multiple Choice

A parent brings a 6-month-old child to the ED.

Health History | Nurses' Notes | Orders | Laboratory Results

1830: Parent reports that the child has been coughing and sneezing, seems to be "breathing funny," and feels warm. Parent reports being single and unhoused. Reports "living on the street, but sleeps in a shelter with the child most nights." Parent states that the child does not have a pediatrician and has not received any child care since birth. Reports still breast-feeding as the child's primary nutritional intake, but child has been refusing to feed.

Health History | Nurses' Notes | Orders | Laboratory Results

1830: T 102°F (38.8°C); HR 176; RR 80; SpO$_2$ 91% on RA
Coughing, sneezing with runny nose
Copious secretions
Color pale, no cyanosis, listless, retractions noted, wheezes noted at lung bases bilaterally
Weight 12.8 lb (5.8 kg), length 22 inches

Health History | Nurses' Notes | Orders | Laboratory Results

1900:
Rapid RSV antigen test
Heated high-flow oxygen 1 L/min via NC
Insert IV, and administer 0.9% NS 25 mL/h
Admit to pediatric unit

Health History | Nurses' Notes | Orders | Laboratory Results

1930:

Test and Reference Range	Result
RSV antigen test negative	Positive

The physician admits the child to the hospital, and the admitting pediatric nurse reviews the ED notes. Select whether the following potential nursing actions are indicated or not indicated for the child at this time.

Potential Nursing Actions	Indicated	Not Indicated
Monitor weight.	☒	☐
Administer oral fluids.	☐	☒
Perform a well-baby assessment.	☒	☐
Suction the airway and nares as needed.	☒	☐
Restrict the parent from holding the child.	☐	☒
Monitor airway status and vital signs.	☒	☐
Assist the parent to pump breast milk.	☒	☐
Institute Contact Precautions and Droplet Precautions.	☒	☐
Contact social services for consultation.	☒	☐
Institute chest percussion and chest physiotherapy for drainage.	☐	☒

Rationale: Respiratory syncytial virus (RSV) is a paramyxovirus infection that affects the epithelial cells of the respiratory tract. It can lead to bronchiolitis. RSV infection occurs more frequently in children who live in crowded conditions and is a frequent cause of hospitalization in children younger than 2 years of age. Initial manifestations of RSV include rhinorrhea, pharyngitis, coughing, sneezing, wheezing, and intermittent fever. With progression of the infection, tachypnea and retractions, copious secretions, and refusal to feed is noted. Severe illness is manifested by tachypnea greater than 70 bpm, listlessness, apneic spells, poor air exchange, and cyanosis. Most uncomplicated cases can be managed at home. However, hospitalization is needed in this scenario because this child is exhibiting signs of severe illness, and the situation is complicated due to homelessness, lack of child care since birth, and the potential inability of the parent to provide adequate care during the child's illness. Hospitalized children with RSV may need a separate room or in some situations may cohort with other RSV children. Contact Precautions and Standard Precautions along with Droplet

Precautions will be instituted. Oral administration of fluids is contraindicated in cases in which the child is tachypneic or listless. If secretions are copious, it may be difficult for the child to take in fluids orally and could present a risk for aspiration. IV fluids may be initiated and continued until the acute stage of the disease has passed. NG tube feeding may also be a consideration if the child is able to tolerate intake. Routine chest percussion and drainage is not recommended if secretions are in the upper airway, but children with copious secretions would benefit from regular suctioning, so the nurse would perform suctioning to assist with airway patency. Heated high-flow nasal cannula (HFNC) oxygen therapy may be prescribed to reduce the work of breathing. The nurse would monitor airway status including vital signs and pulse oximetry because they are abnormal. The nurse would also monitor weight. The average weight of a 6-month-old child is 16.1 lb (7.31 kg) to 17.5 lb (7.95 kg), and the average length is 25.9 to 26.6 inches, based on biological gender. This child is below these norms. These findings along with the report that the child has not had any child care since birth warrants the need for a well-baby assessment to determine the child's health needs, need for immunizations, and a plan for follow-up. The nurse would consult with social services to assist in determining the needs of the child and parent and assist in developing a plan. The parent should be allowed to hold the child while taking the necessary transmission precautions including strict handwashing, and the nurse would encourage and assist the parent to pump milk to store for later use.

Test-Taking Strategy: To answer this question, it is important to use your knowledge regarding the care of a child with RSV and think about the nursing action and its effect on the child regarding promoting improvement in the child's condition. Focus on the manifestations that the child is exhibiting to help determine how the action will or will not be helpful. Create a table as the one below to assist in visualizing the care of the child.

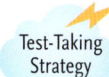

Nursing Action	Helpful in the Care of the Child	Not Helpful in the Care of the Child
Monitor weight.	Helpful: The child's weight and length are below norms.	
Administer oral fluids.		Not helpful: The child is coughing and sneezing and has copious secretions, so it may be difficult to take in oral fluids. The child is listless and tachypneic, so aspiration is a concern. Additionally, the child is refusing intake.
Perform a well-baby assessment.	Helpful: The child has not received child care since birth, and the child's needs require attention. This includes a complete assessment, eye and ear tests, immunizations, and other assessments.	
Suction the airway and nares as needed.	Helpful: Secretions are copious in the upper airway, and this will assist in their removal.	
Restrict the parent from holding the child.		Not helpful: The child needs touch and attention from someone known to the child. If the parent uses appropriate precautions, this should be allowed.

Continued

Nursing Action	Helpful in the Care of the Child	Not Helpful in the Care of the Child
Monitor airway status and vital signs.	Helpful: Needed to monitor status and to detect any deterioration in the child's condition.	
Assist the parent to pump breast milk.	Helpful: Breast-feeding is the child's form of intake so should be continued. It also provides nutritional value.	
Institute Contact Precautions and Droplet Precautions.	Helpful: Prevents transmission to others.	
Contact social services for consultation.	Helpful: Social services can be an important component in planning care for the child and the parent for follow-up needs and living situation.	
Institute chest percussion and chest physiotherapy for drainage.		Not helpful: May be too aggressive for the child's needs. The child's secretions are in the upper airway, and suctioning would be adequate for their removal.

Content Area: Pediatric Nursing
Priority Concept: Gas Exchange, Infection
Reference(s): Hockenberry et al., 2024, pp. 893–895

Practice Question 7.5 — Multiple Response Select All That Apply

The nurse is caring for a 48-year-old client following a laparoscopic cholecystectomy on the surgical outpatient unit.

Nurses' Notes | Vital Signs

1100: Alert and oriented. Dressing dry and intact. IV 5% dextrose/lactated Ringer's infusing at 100 mL/h. Has not voided.

Nurses' Notes | Vital Signs

1100: T 99.2°F (37.3°C); HR 92; RR 16; BP 118/72; SpO$_2$ 97% on RA; Reports pain rated 4/10 (on a 0–10 pain scale)

Which of the following actions would the nurse take in managing this client's care in the immediate postoperative period? **Select all that apply.**

☐ Keep the head of the bed flat.
☒ Assist the client to the bathroom to void.
☒ Assess the incision sites frequently.
☒ Administer antiemetics as needed.
☐ Maintain strict NPO status.
☒ Administer pain medication.
☒ Encourage use of the incentive spirometer.

Rationale: Care of the client in the immediate postoperative period following laparoscopic cholecystectomy includes keeping the head of the bed elevated to avoid aspiration and promote comfort, assisting the client to the bathroom to void, assessing incision sites frequently, administering antiemetics as needed, offering food and water when the client is fully awake, administering pain medication as needed, and encouraging use of an incentive spirometer while awake. Keeping the head of the bed flat would be contraindicated and could result in aspiration, particularly if the client is experiencing nausea and vomiting. In addition, this position causes stress on the abdominal incision sites. It is not necessary to maintain NPO status, but food and water need to be offered after the client is alert to prevent aspiration.

Test-Taking Strategy: Note the strategic word *immediate,* and think about the nursing actions necessary in caring for a client immediately after laparoscopic cholecystectomy as well as general nursing actions for clients undergoing surgery. Using the "Yes/No, Why or Why Not" approach with some thinking processes about the rationale for each option will help you organize the information in a way that will help you answer correctly, as noted in the table.

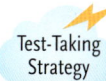

Nursing Actions	Yes	No	Why or Why Not
Keep the head of the bed flat.	☐	☒	Could result in aspiration; postoperative clients often have nausea and vomiting; may cause stress on the incision sites.
Assist the client to the bathroom to void.	☒	☐	Ensuring adequate voiding after surgery is important because urinary retention can occur from anesthesia. Ambulation is also important to prevent respiratory and circulatory complications.
Assess the incision sites frequently.	☒	☐	Monitor for bleeding, drainage, opening of incisions, and infection.
Administer antiemetics as needed.	☒	☐	Nausea and vomiting are common effects of anesthesia.
Maintain strict NPO status.	☐	☒	Would be used prior to surgery but is not needed following surgery. Need to ensure adequate oral intake after surgery and maintain nutrition and hydration when safe to do so.
Administer pain medication.	☒	☐	Pain management in the immediate postoperative period is important in promoting comfort, mobility, and recovery.
Encourage use of the incentive spirometer.	☒	☐	Important in preventing atelectasis and resultant pneumonia.

Remember that test-taking strategies are useful ways to organize information to answer a test question. With Multiple Response questions, the "Yes/No, Why or Why Not" approach is a helpful way to think through each option and rationale and will assist you in choosing the correct answers.

Content Area: Medical-Surgical Nursing
Priority Concept: Inflammation, Tissue Integrity
Reference(s): Ignatavicius et al., 2024, pp. 1244–1245

Practice Question 7.6 — Drop-Down Rationale

The nurse is caring for a hospitalized 70-year-old client who has cellulitis on both lower extremities caused by methicillin-resistant *Staphylococcus aureus* (MRSA) and is being treated with IV vancomycin.

Vital Signs

1100: T 100.8°F (38.2°C); HR 88; RR 18; BP 110/72; SpO$_2$ 96% on RA; Reports pain rated 3/10 (on a 0–10 pain scale)

Laboratory Results

1100:

Test and Reference Range	Result
Vancomycin trough level 10–20 mcg/mL (10.3498–13.7998 µmol/L)	16 mcg/mL (11.3981 µmol/L)
White blood cells (WBCs) 5000–10,000/mm^3 (5–10 × 10^9/L)	11,000/mm^3 (11 × 10^9/L)
Blood urea nitrogen (BUN) 10–20 mg/dL (3.6–7.1 mmol/L)	20 mg/dL (7.1 mmol/L)
Creatinine 0.5–1.2 mg/dL (44–106 µmol/L)	0.6 mg/dL (53 µmol/L)

The next dose of vancomycin is due now, and the nurse checks the laboratory results. Complete the following sentence by selecting from the lists of options provided.

The nurse would **administer the next dose as prescribed** because **the trough level is normal**.

Options for 1	Options for 2
Hold the next dose.	The WBC count is slightly elevated.
Administer a lower dose.	The trough level is normal.
Administer the next dose orally.	The creatinine level indicates toxicity.
Administer the next dose as prescribed.	The BUN level is high but not toxic.

Rationale: Vancomycin is classified as an antimicrobial and works by inhibiting bacterial cell wall synthesis. It is indicated for treatment of serious infections, including infections caused by MRSA. Vancomycin is normally administered orally or intravenously. IV administration is indicated for systemic infections. Dosages need to be reduced in renal impairment, and trough levels need to be monitored for IV vancomycin. The trough level is the lowest concentration of the medication in the client's bloodstream; therefore the specimen should be collected just prior to administration of the vancomycin. The peak level is the highest concentration of the medication in the client's bloodstream. A peak level is drawn 1 hour to several hours as prescribed after the medication is administered, depending on the medication. Vancomycin trough levels of 10 to 20 mcg/mL (10.3498 to 13.7998 µmol/L) are recommended for the most favorable outcomes. A trough level of 16 mcg/mL (11.3981 µmol/L) is normal and in the expected range and indicates that the kidneys are adequately excreting the medication as expected; therefore the nurse can administer the next dose as prescribed based on this information. The reference range for vancomycin peak levels is 20 to 40 mcg/mL (13.7998 to 27.5995 µmol/L). The client's WBC count is slightly elevated, and an elevation is expected if an infection is present. The BUN and creatinine levels are within reference range.

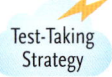

Test-Taking Strategy: First, it is necessary to review the client's laboratory results and note alterations in the levels. From there, it may be helpful to look at the options for the second response column first and determine the appropriate action in terms of dosage adjustment for these findings. This may help you choose the correct answer for the first response column. Refer to the table for an illustration applying this strategy.

Laboratory Result	Action and Rationale
The WBC count is slightly elevated.	No specific action is indicated as the value is expected in infection; this is why the antibiotic is being administered.
The trough level is normal and in expected range.	The same dosage can be administered; the level is in the expected reference range and indicates that the kidneys are adequately excreting the medication as expected.
The creatinine level is normal, not toxic.	No specific action is indicated as the value is in the reference range.
The BUN is normal, not high or toxic.	No specific action is indicated as the value is in the reference range.

Use knowledge to determine that the WBC count is slightly elevated and is expected and the BUN and creatinine level are within reference range. Next, if you can determine that the trough level is in the reference range, you can then decide that the same dosage would be indicated. This will assist in directing you to administer the next dose as prescribed as a safe and appropriate nursing action based on this clinical scenario.

Content Area: Pharmacology
Priority Concept: Elimination, Infection
Reference(s): Lilley et al., 2023, pp. 621, 624

CHAPTER 8

Answers to Practice Questions

Practice Question 8.1 — Matrix Multiple Choice

A 68-year-old client was transferred from the hospital to a rehabilitation center 2 weeks ago following treatment for a right cerebral stroke. The nurse is preparing the client for discharge to home and reviews the admission notes.

Nurses' Notes | Vital Signs | Physician's Orders

1300: Transferred from the hospital. Client is accompanied by spouse, who will be the primary caregiver when the client returns home. Alert and oriented and understands about receiving rehabilitative therapy before returning to home. States does not really have "much to rehab" and is fine, but will do what the doctor says to get home. Has left-sided weakness, and seems impulsive with movements. Able to move right arm and leg with adequate strength noted. Has difficulty focusing, and attention span is short; spouse is assisting with answering questions. Spouse notes that client's judgment is impaired and is concerned about client's safety because of the client's impulsivity. Client exhibits left-sided neglect; lacks proprioception. Has homonymous hemianopsia.

Nurses' Notes | **Vital Signs** | Physician's Orders

1300: T 98.6°F (36°C); HR 92; RR 20; BP 132/78; SpO$_2$ 95% on RA

Nurses' Notes | Vital Signs | **Physician's Orders**

1300:
PT and OT evaluation and initiate a treatment plan as needed
Low-fat diet
Out of bed as much as tolerated
Begin to prepare client and spouse for discharge to home
Referral to case manager to plan discharge
Clopidogrel 75 mg oral daily
Carvedilol 3.125 mg oral twice daily
Docusate 100 mg oral daily
Simvastatin 20 mg oral daily

Collaboration with the client and spouse and the case manager reveals that the spouse will need assistance with the client's personal needs and activities of daily living and with ambulation and physical therapy. A home care aide is scheduled to visit the client for 3 hours daily, and physical therapy is planned for home visits 3 times weekly. The nurse implements a teaching plan and assesses readiness for discharge.

For each client or spouse statement/observation, select whether the home care instruction is either understood or requires further teaching.

Client or Spouse Statement/Observation	Understood	Requires Further Teaching
Client places the right arm into the shirt sleeve first when putting the shirt on.	☐	☒
Spouse states, "It will help vision if I approach my spouse from the right side."	☒	☐
Spouse states, "I will talk to the home care aides when they come to be sure they get all of the care done during the first hour after they arrive."	☐	☒
Client turns the head to the right and then to the left before taking on an activity.	☒	☐
Client states, "I know that I need to call for help if I need to use the bathroom."	☒	☐
Client states, "I can skip the stool softener medication if I have a bowel movement."	☐	☒
Client picks up a washcloth with the left hand to wash the face.	☒	☐

Rationale: A right cerebral stroke occurs in the right side of the brain. The effects of a right cerebral stroke may include left-sided weakness or paralysis and sensory impairment. The client tends to deny deficits such as weakness or paralysis. Visual problems include an inability to see the left visual field of each eye. Unilateral neglect, also known as *unilateral inattention,* occurs most commonly in clients who have had a right cerebral stroke. This problem places the client at risk for injury, especially falls, because of an inability to recognize the physical impairment on one side of the body or a lack of proprioception (body position sense). The client needs to be taught to touch and use both sides of the body. When dressing, the client needs to be reminded to dress the affected side first, which would be the client's left side. In addition, the client should be encouraged to use the affected side so attention is paid to the deficit. The client can use the unaffected side to assist with using the affected (neglected) side. For example, the client can use the unaffected hand to hold the affected hand to perform the activity, such as washing the face. In homonymous hemianopsia, vision is lost on the same side of the visual field in both eyes. The client should be approached from the unaffected visual side so the client can sense someone approaching. In addition, the client is taught to turn the head from side to side to scan the environment and expand the visual field. Because of the client's short attention span, activities should be divided into short steps rather than being performed all at one time. Trying to complete all care and activities in 1 hour can also be very frustrating to the client. Because of the left-sided weakness, the client is at risk for injury, so the client needs to be encouraged to call for assistance when getting out of bed or for other activities that can cause injury. Stool softeners need to be taken on a daily basis as prescribed to assist in promoting bowel elimination because of the risk of constipation caused by decreased mobility. In addition, stool softeners prevent the Valsalva maneuver during defecation to prevent increased intracranial pressure.

Test-Taking Strategy: Begin answering this question by thinking about the physical manifestations following a stroke. Remember that if the stroke affects the right side of the brain, then deficits will be noted on the left side, whereas if the stroke affects the left side of the brain, then deficits will be noted on the right side. Focusing on the fact that this client experienced a right-sided stroke and therefore will exhibit left-sided physical deficits, evaluate each of the statements or observations and consider whether the action will be helpful or not helpful for a client experiencing left-sided physical deficits. Organize your thinking process as illustrated in the table.

Client or Spouse Statement/Observation	Helpful	Not Helpful
Client places the right arm into the shirt sleeve first when putting the shirt on.		X
Spouse states, "It will help vision if I approach my spouse from the right side."	X	
Spouse states, "I will talk to the home care aides when they come to be sure they get all of the care done during the first hour after they arrive."		X
Client turns the head to the right and then to the left before taking on an activity.	X	
Client states, "I know that I need to call for help if I need to use the bathroom."	X	
Client states, "I can skip the stool softener medication if I have a bowel movement."		X
Client picks up a washcloth with the left hand to wash the face.	X	

Caregiving for this client will be helpful by ensuring that others approach the client from the right side, encouraging the client to turn the head to the right and then the left when scanning the environment, and reminding the client to call for help to go to the bathroom. Also recall that both sides need to be used, and the affected side should not be neglected so strength can be regained over time on that side. Looking at the other options, note that it will not be helpful for the client to place the right arm into the right sleeve of the shirt first because of the physical limitations on the left side. Clustering care in the first hour will cause exhaustion and depletion and will also delay recovery. Lastly, recall the pharmacologic concepts surrounding the use of stool softeners, remembering that they work best as a preventive measure, so they should still be taken even with bowel movements occurring.

Content Area: Medical-Surgical Nursing
Priority Concepts: Mobility; Perfusion
Reference(s): Ignatavicius et al., 2024, pp. 948–956

Practice Question 8.2 — Multiple Response Grouping

The nurse performs an admission assessment of a 16-year-old client being admitted to the mental health residential treatment center.

Nurses' Notes

1500: Client is accompanied by parent. Parent consistently interrupts client during the interview. Parent states that client is compulsive and always has to have everything in perfect order or becomes anxious. Parent states, "I was just like my child when I was that age and always had to look perfect and be perfect with everything that I did. I know my child is very skinny, but that is how I was when I was a teenager. I had to starve myself to keep my hourglass figure." Client reports not socializing much because of being too busy exercising and reports constant exercising all day long, at least 10 times a day for 1 hour each session. Reports the need to burn calories and stay in control of weight. States hardly eats because of feeling fat and appearing fat to others. Is very fearful of gaining weight; describes restrictive eating patterns. Loves to collect food recipes and cookbooks and prepare huge meals for other people but does not eat with them. Denies alcohol or drug misuse. Denies suicidal ideation. Denies food binging and purging or use of laxatives or enemas. Reports amenorrhea for the past 3 months. Face is hollowed with sunken eyes. Skin is pale; hair is dry and thin. Growth of lanugo on skin; skin is yellow tinged. Complains of dizziness and skipped heartbeats.

Vital Signs

1500: T 96.4°F (35.7°C); HR 40; RR 16; BP 88/48; SpO$_2$ 92% on RA
Height: 5 ft 6 in
Weight: 88 lb (40 kg)
BMI: 15.99 kg/m^2

An interdisciplinary treatment approach was instituted to treat the client's eating disorder and included nutritional consultation, weight restoration therapy, intensive psychotherapy, and counseling and family therapy. After 70 days of treatment, the interdisciplinary team meets to discuss the client's readiness for discharge to home and use of outpatient support services.

The nurse evaluates for acceptable outcome criteria indicating readiness for discharge. For each factor below, select if the finding indicates readiness for discharge. **Each factor may support more than one finding.**

Factor	Finding
Physiologic	☒ Weight: 102 lb (46.3 kg)
	☒ Eating 80% of each of the 3 meals delivered by the dietary department and 2 snacks
	☐ Laboratory Results:

Test and Reference Range	Result
Potassium 3.5–5.0 mEq/L (3.5–5.0 mmol/L)	3.2 mEq/L (3.2 mmol/L)
Sodium 135–145 mEq/L (135–145 mmol/L)	130 mEq/L (130 mmol/L)
Chloride 98–106 mEq/L (98–106 mmol/L)	95 mEq/L (95 mmol/L)

Factor	Finding
Psychological	Client states:
	☐ "I really need to walk around the nursing unit 10 times a day and do 45 laps each time. I was doing 50 laps each time, but I cut down to 45."
	☐ "I counted the calories I ate for the day, and it came to 950. I think that's more than enough, but I need to keep counting the calories to be sure."
	☒ "I am clear about what triggers my disruptive eating patterns, and I know what alternative behaviors I need to take to help this."
Social	Client states:
	☐ "My best friend asked if I would go to lunch with some of our friends, but I'm not going to go because I have nothing to wear that makes me look good. All my clothes are too tight."
	☒ "My parent is taking me and my siblings to that new movie that just came out; it'll be fun. I'm really looking forward to sharing a big box of popcorn and drinking a cola!"
	☐ "I have no interest in going to my prom this year. I've gained this weight, and people in my class are definitely going to notice that."
Family support	☐ Parent states will be sure that the child eats at least 3 full meals a day and 2 snacks and will remove and throw away any "teen magazines" or other distracting books or magazines that are in the child's bedroom.
	☒ Parent states that all of the children are going to take a 15-minute walk every evening after dinner.
	☒ Parent states, "My child seems to want to stay close to home, but I'm encouraging my child to spend some time with friends from school. I think these peer relationships are important."
Follow-up	☐ Parent states that family therapy sessions are not necessary because the problem is with the one child "and not the family."
	Client states:
	☐ "I have an appointment with the nutrition person in 2 weeks, but I'm thinking that if I maintain my weight and eat like I'm supposed to, then I can cancel it."
	☒ "The nurse at my school says there is a support group for students with eating problems and that they meet weekly. Do you think this will help me?"

Rationale: Individuals with anorexia nervosa, an eating disorder, have intense irrational beliefs about their shape and weight. They engage in self-starvation behaviors and express intense fear of gaining weight. Physiologic outcome criteria for a client with anorexia nervosa include that the client consume a healthy diet and adequate daily calories per kilogram of body weight, demonstrate and maintain an ideal body weight, maintain normal fluid and electrolyte levels, and demonstrate skin turgor and muscle tone that indicate that the nutritional state is proportionate with physiologic and metabolic needs. The client is 102 lb (46.3 kg), which reflects a 14-lb weight gain since admission. A weight less than 90 lb (40.9 kg) can be life-threatening. Although 102 lb (46.3 kg) may not be the ideal weight, it does indicate a gain of 14 lb. Eating 80% of each meal and 2 snacks is a positive outcome for the client. If the client's electrolyte levels are abnormal, this is not a positive outcome and needs to be addressed because of the adverse effects and in some situations life-threatening effects on the body; this does not meet acceptable criteria for discharge. This client's electrolyte levels are low. An extreme regimen of physical exercise in an effort to burn unwanted calories and a focus on counting calories indicate compulsive behavior. In addition, cutting laps from 50 to 45 and thinking that 950 calories a day is sufficient is unhealthy thinking. However, the ability to identify triggers for disruptive eating patterns and strategies that will manage impaired behaviors is positive criterion. These clients express a disturbance in the way their body weight, size, or shape is experienced or viewed and see themselves as fat, although they are grossly underweight. Thinking that clothes are too tight or that classmates will notice a weight gain is a negative outcome. However, viewing a social activity such as a movie as fun and looking forward to sharing popcorn and drinking a cola is a positive outcome. The family's ability to relate to one another and to the client in a meaningful way is important. Clients with anorexia nervosa should not be forced to eat or be punished for not eating because these methods only make them fight more for control. The client should not be controlled in any way because this can disrupt the positive progression. Removing items from the client's room, such as magazines, is controlling and punitive and will not help in the healing process. Rather, giving the client control and responsibility provides the client with the opportunity to grow, develop, and take charge of one's own life. Peer relationships are important and should be encouraged. Taking a 15-minute walk every evening after dinner is a positive activity; the parent shows that exercise in some form is important, acceptable, and healthy. Exercise within limits is important to maintain physical and emotional wellness. Family therapy is helpful to identify strategies to deal with behaviors effectively. Follow-up appointments with a nutritional therapist are important to ensure that adequate progression is made and that weight reaches normal and is maintained because starvation is life-threatening. Any faltering from the plan of care can be identified and addressed early. Support groups provide a safe, supportive setting that gives clients the opportunity to share problems and discuss strategies for management of symptoms.

Test-Taking Strategy: A simple "positive/negative" thinking process can be applied to help you answer this question correctly. Using the table, consider each finding and whether it would be an adaptive or maladaptive outcome for a client with anorexia nervosa.

Finding	Positive (Adaptive)	Negative (Maladaptive)
Weight: 102 lb (46.3 kg)	☒	☐
Eating 80% of each of the 3 meals delivered by the dietary department and 2 snacks	☒	☐
Electrolyte results indicate: Potassium 3.2 mEq/L (3.2 mmol/L); sodium 130 mEq/L (130 mmol/L); chloride 95 mEq/L (95 mmol/L)	☐	☒
"I really need to walk around the nursing unit 10 times a day and do 45 laps each time. I was doing 50 laps each time but cut down to 45."	☐	☒
"I counted my calories that I ate for the day and it came to 950. I think that's more than enough, but I need to keep counting the calories to be sure."	☐	☒
"I am clear about what triggers my disruptive eating patterns, and I know what alternative behaviors I need to take to help this."	☒	☐
"My best friend asked if I would go to lunch with some of our friends, but I'm not going to go because I have nothing to wear that makes me look good. All my clothes are too tight."	☐	☒
"My parent is taking me and my siblings to that new movie that just came out; it'll be fun. I'm really looking forward to sharing a big box of popcorn and drinking a cola!"	☒	☐
"I have no interest in going to my prom this year. I've gained this weight, and people in my class are definitely going to notice that."	☐	☒
Parent states will be sure that the child eats at least 3 full meals a day and 2 snacks and will remove and throw away any "teen magazines" or other distracting books or magazines that are in the child's bedroom.	☐	☒
Parent states that all of the children are going to take a 15-minute walk every evening after dinner.	☒	☐
Parent states, "My child seems to want to stay close to home, but I'm encouraging my child to spend some time with friends from school. I think these peer relationships are important."	☒	☐
Parent states that family therapy sessions are not necessary because the problem is with the one child "and not the family."	☐	☒
"I have an appointment with the nutrition person in 2 weeks, but I'm thinking that if I maintain my weight and eat like I'm supposed to, then I can cancel it."	☐	☒
"The nurse at my school says there is a support group for students with eating problems and that they meet weekly. Do you think this will help me?"	☒	☐

In evaluating each of these findings, look for words or indicators that indicate progression toward a successful outcome. Consider negative words, such as "I have no interest," and associate these with a negative or maladaptive outcome. On the other hand, evaluate positive words, such as "support groups," as being aligned with a positive or adaptive outcome. Using this thinking process will help you organize your evaluation and answer this question correctly.

Content Area: Mental Health Nursing
Priority Concepts: Mood and Affect; Stress and Coping
Reference(s): Halter, 2022, pp. 332–337

Practice Question 8.3 — Multiple Response Select N

A 68-year-old unhoused client was brought to the ED by EMS, who reports that the client was found lying in an alley. The client is diagnosed with atrial fibrillation and rapid ventricular response. Intravenous amiodarone is prescribed to treat the dysrhythmia.

History and Physical

1215: A 68-year-old unhoused client is brought to the ED by EMS. Reports "heart fluttering" and shortness of breath that started this morning. Associated with fatigue and dizziness; worsened by activity. No alleviating factors; symptoms are constant. Denies chest pain, losing consciousness, and difficulty breathing while lying down. Reports past medical history of hypertension, hyperlipidemia, and type 2 diabetes mellitus. States that family history is negative for cardiac events. Speaks in short sentences; appears short of breath while talking. Skin is warm, dry, and intact throughout. Rapid, irregular HR, 120–140 on auscultation. Lung sounds clear on auscultation in all fields. No peripheral edema.

Nurses' Notes

1215: Client admitted to ED. Received orders for IV amiodarone.

1230: Admission assessment completed. Amiodarone started. Continuous VS monitoring and cardiac monitor in place. Cardiac monitor shows shortened PR interval, narrowed QRS complex, atrial fibrillation with an irregular rate of 120–140.

1300: Follow-up VS and assessment completed. Client reports tremors, light sensitivity, lack of appetite with nausea, vomiting × 1 undigested food, no hematemesis. HR 102 and regular; BP 90/56. Cardiac monitor shows prolongation of previously shortened PR interval, widening of previously narrowed QRS complex, atrial fibrillation converted to sinus rhythm. 2+ pitting peripheral edema.

Vital Signs

1215: T 98.8°F (37.1°C); HR 120–140 and irregular; RR 22; BP 128/76; SpO₂ 95% on RA

1230: HR 120–140 and irregular; RR 22; BP 128/76; SpO₂ 95% on RA

1300: HR 102 and regular; RR 22; BP 90/56; SpO₂ 95% on RA

---

*Select the **4** client findings that indicate a therapeutic outcome of medication therapy.*

- ☐ Reports of tremors
- ☐ Reports of photosensitivity
- ☐ BP 90/56
- ☒ HR 102 and regular
- ☒ Prolonged PR interval
- ☒ Widened QRS complex
- ☐ 2+ peripheral edema pitting bilaterally
- ☐ Reports of anorexia, nausea, and vomiting
- ☒ Atrial fibrillation converted to sinus rhythm

Rationale: Amiodarone is an antidysrhythmic used for treatment and prevention of atrial fibrillation and other cardiac dysrhythmias. For this client experiencing atrial fibrillation with rapid ventricular response, IV therapy is a lifesaving measure. The client comes to the ED with elevated heart rate, shortened PR interval, narrowed QRS complex, and atrial fibrillation, as noted on the cardiac monitor. Amiodarone primarily affects the atrioventricular node and slows conduction; therefore, on follow-up assessment after starting the medication, client findings that indicate a therapeutic outcome include heart rate regular at 102 (previously irregular at 120 to 140), prolongation of the PR interval (previously shortened), widening of the QRS complex (previously narrowed), and conversion of the rhythm from atrial fibrillation to sinus rhythm. Reports of tremors; photosensitivity; and anorexia, nausea, and vomiting are adverse (as opposed to therapeutic) outcomes associated with amiodarone use. Blood pressure of 90/56 (previously 128/76) indicates hypotension, which can occur as an adverse outcome (not therapeutic) in some clients receiving this medication. Peripheral edema is an abnormal finding and may be associated with cardiotoxicity and heart failure, which is another possible adverse outcome (not therapeutic) of this medication.

Test-Taking Strategy: Evaluate each of the options in this question, thinking about whether the finding is consistent with a therapeutic outcome or an adverse outcome, recalling that amiodarone is used for its antidysrhythmic properties. Also think about the normal and abnormal findings. Using the table, consider each finding and whether it would be a therapeutic or normal and expected outcome or an adverse or abnormal and unexpected outcome.

Finding	Therapeutic Outcome	Adverse Outcome
Reports of tremors	☐	✗
Reports of photosensitivity	☐	✗
BP 90/56	☐	✗
HR regular at 102	✗	☐
Prolonged PR interval	✗	☐
Widened QRS complex	✗	☐
2+ peripheral edema pitting bilaterally	☐	✗
Reports of anorexia, nausea, and vomiting	☐	✗
Atrial fibrillation converted to sinus rhythm	✗	☐

Think about cardiac monitoring findings when a client is experiencing atrial fibrillation with rapid ventricular response. The heart rate will be elevated, the PR interval shortened, the QRS complex narrowed, and morphology reflective of fibrillation in the atria. Knowing that amiodarone is used to address the problems with cardiac conduction, consider these options as the answers, and then further evaluate them to determine whether they indicate a therapeutic outcome. Also recall that, although amiodarone can be very beneficial and in some cases lifesaving, there are adverse outcomes; therefore monitoring the client and evaluating for therapeutic as well as adverse outcomes is integral to promoting safe client care. The incorrect options are not specifically related to cardiac conduction and would be good options to consider as possible adverse outcomes of amiodarone.

Content Area: Pharmacology
Priority Concepts: Gas Exchange; Perfusion
Reference(s): Ignatavicius et al., 2024, pp. 673–679

Practice Question 8.4 — Matrix Multiple Choice

A 39-year-old client is being seen in the outpatient pain management clinic for follow-up evaluation.

History and Physical | Vital Signs

0900: Client sustained an injury to the cervical and lumbar spine in a motor vehicle accident 1 year ago and has been experiencing neck and back pain since the injury. Client has tried conservative measures, including ice and heat, massage, and PT. Client has also tried acetaminophen, NSAIDs, muscle relaxants, and opioid analgesics, and the pain has become intolerable again, even with these measures. Client was seen in clinic 1 month ago, and amitriptyline was added to the treatment plan. Visit to the clinic today for a 1-month follow-up evaluation.

History and Physical | **Vital Signs**

0900: T 98.8°F (37.1°C); HR 80; RR 22; BP 138/92; SpO$_2$ 95% on RA; reports pain rated 2/10 (on a 0–10 pain scale)

For each client statement/observation, select whether the statement/observation indicates that treatment with amitriptyline is effective or ineffective.

Statement/Observation	Effective	Ineffective
Client states, "My back and neck are sore after PT."	X	
Client states, "I have been walking a mile each day before going to work."	X	
Client states, "I need to wear my neck collar all the time because I need it for added support."		X
Client ambulates to the examination room and is limping and leaning a hand on the wall while walking.		X
Client states, "I know that new medication is used for depression, but it has helped my pain too."	X	

Rationale: Amitriptyline is a tricyclic antidepressant that can reduce pain of neuropathic origin. It can be used either on its own or in conjunction with opioid analgesics for chronic pain. This medication works by inhibiting norepinephrine uptake, thereby reducing pain. This medication is particularly helpful in the management of chronic back pain and neuropathic pain. PT is often used in conjunction with medication therapy for chronic pain management. It is normal and expected for there to be some pain or discomfort after PT because of exercising muscles associated with the injury and would be an indicator of effectiveness of the treatment plan. The client's ability to walk a mile before going to work and the ability to continue working are both indicators of effectiveness as well. The client statement that the medication has helped the pain also provides evidence of an effective treatment plan. The need to wear a neck collar all the time for support along with limping and leaning on the wall during ambulation are signs that the treatment plan may be inadequate or ineffective and would need to be addressed further.

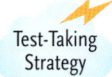

Test-Taking Strategy: Note that this question is asking about evidence of an effective treatment plan for a client with chronic pain. You need to look for signs that pain management interventions are indicating either an improvement and an expected outcome or no improvement and an unexpected outcome. Organize your thinking process as illustrated in the table.

Observation	Improving/ Expected	Not Improving/ Unexpected
Client states, "My back and neck are sore after PT."	☒	☐
Client states, "I have been walking a mile each day before going to work."	☒	☐
Client states, "I need to wear my neck collar all the time because I need it for added support."	☐	☒
Client ambulates to the examination room and is limping and leaning the hand on the wall while walking.	☐	☒
Client states, "I know that new medication is used for depression, but it has helped my pain too."	☒	☐

You may think that soreness in the neck and back after PT is not an improvement; however, continued adherence to the treatment plan is important, and some soreness is expected after these activities because the affected muscles are targeted during therapy. Increased activity and functionality, such as walking and going to work, are signs of improvement as well. Any client statement regarding relief of pain is also an indication of improvement. The report of using the neck collar all the time is an indication that the pain is not adequately controlled with other measures; a neck collar should not be needed all the time or on a long-term basis. Objective signs such as limping are indicators of a lack of improvement or a decline in the client's progress and therefore may indicate that the treatment plan is inadequate or ineffective.

Content Area: Pharmacology
Priority Concepts: Mobility; Tissue Integrity
Reference(s): Halter, 2022, pp. 258–259; Ignatavicius et al., 2024, pp. 930–932

Practice Question 8.5 — Drop-Down Cloze

A 58-year-old client is admitted to the medical-surgical unit from the ED with abdominal pain, fatigue, dizziness, and bright-red blood in the stool and is diagnosed with gastrointestinal hemorrhage.

History and Physical | Physician's Orders | Nurses' Notes | Lab Results

0600: History of diabetes mellitus, osteoarthritis, and depression. Smokes cigarettes 1 pack per day for 10 years, drinks 3 glasses of wine nightly, denies other recreational drug use. Medications include metformin 500 mg twice daily, ibuprofen 800 mg three times daily for joint pain, citalopram 10 mg daily

History and Physical | **Physician's Orders** | Nurses' Notes | Lab Results

0700:
Complete blood count (CBC)
Prothrombin time (PT)
Partial thromboplastin time (aPTT)
International normalized ratio (INR)
Type and crossmatch
1 unit PRBCs if hemoglobin is less than 8.0 g/dL (80 g/L), repeat hemoglobin and hematocrit level 2 hours after transfusion is complete
Bowel preparation (polyethylene glycol as directed) for colonoscopy
Obtain consent for colonoscopy
Pantoprazole 40 mg IV every 8 hr
Bowel rest, NPO
Normal saline IV maintenance fluids at 125 mL/h
Hydromorphone 1 mg IV push every 3 hr as needed for pain
GI specialist consultation

History and Physical | Physician's Orders | **Nurses' Notes** | Lab Results

0630: T 98.8°F (37.1°C); HR 100; RR 20; BP 102/68; SpO$_2$ 93% on RA; reports pain 5/10.

0800: Received and reviewed laboratory results. Started blood transfusion per protocol. Administering 1 unit PRBCs. Client reports continued abdominal pain, fatigue, dizziness. VS stable.

1200: 1 unit PRBCs completed. VS stable throughout transfusion. Client reports abdominal pain is unchanged. States no longer feels dizzy and feels less fatigued.

1400: Hemoglobin and hematocrit result updated. T 98.8°F (37.1°C); HR 82; RR 18; BP 122/74; SpO$_2$ 95% on RA.

History and Physical | Physician's Orders | Nurses' Notes | **Lab Results**

0745:

Test and Reference Range	Result
Red blood cells (RBCs) 4.2–6.2 × 10^{12}/L (4.2–6.2 × 10^{12}/L)	4.5 (4.5 × 10^{12})
White blood cells (WBCs) 5000–10,000/mm^3 (5–10 × 10^9/L)	8000/mm^3 (8 × 10^9/L)
Platelets 150,000–400,000/mm^3 (150–400 × 10^9/L)	180,000/mm^3 (180 × 10^9/L)
Hemoglobin (Hgb) 12–18 g/dL (120–180 g/L)	7.6 g/dL (76 g/L)
Hematocrit (Hct) 37%–52% (0.37–0.52)	32% (0.32)
aPTT 30–40 seconds	32 seconds
PT 11–12.5 seconds	12.5 seconds
INR 0.81–1.2	1.0
Occult blood Negative	Detected
Type and crossmatch	O positive, No antibodies detected

1400:

Test and Reference Range	Result
Hemoglobin (Hgb) 12–18 g/dL (120–180 g/L)	10.0 g/dL (100 g/L)
Hematocrit (Hct) 37%–52% (0.37–0.52)	39% (0.39)

Based on the client findings, complete the following sentence by selecting from the lists of options provided.

The nurse determines that the **blood transfusion** was effective, as evidenced by the **hemoglobin and hematocrit level** and the **report about fatigue and dizziness**.

Options for 1	Options for 2	Options for 3
Pantoprazole	Hemoglobin and hematocrit level	Vital signs
Hydromorphone	Coagulation studies result	Abdominal pain
Blood transfusion	Fecal occult blood test result	Report about fatigue and dizziness

Rationale: Gastrointestinal bleeding can occur in the upper or lower gastrointestinal tract. In this clinical scenario, the location of bleeding would be determined once the client undergoes the colonoscopy. Certain risk factors increase the likelihood of this health problem, such as smoking, use of NSAIDs and selective serotonin reuptake inhibitors, alcohol consumption, and a history of diabetes mellitus. The client's subjective complaints of abdominal pain, dizziness, and fatigue are supportive of GI bleeding. The client's laboratory results, specifically the hemoglobin and hematocrit levels, are below normal range and are consistent with anemia, likely secondary to the bleeding. The physician ordered PRBCs to be administered, and the client's hemoglobin level necessitates this order. In addition, the physician ordered pantoprazole, which is a proton pump inhibitor. This is an important part of the treatment plan for a client with gastrointestinal bleeding. Pain management is also often necessary for the client with this problem, and hydromorphone is the treatment for this, as well as bowel rest (NPO status). Based on this clinical scenario, the nurse determines that interventions were effective, specifically the blood transfusion, as evidenced by the improved hemoglobin and hematocrit levels and the reports of dizziness and fatigue being improved. Although pantoprazole and hydromorphone have been administered, the evidence does not exist to support these interventions as being effective at this time. The client's abdominal pain is still present; this does not provide information to confirm these interventions as being effective. The coagulation studies results were normal and unrelated to these interventions, and the fecal occult blood test result does not provide additional evaluative information for these interventions.

Test-Taking Strategy: Note that this question is asking you to evaluate whether certain interventions (blood transfusion, medications) were effective and to decide based on the evidence of that evaluation. Recall that blood transfusions are used to treat acute blood loss and anemia. Also remember that pantoprazole and hydromorphone are components of the treatment plan for GI bleeding. Look at the answer options for all three columns in the question. Then connect the evidence (option columns 2 and 3 in the question) with the interventions (option column 1), as illustrated in the table.

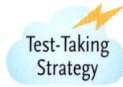

Evidence	Intervention
Hemoglobin and hematocrit level improved	Blood transfusion
Coagulation studies results—normal	Not specific to a listed intervention
Fecal occult blood test result—positive	Not specific to a listed intervention
VS—normal	Hydromorphone (nonspecific)
Abdominal pain unchanged	Hydromorphone and pantoprazole
Reports about dizziness—no longer feels dizzy and is less fatigued	Blood transfusion

Note that the question is asking for an intervention that is supported by two different sources of evidence. Consider the evidence first: The improved hemoglobin and hematocrit level and the report that the client no longer feels dizzy provide specific information about the client's anemia and the effectiveness of the blood transfusion. The results of the coagulation studies and the fecal occult blood test do not provide information specific to the blood transfusion, the hydromorphone, or the pantoprazole. The vital signs (noted as stable and are normal) may provide information about the effectiveness of the hydromorphone, but this information is nonspecific. The abdominal pain would provide evidence for the effectiveness of hydromorphone and pantoprazole, but the client's pain is unchanged. Note that the only intervention that is supported by two sources of evidence is the blood transfusion, which may be another strategy to assist you in choosing the correct options.

Content Area: Medical-Surgical Nursing
Priority Concepts: Perfusion; Tissue Integrity
Reference(s): Ignatavicius et al., 2024, pp. 1159–1160, 1203–1204

Practice Question 8.6 — Highlight-in-Text

A 3-day-old newborn is seen at the outpatient pediatric clinic for a posthospital follow-up appointment.

Highlight the findings that indicate the need for follow-up in the 3-day-old newborn.

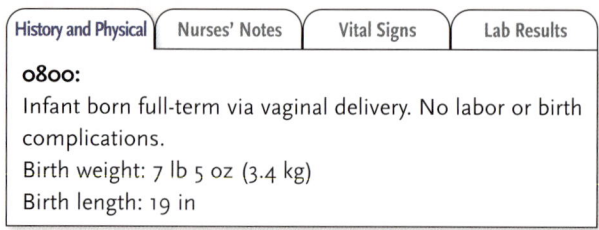

History and Physical | Nurses' Notes | Vital Signs | Lab Results

0800:
Infant born full-term via vaginal delivery. No labor or birth complications.
Birth weight: 7 lb 5 oz (3.4 kg)
Birth length: 19 in

History and Physical | **Nurses' Notes** | Vital Signs | Lab Results

0800: Breast-feeding every 2 to 3 hours without difficulty. Parents report infant urinates 12 to 15 times per day and has a bowel movement 5 to 6 times per day. They report that stool is greenish brown to yellowish brown, thin, and less sticky in consistency than it has been. ==Newborn skin is tan in color, and the sclera of the eyes is yellow. Parents state that the tan skin and yellow eyes first appeared this morning.== Blood specimen sent to lab for evaluation of bilirubin level.

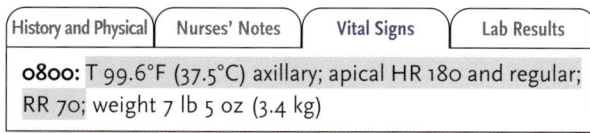

History and Physical | Nurses' Notes | **Vital Signs** | Lab Results

0800: T 99.6°F (37.5°C) axillary; apical HR 180 and regular; RR 70; weight 7 lb 5 oz (3.4 kg)

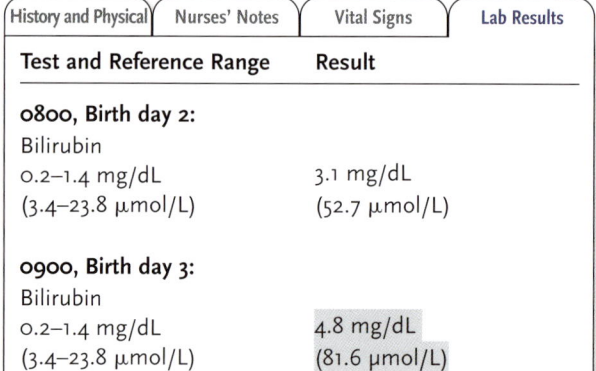

History and Physical | Nurses' Notes | Vital Signs | **Lab Results**

Test and Reference Range	Result
0800, Birth day 2:	
Bilirubin	
0.2–1.4 mg/dL	3.1 mg/dL
(3.4–23.8 μmol/L)	(52.7 μmol/L)
0900, Birth day 3:	
Bilirubin	
0.2–1.4 mg/dL	==4.8 mg/dL==
(3.4–23.8 μmol/L)	==(81.6 μmol/L)==

Rationale: Hyperbilirubinemia occurs when an excessive amount of bilirubin accumulates in the blood. The most common evidence of hyperbilirubinemia is the relatively mild and self-limited physiologic jaundice, or icterus neonatorum. Physiologic jaundice is not associated with any pathologic process. Although almost all newborns experience elevated bilirubin levels, only about half demonstrate observable signs of jaundice. An elevated bilirubin on birth day 2 is not a concern as long as jaundice is not present. In all newborns, levels need to exceed 5 mg/dL (85 μmol/L) before jaundice is observable. Because this 3-day-old has a serum bilirubin level of 4.8 mg/dL (81.6 μmol/L), signs of jaundice such as tan-colored skin and yellow eyes are not expected and are a concern requiring follow-up for evaluation of pathologic jaundice associated with a disease process. Newborns will urinate up to 20 times a day because the bladder involuntary empties when stretched by a volume of 15 mL. Transitional stools appear by the third day after initiation of feeding and are greenish brown to yellowish brown, thin, and less sticky than meconium. A bowel movement 5 to 6 times a day is expected depending on the frequency of feeding. Normal vital signs are temperature 97.7°F to 98°F (36.5°C to 37°C) axillary, apical heart rate 120 to 140, and respiratory rate 30 to 60. The temperature, apical heart rate, and respiratory rate are elevated, warranting follow-up. The serum bilirubin level of 4.8 mg/dL (81.6 μmol/L) requires follow-up because of observable signs of jaundice in this newborn. The bilirubin level will rise and peak before it returns to a normal level in physiologic jaundice. Depending on age, it could peak as high as 12 mg/dL (204 μmol/L) before dropping to a normal range.

Test-Taking Strategy: This question is asking you to evaluate the findings that indicate the need for follow-up in the 3-day-old newborn. You need to use knowledge and recall normal findings in a newborn infant and expected progression of the jaundice that occurs, differentiating physiologic from pathologic jaundice. Create a table, and organize your thinking process by considering findings that are consistent with expected outcomes or outcomes that are abnormal and/or indicate the need for follow-up.

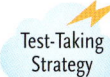
Test-Taking Strategy

Finding	Expected/ Normal Outcome	Unexpected Outcome/ Requires Follow-up
Breast-feeding every 2 to 3 hours without difficulty	X	☐
Urinates 12 to 15 times per day	X	☐
Has a bowel movement 5 to 6 times per day	X	☐
Stool is greenish brown to yellowish brown, thin, and less sticky in consistency than it has been	X	☐
Skin looks tan, and eyes look yellow	☐	X
Temperature 99.6°F (37.5°C) axillary	☐	X
Apical HR 180	☐	X
RR 70	☐	X
Weight 7 lb 5 oz (3.4 kg)	X	☐
Serum bilirubin level 4.8 mg/dL (81.6 mcmol/L)	☐	X

Content Area: Obstetric-Newborn Nursing
Priority Concept: Elimination; Tissue Integrity
Reference(s): Hockenberry et al., 2024, pp. 253–259

CHAPTER 10

Answers to Practice Questions

Unfolding Case Study 1

Content Area: Mental Health Nursing
Priority Concepts: Stress and Coping; Mood and Affect
Reference(s): Halter et al., 2022, pp. 52–53, 242–251, 258, 275, 299–300

Practice Question 10.1 Unfolding Case Study 1

The nurse is caring for a 56-year-old client in the ED.

*Highlight the findings that require **immediate** follow-up.*

Nurses' Notes

2215: Spouse brought client to ED after finding a suicide note and their gun cabinet unlocked. Reports that client is "not the same person" after being hospitalized 3 months ago with severe COVID-19 and mechanically ventilated for over 2 weeks. Client states that since being discharged from the hospital, has periods of heart palpitations, insomnia, apathy, depressed mood, and anorexia. Reports that drinking alcohol every night helps to relax, but still becomes anxious and depressed at times. Is very worried about getting COVID again because the client's sibling, whom the client recently visited, tested positive yesterday. Has frequent nightmares about the hospital experience because the client nearly died. Lost 35 lb (15.9 kg) during the hospital stay, but states still weighs more than 260 lb (117.9 kg). Was considering suicide this evening because the client was afraid of possibly "being reinfected and dying this time." Recently diagnosed with type 2 diabetes mellitus controlled by diet and metformin.

Rationale: The client was brought to the hospital because the client was planning suicide, a life-threatening problem that requires immediate follow-up. Because of the client's near-death experience with COVID-19, the client is having physical, psychological, and emotional manifestations that are likely contributing to suicide risk, including palpitations, depressed mood, insomnia, anorexia, apathy, anxiety, and frequent nightmares. Therefore these symptoms and behaviors are also of immediate concern to the nurse. Although alcohol is an ineffective coping strategy for the client, the nurse is not concerned about this behavior at this time because it is not immediately life threatening. The client's weight and diabetes are important for overall health but are not necessarily related to suicide risk. Therefore these client findings do not require follow-up at this time.

Test-Taking Strategy: Remember to first identify normal/usual or abnormal and expected (not relevant) client findings versus abnormal and not expected (relevant) findings to determine which findings require immediate follow-up by the nurse. The client findings in the Nurses' Notes can be categorized as shown in the table to help *Recognize Cues* in this case study.

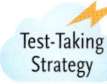

Client Finding	Abnormal and Not Expected (Relevant) and Requiring Immediate Follow-up	Normal/Usual or Abnormal but Expected (Not Relevant) and Not Requiring Immediate Follow-up
Insomnia	X	☐
Heart palpitations	X	☐
Anxiety	X	☐
Anorexia	X	☐
Depressed mood	X	☐
Apathy	X	☐
Drinks alcohol every night	☐	X
Frequent nightmares	X	☐
Overweight	☐	X
Type 2 diabetes mellitus	☐	X
Planned suicide earlier today	X	☐

Review the factors that contribute to the client's risk for suicide. The client's reported physical, psychological, and emotional behaviors place the client at current risk for suicide and therefore require immediate follow-up.

CJ Cognitive Skill: Recognize Cues

Practice Question 10.2 — Unfolding Case Study 1

The nurse is caring for a 56-year-old client in the ED.

Nurses' Notes

2215: Spouse brought client to ED after finding a suicide note and their gun cabinet unlocked. Reports that client is "not the same person" after being hospitalized 3 months ago with severe COVID-19 and mechanically ventilated for over 2 weeks. Client states that since being discharged from the hospital, has periods of heart palpitations, insomnia, apathy, depressed mood, and anorexia. Reports that drinking alcohol every night helps to relax, but still becomes anxious and depressed at times. Is very worried about getting COVID again because the client's sibling, whom the client recently visited, tested positive yesterday. Has nightmares about the hospital experience because the client nearly died. Lost 35 lb (15.9 kg) during the hospital stay, but states still weighs more than 260 lb (117.9 kg). Was considering suicide this evening because the client was afraid of possibly "being reinfected and dying this time." Recently diagnosed with type 2 DM controlled by diet and metformin.

For each client finding, select which finding is associated with which client condition. Some findings may be consistent with more than one condition.

Client Findings	Generalized Anxiety Disorder	Major Depressive Disorder	Posttraumatic Stress Disorder (PTSD)
Had recent near-death experience	☒	☒	☒
Anorexia	☒	☒	☐
Depressed mood	☐	☒	☒
Apathy	☐	☒	☒
Frequent nightmares	☐	☐	☒
Potential suicide risk	☐	☒	☒
Excessive worry	☒	☐	☐
Insomnia	☒	☒	☒

Rationale: The nurse analyzes the client findings to determine which mental health conditions the client is likely experiencing. Posttraumatic stress disorder (PTSD) can occur after any traumatic event that is not part of one's usual life experience. Clients who experience a highly traumatic event that has the potential for actual or threatened death often respond with fear similar to what this client expressed. Adults who have PTSD often have comorbidities including anxiety disorders, major depressive disorder, and/or dissociative disorders. In this client's case, the near-death experience as a result of a severe COVID-19 infection most likely led to PTSD, major depressive disorder, and generalized anxiety disorder.

Clients who have generalized anxiety disorder display excessive worry, which can affect their sleep patterns and appetite. Some clients have anorexia, whereas others respond to excessive stress by eating more than usual. Clients who have major depressive disorder can also be anorexic or overeat. They tend to lack energy, are apathetic, and experience a negative or depressed mood, often every day. These negative and depressed thoughts place them at risk for suicide. Clients who have PTSD have many of the same physical and emotional behaviors that are common in clients with anxiety and depressive disorders yet are more likely to binge-eat rather than experience anorexia. Two additional common behaviors seen in clients with PTSD are frequent nightmares and flashbacks. Flashbacks are intense, repeated episodes of reliving the traumatic experience while a client is fully awake. Nightmares and flashbacks are very frightening for the client and can lead to thoughts of suicide as an escape.

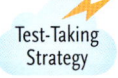

Test-Taking Strategy: Many of the client findings are common behaviors associated with more than one mental health condition. To add to that challenge in answering this test item, many clients who have PTSD also have other mental health conditions, including anxiety and clinical depression. Use the table to help you decide which client findings represent supporting data for each mental health condition in this test item measuring *Analyze Cues.*

Client Finding (Assessment Data)	Supporting Data for Generalized Anxiety Disorder? Yes or No	Supporting Data for Major Depressive Disorder? Yes or No	Supporting Data for Posttraumatic Stress Disorder? Yes or No
Had recent near-death experience	Yes	Yes	Yes
Anorexia	Yes	Yes	No
Depressed mood	No	Yes	Yes
Apathy	No	Yes	Yes
Nightmares	No	No	Yes
Potential suicide risk	No	Yes	Yes
Excessive worry	Yes	No	No
Insomnia	Yes	Yes	Yes

Recall and retrieve nursing knowledge about the characteristics and assessment findings for each condition. Once you review these data in the table, you can more easily determine which mental health conditions the client *may be* experiencing to answer the test item.

CJ Cognitive Skill: Analyze Cues

Practice Question 10.3 — Unfolding Case Study 1

The nurse is caring for a 56-year-old client in the ED.

Nurses' Notes

2215: Spouse brought client to ED after finding a suicide note and their gun cabinet unlocked. Reports that client is "not the same person" after being hospitalized 3 months ago with severe COVID-19 and mechanically ventilated for over 2 weeks. Client states that since being discharged from the hospital, has periods of heart palpitations, insomnia, apathy, depressed mood, and anorexia. Reports that drinking alcohol every night helps to relax, but still becomes anxious and depressed at times. Is very worried about getting COVID again because the client's sibling, whom the client recently visited, tested positive yesterday. Has frequent nightmares about the hospital experience because the client nearly died. Lost 35 lb (15.9 kg) during the hospital stay, but states still weighs more than 260 lb (117.9 kg). Was considering suicide this evening because the client was afraid of possibly "being reinfected and dying this time." Recently diagnosed with type 2 DM controlled by diet and metformin.

2330: Social worker (SW) interviewed client and administered several screening assessments for selected mental health conditions. Client admitted to flashbacks about hospitalization and feels guilty about putting family through that experience. States was "lazy" and did not wear a mask or social distance at an important corporate meeting. As a result, the client developed a COVID-19 infection, which worsened and led to the hospital stay and mechanical ventilation. Expressed remorse for upsetting spouse and apologized to both the client's spouse and SW.

Complete the following sentence by selecting from the lists of options provided.

The **priority** for the client's care is to **ensure personal safety** because the client most likely has **posttraumatic stress disorder.**

Options for 1	Options for 2
Begin intensive counseling	Paranoid personality disorder
Ensure personal safety	Dissociative identity disorder
Start drug therapy	Posttraumatic stress disorder
Refer the client to a spiritual advisor	Generalized anxiety disorder

Rationale: Safety is always the priority for any client. This client was planning suicide, but the suicide note and unlocked gun cabinet were found before the client could actually commit this action. The priority for the client, then, is to keep the client safe at all times. Once safety is ensured, the client may start drug therapy, begin counseling, and/or need a spiritual advisor. The client likely has several mental health conditions. However, the primary life-threatening mental health condition is PTSD due to the client's history of a near-death experience as a result of having severe COVID-19 infection. The client expresses being afraid of getting the infection again and perhaps not surviving a second event. Although the client displays excessive worry, generalized anxiety disorder is typically not a threat to the client's safety or safety of others. The client does not demonstrate lack of trust or having multiple personalities. Therefore there is no evidence supporting the conditions of paranoid personality disorder or dissociative identity disorder.

Test-Taking Strategy: To answer this test item measuring the CJ cognitive skill *Prioritize Hypotheses*, first determine what the client's priority need is at this time. Safety is the priority for all clients and is ensured by using a variety of nursing and collaborative interventions. Use the table to help you decide which condition can cause a personal safety risk.

Client Conditions	Personal Safety Risk? Yes or No
Paranoid personality disorder	No
Dissociative identity disorder	No
Posttraumatic stress disorder	Yes
Generalized anxiety disorder	No

CJ Cognitive Skill: Prioritize Hypotheses

Practice Question 10.4 — Unfolding Case Study 1

The nurse is caring for a 56-year-old client in the ED.

Nurses' Notes

2215: Spouse brought client to ED after finding a suicide note and their gun cabinet unlocked. Reports that client is "not the same person" after being hospitalized 3 months ago with severe COVID-19 and mechanically ventilated for over 2 weeks. Client states that since being discharged from the hospital, has periods of heart palpitations, insomnia, apathy, depressed mood, and anorexia. Reports that drinking alcohol every night helps to relax, but still becomes anxious and depressed at times. Is very worried about getting COVID again because the client's sibling, whom the client recently visited, tested positive yesterday. Has frequent nightmares about the hospital experience because the client nearly died. Lost 35 lb (15.9 kg) during the hospital stay, but states still weighs more than 260 lb (117.9 kg). Was considering suicide this evening because the client was afraid of possibly "being reinfected and dying this time." Recently diagnosed with type 2 DM controlled by diet and metformin.

2330: Social worker (SW) interviewed client and administered several screening assessments for selected mental health conditions. Client admitted to flashbacks about hospitalization and feels guilty about putting family through that experience. States was "lazy" and did not wear a mask or social distance at an important corporate meeting. As a result, the client developed a COVID-19 infection, which worsened and led to the hospital stay and mechanical ventilation. Expressed remorse for upsetting spouse and apologized to both the client's spouse and SW.

Which of the following orders would the nurse anticipate for the client at this time? **Select all that apply.**

- ☒ Begin antidepressant drug therapy.
- ☒ Admit to the acute psychiatric unit.
- ☐ Refer to a case manager.
- ☐ Refer to a spiritual advisor.
- ☒ Begin intensive psychotherapy.
- ☒ Place on suicide precautions.
- ☒ Limit visitors to immediate family.

Rationale: The desired outcome for this client's care is to ensure safety because of potential suicide. The orders would be focused on ways to keep the client safe, including admission to the acute psychiatric unit for one-on-one observation and treatment with medication and psychotherapy. The client would also be placed on suicide precautions, which usually include:

- Observing the client swallow each dose of medication
- Removing glass and knives from meal trays to prevent self-injury
- Removing any unsafe objects from the client's environment
- Providing one-on-one observation of the client at all times
- Documenting the client's behavior and verbal statements every 15 to 30 minutes

Visitors would likely be limited to a small number of immediate family members to prevent the client from inadvertently obtaining devices from others that could cause self-harm. Immediate family members could provide support and encouragement for the client during the hospital stay. A case manager can help plan for the client's discharge to ensure continuity of care to keep the client safe at home or in another setting but would not help ensure immediate safety. A spiritual advisor may be requested by the client but is not typically ordered for this type of situation unless the client requests it.

Test-Taking Strategy: To answer this question measuring *Generate Solutions*, remember that the *priority* desired outcome is to ensure the client's safety. Therefore review each choice in the test item to determine if the intervention or order would promote the client's immediate safety. Use the table to help you decide.

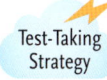

Potential Orders	Promotes Client's Immediate Safety? Yes or No
Begin antidepressant drug therapy.	Yes
Admit to the acute psychiatric unit.	Yes
Refer to a case manager.	No
Refer to a spiritual advisor.	No
Begin intensive psychotherapy.	Yes
Place on suicide precautions.	Yes
Limit visitors to immediate family.	Yes

Note that this question asks you to identify the orders that you would anticipate for the client at this time. Think about the client's conditions and immediate needs. The potential orders that promote the client's immediate safety and are marked by "Yes" are the correct responses to the test item.

CJ Cognitive Skill: Generate Solutions

Practice Question 10.5 — Unfolding Case Study 1

The nurse is caring for a 56-year-old client in the ED.

Nurses' Notes

2215: Spouse brought client to ED after finding a suicide note and their gun cabinet unlocked. Reports that client is "not the same person" after being hospitalized 3 months ago with severe COVID-19 and mechanically ventilated for over 2 weeks. Client states that since being discharged from the hospital, has periods of heart palpitations, insomnia, apathy, depressed mood, and anorexia. Reports that drinking alcohol every night helps to relax, but still becomes anxious and depressed at times. Is very worried about getting COVID again because the client's sibling, whom the client recently visited, tested positive yesterday. Has frequent nightmares about the hospital experience because the client nearly died. Lost 35 lb (15.9 kg) during the hospital stay, but states still weighs more than 260 lb (117.9 kg). Was considering suicide this evening because the client was afraid of possibly "being reinfected and dying this time." Recently diagnosed with type 2 DM controlled by diet and metformin.

2330: Social worker (SW) interviewed client and administered several screening assessments for selected mental health conditions. Client admitted to flashbacks about hospitalization and feels guilty about putting family through that experience. States was "lazy" and did not wear a mask or social distance at an important corporate meeting. As a result, the client developed a COVID-19 infection, which worsened and led to the hospital stay and mechanical ventilation. Expressed remorse for upsetting spouse and apologized to both the client's spouse and SW.

0150: Client admitted to the acute psychiatric unit for one-on-one observation; started on sertraline and psychotherapy.

The nurse plans health teaching about sertraline before administering the first dose to the client. Select the 5 statements the nurse would include in the health teaching about this medication.

- ☒ "This drug is one of the most effective ways to treat PTSD and depression."
- ☐ "We will be monitoring you for sedation effects while you are here."
- ☐ "Let me know if you have trouble urinating or having a bowel movement."
- ☒ "Let me know if you have trouble sleeping or feel nervous while on the drug."
- ☒ "We will be monitoring you carefully for changes in your vital signs."
- ☒ "You might experience mild nausea and feel agitated when you start this drug."
- ☒ "Your liver and kidney function will need to be monitored by lab testing."

Rationale: Sertraline is a selective serotonin reuptake inhibitor (SSRI) that can be very effective in managing clinical depression and/or PTSD. Side effects of the drug include insomnia, nervousness, anxiety, agitation, and mild nausea. Although not common, like most antidepressants, this drug can affect liver and kidney function, which should be monitored through frequent laboratory testing. The nurse would monitor vital signs to help assess for a rare adverse drug reaction called *serotonin syndrome*. This syndrome is likely due to overaction of central nervous system receptors and is usually dose related or the result of drug interactions. Symptoms include elevated temperature, heart rate, and blood pressure; delirium; muscle spasms; abdominal pain; diarrhea; and possible seizures. Severe manifestations can lead to shock or possibly death. Urinary retention, constipation, and sedation more commonly occur in clients who take other classes of antidepressants, especially tricyclic antidepressants.

Test-Taking Strategy: Remember that health teaching about side effects and adverse effects is particularly important for clients starting new drug therapy. If the client responds to and tolerates the medication, the client will likely continue taking it after being discharged. Also recall that sertraline is classified as an SSRI. Apply knowledge of antidepressant drug therapy as shown in the table to help delineate which side effects or adverse effects can occur when clients are prescribed SSRIs.

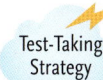

Potential Drug Side Effects or Adverse Effects	Can Occur in Clients Taking SSRIs? Yes or No
Sedation effects	No
Urinary retention and constipation	No
Insomnia and nervousness	Yes
Increased vital signs	Yes
Mild nausea	Yes
Agitation	Yes
Liver and/or kidney impairment	Yes

Based on the side effects or adverse effects for which you responded with "Yes" for SSRIs such as sertraline, you can then select the appropriate options in the test item that would be included in health teaching to measure *Take Actions*.

CJ Cognitive Skill: Take Actions

Practice Question 10.6 — Unfolding Case Study 1

The nurse is interviewing a 56-year-old client at the ambulatory mental health clinic.

Nurses' Notes

2215: Spouse brought client to ED after finding a suicide note and their gun cabinet unlocked. Reports that client is "not the same person" after being hospitalized 3 months ago with severe COVID-19 and mechanically ventilated for over 2 weeks. Client states that since being discharged from the hospital, has periods of heart palpitations, insomnia, apathy, depressed mood, and anorexia. Reports that drinking alcohol every night helps to relax, but still becomes anxious and depressed at times. Is very worried about getting COVID again because the client's sibling, whom the client recently visited, tested positive yesterday. Has frequent nightmares about the hospital experience because the client nearly died. Lost 35 lb (15.9 kg) during the hospital stay, but states still weighs more than 260 lb (117.9 kg). Was considering suicide this evening because the client was afraid of possibly "being reinfected and dying this time." Recently diagnosed with type 2 DM controlled by diet and metformin.

2330: Social worker (SW) interviewed client and administered several screening assessments for selected mental health conditions. Client admitted to flashbacks about hospitalization and feels guilty about putting family through that experience. States was "lazy" and did not wear a mask or social distance at an important corporate meeting. As a result, the client developed a COVID-19 infection, which worsened and led to the hospital stay and mechanical ventilation. Expressed remorse for upsetting spouse and apologized to both the client's spouse and SW.

0150: Client admitted to the acute psychiatric unit for one-on-one observation; started on sertraline and psychotherapy.

Ambulatory Mental Health Clinic—6 Weeks Later

0900: Has history of PTSD, anxiety, and suicide risk for which client was admitted for short stay in acute psychiatric unit. Today client reports having a more positive outlook without depressed moods and having a good appetite. Sleeps most nights for 7 to 8 hours, and no longer has heart palpitations. Has not consumed alcohol since hospital discharge. Continues to have flashbacks and nightmares about once a week and usually in the evening. Has been following the treatment plan taking sertraline as prescribed and attending psychotherapy sessions twice a week.

For each current client finding, indicate if the client's condition is improving or not improving.

Client Findings	Improving	Not Improving
Has not consumed any alcohol since hospital discharge	☒	☐
States has a more positive outlook without depressed moods and has a good appetite	☒	☐
Has flashbacks and nightmares about once a week	☐	☒
Sleeps most nights for 7 to 8 hours	☒	☐
States no longer has heart palpitations	☒	☐

Rationale: Prior to the psychiatric hospital stay, the client consumed alcohol every night to help relax. However, since discharge, the client states has not consumed alcohol to help cope with the situation. Today the client does not have insomnia or palpitations, has a good appetite, and reports not experiencing the depressed moods experienced prior to hospitalization. All of these client findings show that the client has improved and is progressing. The client still reports flashbacks and nightmares, which does not indicate improvement, but the client is sleeping better.

Test-Taking Strategy: This test item requires you to compare the client's initial findings before the inpatient psychiatric unit stay with current findings during this postdischarge follow-up visit. Use the table to help you decide if the client has improved, and is therefore progressing, to answer this test item measuring *Evaluate Outcomes*.

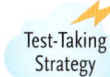

Client Finding Before Psychiatric Unit Stay	Client Finding During Current Postdischarge Visit	Current Finding Demonstrates Client Is Progressing or Improving? Yes or No
Reports that drinking alcohol every night helps to relax	States has not consumed alcohol since hospital discharge	Yes
Has anorexia and is depressed at times	States has a more positive outlook without depressed moods and has a good appetite	Yes
Has flashbacks and nightmares	Has flashbacks and nightmares at least once a week	No
Has insomnia	Sleeps most nights for 7 to 8 hours	Yes
Has heart palpitations	States no longer has heart palpitations	Yes

Creating a table as illustrated will help you organize your thoughts to help answer the question. Use the findings that are answered with "Yes" as the correct responses for the test item.

CJ Cognitive Skill: Evaluate Outcomes

Unfolding Case Study 2

Content Area: Medical-Surgical Nursing
Priority Concepts: Clotting; Gas Exchange
Reference(s): Lilley, et al., 2023, pp. 413–414; Ignatavicius et al., 2024, pp. 597–603, 1055–1061

Practice Question 10.7 — Unfolding Case Study 2

The nurse is caring for a 68-year-old client in the inpatient surgical suite.

Nurses' Notes

0645: Admitted to surgical suite preoperative area for right anterior total hip arthroplasty (THA). History of several surgeries including hysterectomy, appendectomy, and cholecystectomy. 52–pack-year smoking history, but quit 2 years ago; BMI of 30.1. History of deep vein thrombosis (DVT) × 2, hypertension controlled by diet and drug therapy, high cholesterol controlled by statins, and gastroesophageal reflux disorder (GERD) controlled by antacid PRN. Bilateral hip osteoarthritis with right hip more painful than left. Lives in a second-floor apartment in a rural town. Has no transportation, and depends on family and friends to obtain food and get to medical appointments. Family and friends are willing to help with postoperative recovery and transportation. Advance directive on file. Prepped for surgery.

Which of the following assessment findings place the client at high risk for postoperative venous thromboembolism? **Select all that apply.**

- ☐ History of hypertension
- ☒ 52–pack-year smoking history
- ☒ BMI of 30.1
- ☐ History of high cholesterol
- ☒ Having a THA
- ☐ History of cholecystectomy
- ☐ History of bilateral hip osteoarthritis
- ☒ History of DVT × 2

Rationale: Venous thromboembolism (VTE) is the development of one or more blood clots and includes deep vein thrombosis (DVT) and pulmonary embolism (PE). The nurse must recognize that the client has multiple risk factors for developing VTE, which can be potentially life threatening. The client has a 52–pack-year smoking history, but quit 2 years ago. However, long-term smoking exposure causes vasoconstriction and vessel damage, which predispose the client to clot development. A BMI of over 30 indicates that the client is obese; clients who are obese are at higher risk for developing VTE and other postoperative complications than clients who are within a normal weight range. For unknown reasons, orthopedic injuries and surgery increase VTE risk. Clients who have a history of VTE are at higher risk for recurrence than clients who do not have a history.

Hypertension is an arterial health condition that affects peripheral vessels and would not likely contribute to developing a peripheral venous or pulmonary clot. High cholesterol can contribute to hypertension and atherosclerosis development in small arterial vessels. A surgical history of cholecystectomy, GERD, and current bilateral osteoarthritis are unrelated to one's risk for VTE.

Test-Taking Strategy: Recall that all clients who have major orthopedic surgery are at risk for VTE. However, this client has additional findings, making the client especially prone to this postoperative complication. Use the table to help you decide which assessment findings to select to *Recognize Cues* that should concern the nurse.

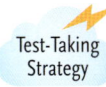

Client Assessment Findings	Can Contribute to Developing Venous Thromboembolism	Does Not Typically Contribute to Developing Venous Thromboembolism
History of hypertension	☐	☒
52–pack-year smoking history	☒	☐
BMI of 30.1	☒	☐
History of high cholesterol	☐	☒
Having a THA	☒	☐
History of cholecystectomy	☐	☒
History of bilateral hip osteoarthritis	☐	☒
History of DVT × 2	☒	☐

Apply your knowledge of VTE pathophysiology to help you determine the correct responses. Based on this table, select all of the client findings that are marked with an X under "Can Contribute to Developing Venous Thromboembolism" to correctly answer the test item.

CJ Cognitive Skill: Recognize Cues

Practice Question 10.8 — Unfolding Case Study 2

The nurse is caring for a 68-year-old client in the acute orthopedic unit.

Nurses' Notes | Orders

0645: Admitted to surgical suite preoperative area for right anterior total hip arthroplasty (THA). History of several surgeries including hysterectomy, appendectomy, and cholecystectomy. 52–pack-year smoking history but quit 2 years ago; BMI of 30.1. History of deep vein thrombosis (DVT) × 2, hypertension controlled by diet and drug therapy, high cholesterol controlled by statins, and gastroesophageal reflux disorder (GERD) controlled by antacid PRN. Bilateral hip osteoarthritis with right hip more painful than left. Lives in a second-floor apartment in a rural town. Has no transportation, and depends on family and friends to obtain food and get to medical appointments. Family and friends are willing to help with postoperative recovery and transportation. Advance directive on file. Prepped for surgery.

1510: Had a right THA 2 days ago, and recovering on the acute orthopedic unit; client's pain being managed with oral opioids and gabapentin. Possible discharge tomorrow. Client will continue taking apixaban 5 mg orally twice a day and ambulating with assistance at least 4 to 5 times each day with a walker at home. Follow up with outpatient PT.

1935: Client reports was unable to ambulate this evening because of sharp chest pain that worsens when taking a deep breath. States has been "belching" since dinner because of eating onions and peppers on a steak. Restless and anxious about pain, but no acute confusion. T 100°F (37.8°C); HR 104 and irregular; RR 20 with dyspnea; BP 114/62; SpO$_2$ 88% on RA. Right THA incision dry and intact without redness. Right pedal pulses nonpalpable but detected on Doppler; foot warm and not swollen. Posterior tibial and popliteal pulses +2 bilaterally. Able to flex both feet equally; cap refill <3 seconds.

For each client finding, select which finding is associated with which potential client condition. Some findings may be consistent with more than one condition.

Client Findings	Pulmonary Embolism	GERD	Respiratory Infection
Chest pain	☒	☒	☒
Belching	☐	☒	☐
Restlessness	☒	☐	☒
Anxiety	☒	☐	☒
T 100°F (37.8°C)	☐	☐	☒
HR 104 and irregular	☒	☐	☒
RR 20 with dyspnea	☒	☐	☒
SpO$_2$ 88% on RA	☒	☐	☒

Rationale: The client is at risk for postoperative complications including VTE and respiratory infection because of age, decreased mobility, smoking history, DVT history, and obesity. The client has a history of GERD, which can cause eructation (belching) and chest discomfort or pain after eating foods that are spicy or highly seasoned. However, none of the other client findings are associated with GERD. Chest pain can also occur in clients who are experiencing PE or respiratory infection such as pneumonia. PEs can be massive or small, but they most often result when a piece of clot dislodges from a DVT and occludes one or more pulmonary blood vessels. In many cases, the DVT is undetected or not diagnosed. PE typically results in obstructed pulmonary blood flow, which leads to hypoxia. This hypoxia may manifest with tachypnea, dyspnea, restlessness, anxiety, and decreased oxygen saturation. As a compensatory mechanism, the heart rate increases (tachycardia) to circulate blood more rapidly throughout the body. These same pulmonary and cardiac findings may be seen in clients with a respiratory infection. Infection is also usually accompanied by fever, which increases the body's metabolic rate. Anxiety may be present in clients with PE and respiratory infection because of dyspnea and chest pain. Increased temperature in clients with respiratory infection occurs as the body attempts to reduce or destroy the microorganisms that are causing the infection. Fever is not common in clients who have either a PE or GERD.

Test-Taking Strategy: To answer this test item, you need to recall the pathophysiology and typical clinical manifestations associated with three health problems—PE, GERD, and respiratory infection, such as pneumonia. Use the table to help organize the information you will need to *Analyze Cues*. Review each client finding, and decide if it provides supporting evidence for PE, GERD, and/or respiratory infection.

Client Findings	Supporting Evidence for Pulmonary Embolism? Yes or No	Supporting Evidence for GERD? Yes or No	Supporting Evidence for Respiratory Infection? Yes or No
Chest pain	Yes	Yes	Yes
Belching	No	Yes	No
Restlessness	Yes	No	Yes
Anxiety	Yes	No	Yes
T 100°F (37.8°C)	No	No	Yes
HR 104 and irregular	Yes	No	Yes
RR 20 with dyspnea	Yes	No	Yes
SpO$_2$ 90% on RA	Yes	No	Yes

As you likely noted, some client findings such as chest pain support several client conditions or health problems. In other cases, the client finding supports only one of the client conditions. For example, belching (also called *eructation*) supports only GERD. This gastrointestinal symptom is not associated with pulmonary conditions. An elevated temperature can occur in clients with infection but is not associated with PE or GERD.

CJ Cognitive Skill: Analyze Cues

Practice Question 10.9 — Unfolding Case Study 2

The nurse is caring for a 68-year-old client in the acute orthopedic unit.

Nurses' Notes

0645: Admitted to surgical suite preoperative area for right anterior total hip arthroplasty (THA). History of several surgeries including hysterectomy, appendectomy, and cholecystectomy. 52–pack-year smoking history, but quit 2 years ago; BMI of 30.1. History of deep vein thrombosis (DVT) × 2, hypertension controlled by diet and drug therapy, high cholesterol controlled by statins, and gastroesophageal reflux disorder (GERD) controlled by antacid PRN. Bilateral hip osteoarthritis with right hip more painful than left. Lives in a second-floor apartment in a rural town. Has no transportation, and depends on family and friends to obtain food and get to medical appointments. Family and friends are willing to help with postoperative recovery and transportation. Advance directive on file. Prepped for surgery.

1510: Had a right THA 2 days ago, and recovering on the acute orthopedic unit; client's pain being managed with oral opioids and gabapentin. Possible discharge tomorrow. Client will continue taking apixaban 5 mg orally twice a day and ambulating with assistance at least 4 to 5 times each day with a walker at home. Follow up with outpatient PT.

1935: Client reports was unable to ambulate this evening because of sharp chest pain that worsens when taking a deep breath. States has been "belching" since dinner because of eating onions and peppers on a steak. Restless and anxious about pain, but no acute confusion. T 100°F (37.8°C); HR 104 and irregular; RR 20 with dyspnea; BP 114/62; SpO$_2$ 88% on RA. Right THA incision dry and intact without redness. Right pedal pulses nonpalpable, but detected on Doppler; foot warm and not swollen. Posterior tibial and popliteal pulses +2 bilaterally. Able to flex both feet equally; cap refill <3 seconds.

Complete the following sentence by selecting from the lists of options provided.

The **priority** for the client's care is to **promote oxygenation** because the client most likely has **pulmonary embolism**.

Options for 1	Options for 2
Reduce surgical pain	GERD
Decrease stomach pH	Pneumonia
Promote oxygenation	Right leg neurovascular compromise
Prevent bleeding	Pulmonary embolism

Rationale: The client had orthopedic surgery 2 days ago and is at risk for a number of postoperative complications. The risk is further increased by obesity and a smoking history. Although the client may be at risk for or have findings associated with the four client conditions listed for option 2, the potentially life-threatening condition is PE. Because the classic manifestations of a PE are sudden onset of chest pain and dyspnea, and the client has an SpO_2 well below the desired level of 95% or higher, the *priority* need for client care is to promote oxygenation. There is no indication that the client is experiencing surgical pain, and the PRN antacid reduces the pH of the stomach to help control GERD. The client is receiving an anticoagulant to help prevent VTE, and although bleeding is a potential adverse effect, it is not a priority.

A respiratory infection such as pneumonia could possibly be life threatening if not treated, but neurovascular compromise in the surgical leg and GERD are not life threatening unless they progress over time. A long-term diagnosis of GERD that is not well managed can cause Barrett esophageal cell changes, which can predispose the client to esophageal or gastric cancer. Neurovascular compromise may result in compartment syndrome, which can cause irreversible tissue damage due to impaired perfusion. Clients who have pneumonia may also have chest discomfort, but onset tends to be more gradual and may be described as discomfort rather than sharp pain. The client does not have hypotension, bradycardia, or tachypnea, but does have dyspnea, which can be associated with PE or pneumonia. Nonpalpable pedal pulses may not be significant as long as there are other indicators of adequate perfusion. The client has adequate capillary refill and the affected foot is warm, indicating that there is no problem with perfusion. Therefore there is no evidence that the client has neurovascular compromise.

Test-Taking Strategy

Test-Taking Strategy: This test item requires you to determine the priority for client care based on the priority client condition. First, you need to determine the priority client condition. In this client's case, the amount of risk is the key factor in deciding the priority because one of the four choices in the options for 2 is potentially immediately life threatening, and the others are not immediately life threatening. Therefore PE is the client condition that takes priority over the other conditions because it can affect perfusion and causes hypoxia. Once you make this decision, you need to determine the client's *priority for care* at this time. Recall from Chapter 5 that factors such as complexity, urgency, risk, and difficulty affect how you decide on the client's priority for care. Use the tables to help make these decisions. The first table will help you identify the supporting evidence for the client's condition of pulmonary embolism. The second table will help you determine the client's priority for care based on that condition.

Client Findings	Supporting Evidence for Pulmonary Embolism? Yes or No	Finding Present in This Client? Yes or No
Chest pain	Yes	Yes
Hypotension	Yes	No
Bradycardia	No	No
Nonpalpable right pedal pulses	No	Yes
Tachypnea	Yes	No
Belching	No	Yes
Decreased capillary refill	No	No
Dyspnea	Yes	Yes

Potential Priority for Client Care	Appropriate for Care of Client with Pulmonary Embolism	Not Appropriate for Care of Client with Pulmonary Embolism
Reduce surgical pain	☐	☒
Decrease stomach pH	☐	☒
Promote oxygenation	☒	☐
Prevent bleeding	☐	☒

CJ Cognitive Skill: Prioritize Hypotheses

Practice Question 10.10 — Unfolding Case Study 2

The nurse is caring for a 68-year-old client in the acute orthopedic unit.

Nurses' Notes | **Orders**

0645: Admitted to surgical suite preoperative area for right anterior total hip arthroplasty (THA). History of several surgeries including hysterectomy, appendectomy, and cholecystectomy. 52–pack-year smoking history, but quit 2 years ago; BMI of 30.1. History of deep vein thrombosis (DVT) × 2, hypertension controlled by diet and drug therapy, high cholesterol controlled by statins, and gastroesophageal reflux disorder (GERD) controlled by antacid PRN. Bilateral hip osteoarthritis with right hip more painful than left. Lives in a second-floor apartment in a rural town. Has no transportation, and depends on family and friends to obtain food and get to medical appointments. Family and friends are willing to help with postoperative recovery and transportation. Advance directive on file. Prepped for surgery.

1510: Had a right THA 2 days ago, and recovering on the acute orthopedic unit; client's pain being managed with oral opioids and gabapentin. Possible discharge tomorrow. Client will continue taking apixaban 5 mg orally twice a day and ambulating with assistance at least 4 to 5 times each day with a walker at home. Follow up with outpatient PT.

1935: Client reports was unable to ambulate this evening because of sharp chest pain that worsens when taking a deep breath. States has been "belching" since dinner because of eating onions and peppers on a steak. Restless and anxious about pain, but no acute confusion. T 100°F (37.8°C); HR 104 and irregular; RR 20 with dyspnea; BP 114/62; SpO_2 88% on RA. Right THA incision dry and intact without redness. Right pedal pulses nonpalpable, but detected on Doppler; foot warm and not swollen. Posterior tibial and popliteal pulses +2 bilaterally. Able to flex both feet equally; cap refill <3 seconds.

The nurse develops a plan of care to manage the client findings. Select the **6** actions that would be appropriate for the nurse to include in the plan of care at this time.

☒ Obtain peripheral venous access.
☐ Place the client in a flat supine position.
☒ Connect the client to a continuous cardiac monitor.
☒ Prepare the client for computed tomography pulmonary angiography.
☒ Apply oxygen by nasal cannula (NC) or mask.
☐ Increase the client's oral apixaban dosage from 5 mg to 10 mg.
☒ Draw blood for laboratory testing, including complete blood count and coagulation studies.
☒ Place the client on continuous oxygen saturation monitoring.

Rationale: The client most likely has PE with one or more emboli obstructing pulmonary blood flow. Computed tomography (CT) pulmonary angiography or helical CT is usually used to confirm this potentially life-threatening condition. In some settings, magnetic resonance angiography (MRA) may be used instead of either CT scan procedure. As a result of PE, the client develops hypoxia with either normal breath sounds or adventitious sounds such as crackles and wheezes. Therefore the nurse would place the client in a sitting (high-Fowler) position rather than a flat (supine) position to facilitate breathing and would apply oxygen therapy and continuous pulse oximetry to monitor SpO_2. If the PE is not treated or is large, cardiac symptoms such as hypotension and tachycardia can occur as a result of decreased tissue perfusion. Electrocardiography changes such as transient T-wave and ST-segment changes can also occur, so the nurse would provide continuous cardiac monitoring. Peripheral venous access is needed for administering drug therapy or fluids as indicated. The client needs therapeutic anticoagulant therapy if PE is confirmed to prevent the clot(s) from becoming larger. Laboratory testing to check the platelet count, serum creatinine, CBC, and coagulation studies provide a baseline before drug therapy is initiated. Increasing the dosage of the client's current oral anticoagulant, apixaban, would not be effective in managing this potentially life-threatening condition because it does not act immediately or prevent a clot from becoming larger. Instead, apixaban helps prevent the formation of a VTE.

Test-Taking Strategy: To help you decide on possible actions to include in the client's care, first recall the pathophysiology of PE. This acute health problem causes respiratory and cardiovascular compromise, which can be potentially life threatening. Therefore nursing interventions would be planned to provide respiratory and/or cardiovascular assessment data or support. Use the table to help you decide which actions would be indicated for this client.

Potential Nursing Action	Action Provides Respiratory Assessment Data or Support? Yes or No	Action Provides Cardiovascular Assessment Data or Support? Yes or No
Obtain venous access.	No	Yes
Place the client in a flat supine position.	No	No
Connect the client to a continuous cardiac monitor.	No	Yes
Prepare the client for computed tomography pulmonary angiography.	Yes	Yes
Apply oxygen by nasal cannula (NC) or mask.	Yes	Yes
Increase the client's oral apixaban dosage from 5 mg to 10 mg.	No	No
Draw blood for laboratory testing including CBC and coagulation studies.	No	Yes
Place the client on continuous oxygen saturation monitoring.	Yes	Yes

Once you review the table, select all of the nursing actions that provide assessment data regarding the status of the client's cardiopulmonary system *and/or* support the function of the cardiopulmonary system to *Generate Solutions*.

CJ Cognitive Skill: Generate Solutions

Practice Question 10.11 — Unfolding Case Study 2

The nurse is caring for a 68-year-old client on the acute orthopedic unit.

Nurses' Notes

0645: Admitted to surgical suite preoperative area for right anterior total hip arthroplasty (THA). History of several surgeries including hysterectomy, appendectomy, and cholecystectomy. 52–pack-year smoking history, but quit 2 years ago; BMI of 30.1. History of deep vein thrombosis (DVT) × 2, hypertension controlled by diet and drug therapy, high cholesterol controlled by statins, and gastroesophageal reflux disorder (GERD) controlled by antacid PRN. Bilateral hip osteoarthritis with right hip more painful than left. Lives in a second-floor apartment in a rural town. Has no transportation, and depends on family and friends to obtain food and get to medical appointments. Family and friends are willing to help with postoperative recovery and transportation. Advance directive on file. Prepped for surgery.

1510: Had a right THA 2 days ago and recovering on the acute orthopedic unit; client's pain being managed with oral opioids and gabapentin. Possible discharge tomorrow. Client will continue taking apixaban 5 mg orally twice a day and ambulating with assistance at least 4 to 5 times each day with a walker at home. Follow up with outpatient PT.

1935: Client reports was unable to ambulate this evening because of sharp chest pain that worsens when taking a deep breath. States has been "belching" since dinner because of eating onions and peppers on a steak. Restless and anxious about pain, but no acute confusion. T 100°F (37.8°C); HR 104 and irregular; RR 20 with dyspnea; BP 114/62; SpO$_2$ 88% on RA. Right THA incision dry and intact without redness. Right pedal pulses nonpalpable, but detected on Doppler; foot warm and not swollen. Posterior tibial and popliteal pulses +2 bilaterally. Able to flex both feet equally; cap refill <3 seconds.

1955: Reports mild chest pain and occasional dyspnea. Supplemental oxygen started at 4 L/min via NC. Orthopedic surgeon notified.

2100: Computed tomography pulmonary angiography (CTPA) confirmed diagnosis of a submassive PE. Orders received.

Orders

2300:
Discontinue apixaban
Fondaparinux 7.5 mg/day subcutaneously
Warfarin 5 mg/day orally
Supplemental oxygen at 5 L/min via NC
Continuous pulse oximetry monitoring
Continuous cardiac monitoring

The nurse revises the plan of care for the client with a confirmed diagnosis of pulmonary embolism. Select whether the following potential nursing actions are indicated or not indicated for the client at this time.

Potential Nursing Actions	Indicated	Not Indicated
Monitor the client's platelet count.	X	☐
Monitor the client's activated partial thromboplastin time (aPTT).	☐	X
Assess the client for bleeding or excessive bruising.	X	☐
Monitor the client's international normalized ratio (INR).	X	☐
Monitor the client's hematocrit.	X	☐
Check for availability of protamine sulfate.	☐	X
Check for availability of phytonadione (vitamin K).	X	☐

Rationale: Fondaparinux is a synthetic anticoagulant that increases the activity of antithrombin to cause selective inhibition of factor Xa. Unlike heparin, this drug does not affect thrombin and therefore has no effect on prothrombin time or aPTT. However, it can lower platelet counts. Warfarin affects multiple vitamin K–dependent clotting factors in the liver. The drug's effectiveness is measured by monitoring the INR. Therefore the nurse would monitor the client's platelets (for fondaparinux) and INR (for warfarin), but there is no need to monitor the aPTT. Both drugs can cause bleeding, therefore the nurse would monitor the client for bleeding and excessive bruising. The client's hematocrit would decrease if the client experiences internal bleeding and would also need to be monitored. Unlike heparin, the antidote for fondaparinux is not protamine sulfate, but vitamin K is the antidote for warfarin overdose. The nurse would ensure that vitamin K is readily available if needed.

Test-Taking Strategy: To correctly answer this test item, you will need to differentiate fondaparinux from heparin, although both drugs are fast-acting anticoagulants used for DVT and PE and given parenterally to prevent clots from enlarging. Fondaparinux is administered as a fixed dose, but IV heparin must be titrated based on the client's laboratory values. Warfarin is an oral anticoagulant that works slowly in the liver and takes several days to provide a therapeutic effect. Both drugs that are ordered for the client can cause bleeding. There is no antidote for fondaparinux, but vitamin K is the antidote for warfarin. The remaining nursing actions are primarily focused on laboratory test monitoring. Use the table to help you decide which laboratory tests are appropriate based on the mechanism of drug actions.

Laboratory Test	Appropriate to Monitor When Client Receives Fondaparinux? Yes or No	Appropriate to Monitor When Client Receives Warfarin? Yes or No?
aPTT	No	No
Prothrombin time	No	Yes
INR	No	Yes
Hematocrit	Yes	Yes
Platelet count	Yes	No

Review the table to determine which laboratory tests are appropriate to monitor for each of the two drugs, and select the laboratory tests that match the choices provided in the test item to measure *Take Actions*.

CJ Cognitive Skill: Take Actions

Practice Question 10.12 — Unfolding Case Study 2

The nurse is assessing a 68-year-old client at the orthopedic surgeon's office.

Nurses' Notes

0645: Admitted to surgical suite preoperative area for right anterior total hip arthroplasty (THA). History of several surgeries including hysterectomy, appendectomy, and cholecystectomy. 52–pack-year smoking history, but quit 2 years ago; BMI of 30.1. History of deep vein thrombosis (DVT) × 2, hypertension controlled by diet and drug therapy, high cholesterol controlled by statins, and gastroesophageal reflux disorder (GERD) controlled by antacid PRN. Bilateral hip osteoarthritis with right hip more painful than left. Lives in a second-floor apartment in a rural town. Has no transportation, and depends on family and friends to obtain food and get to medical appointments. Family and friends are willing to help with postoperative recovery and transportation. Advance directive on file. Prepped for surgery.

1510: Had a right THA 2 days ago, and recovering on the acute orthopedic unit; client's pain being managed with oral opioids and gabapentin. Possible discharge tomorrow. Client will continue taking apixaban 5 mg orally twice a day and ambulating with assistance at least 4 to 5 times each day with a walker at home. Follow up with outpatient PT.

1935: Client reports was unable to ambulate this evening because of sharp chest pain that worsens when taking a deep breath. States has been "belching" since dinner because of eating onions and peppers on a steak. Restless and anxious about pain, but no acute confusion. T 100°F (37.8°C); HR 104 and irregular; RR 20 with dyspnea; BP 114/62; SpO_2 88% on RA. Right THA incision dry and intact without redness. Right pedal pulses nonpalpable, but detected on Doppler; foot warm and not swollen. Posterior tibial and popliteal pulses +2 bilaterally. Able to flex both feet equally; cap refill <3 seconds.

1955: Reports mild chest pain and occasional dyspnea. Supplemental oxygen started at 4 L/min via NC. Orthopedic surgeon notified.

2100: Computed tomography pulmonary angiography (CTPA) confirmed the diagnosis of a submassive PE. Orders received.

Surgeon's Office—6 Weeks Later

1015: Walking independently with a cane with full weight bearing; states is able to perform ADLs without assistance. Right hip incision healed with hairline scar and slight distal bruising. Taking warfarin as prescribed, and following up on INR testing, but depends mostly on family and friends for transportation to the lab. Right arm bruised, but reports no other bleeding. T 97.9°F (36.6°C); HR 86; RR 18; BP 126/74; SpO_2 95% on RA. No adventitious breath sounds; no new report of shortness of breath or chest pain. States a loss of 27 lb (12.2 kg) since hospitalization as part of a new weight-loss program. Also reports that left nonsurgical hip is increasingly painful.

Based on the nurse's focused assessment, which findings indicate that the client is improving or progressing? **Select all that apply.**

- ☒ No new report of shortness of breath or chest pain
- ☒ Hip incision healed with hairline scar
- ☒ SpO_2 of 95% on RA
- ☐ Right arm badly bruised
- ☒ Recent weight loss of 27 lb (12.2 kg)
- ☐ Left hip becoming more painful
- ☒ Walking independently with a cane
- ☒ Performing ADLs without assistance

Rationale: The client was treated for PE on the second postoperative day while recovering from hip surgery 6 weeks ago. At that time, the client was able to ambulate with assistance and a walker but likely needed help with selected ADLs. Today the client is independent in both ADLs and ambulation and has progressed from walking with a walker to walking with a cane, which provides less support for the client and shows improvement. The client does not currently have chest pain or dyspnea, and the SpO_2 has increased from 90% to 95%. The desired SpO_2 is 95% or greater for adults without chronic pulmonary problems. The client's incision has healed normally with minimal bruising or scarring, which is a desired outcome. However, the client's right arm is bruised, which is likely an adverse effect of warfarin therapy. When admitted for hip arthroplasty, the client's BMI was 30.1, indicating that the client was obese. Obesity likely contributed to hip arthritis and PE. The increased pain in the client's left hip demonstrates that the arthritis is worsening rather than improving. After discharge, the client apparently entered a new weight-loss program and has already lost 27 lb (12.2 kg) in about 6 weeks. This weight loss will help the client continue to become more mobile, decrease left hip pain, and place the client at less risk for additional medical complications.

Test-Taking Strategy: To correctly answer this test item, you will need to compare the client findings in the most recent Nurses' Notes with those documented in the hospital Nurses' Notes. Use the table to make this comparison, and then determine if the most current findings show improvement in the client's condition to *Evaluate Outcomes*.

Client Findings During Hospitalization	Current Client Findings	Client Condition Improving or Progressing? Yes or No
Acute onset of dyspnea and chest pain	No new report of shortness of breath or chest pain	Yes
Incision only a few days old and likely not healed	Hip incision healed with hairline scar	Yes
Oxygen saturation of 90% on RA	SpO_2 of 95% on RA	Yes
No noted arm bruising	Right arm bruised	No
Weight not noted, but client obese as evidenced by BMI over 30	Recent weight loss of 27 lb	Yes
Right hip pain was worse than left and was therefore replaced during first THA	Left hip is becoming more painful	No
Ambulated with walker four times a day until onset of chest pain and dyspnea	Walking independently with a cane	Yes
Was receiving drug therapy to manage pain and likely needed assistance with selected ADLs such as dressing or bathing lower extremities	Performing ADLs without assistance	Yes

To answer this test item, review the table and select all of the findings for which you indicated "yes" for improvement in the client's condition in the right column.

CJ Cognitive Skill: Evaluate Outcomes

Unfolding Case Study 3

CJ Cognitive Skill: Medical-Surgical Nursing
Priority Concept: Fluid and Electrolyte Balance; Glucose Regulation
Reference(s): Ignatavicius et al., 2024, pp. 280–281; 576–577; 597; 606–610; 747; 1326–1329; 1351–1352; 1370–1372

Practice Question 10.13 — Unfolding Case Study 3

A 64-year-old client presents to the ED and reports a 2-week history of fever and chills, nausea and abdominal pain, sore throat, cough, fatigue and lethargy, and muscle aches.

History and Physical

1000: History of type 1 diabetes mellitus, hypertension, hyperlipidemia, and hypothyroidism. Denies chest pain or shortness of breath. Nonproductive cough, coarse crackles heard in lower lobes bilaterally. Blood glucose levels have been well controlled, but this morning the client reports a level of 375 mg/dL (20.8 mmol/L), prompting the visit to the ED. States recent glycated hemoglobin (A1c) level performed 2 months ago was 7%. Unable to eat, and reports discontinuing medications 3 days ago because of nausea and abdominal pain. Reports increased urination despite inability to tolerate food or fluids. Reports weakness and muscle aches and being confined to the bed for the past 3 weeks. Fruity breath odor noted. POC glucose 400 mg/dL (22.2 mmol/L).
VS: T 100.4°F (38°C); HR 96; RR 24; BP 142/90; SpO$_2$ 91% on RA. Weight 175 lb (79.37 kg), height 5 feet 9 inches (stated). Voided: 250 mL.

Medications:
Levothyroxine 125 mcg/day orally
Lisinopril 2.5 mg/day orally
Simvastatin 20 mg/day orally
Insulin glargine 28 units/day subcutaneously
Semaglutide 1 mg/week subcutaneously

Laboratory Results

1120: The nurse reviews the recent laboratory and diagnostic results.

Test and Reference Range	Results
Glucose 74–106 mg/dL (3.9–6.1 mmol/L)	440 mg/dL (24.4 mmol/L)
Ketones <0 mg/dL (0.0–0.27 mmol/L)	86.4 mg/dL (4.8 mmol/L)
White blood cells (WBCs) 5000–10,000/mm^3 (5–10 × 10^9/L)	9900/mm^3 (9 × 10^9/L)
Blood urea nitrogen (BUN) 10–20 mg/dL (2.9–8.2 mmol/L)	22 mg/dL (9.0 mmol/L)
Creatinine 0.6–1.2 mg/dL (53–106 µmol/L)	1.0 mg/dL (88.3 µmol/L)
Potassium 3.5–5.0 mEq/L (3.5–5.0 mmol/L)	5.9 mEq/L (5.9 mmol/L)
Sodium 136–145 mEq/L (136–145 mmol/L)	150 mEq/L (150 mmol/L)
Thyroid-stimulating hormone (TSH) 2–10 mIU/mL (0.4–4.8 mIU/L)	4.0 mIU/mL (4.0 mIU/L)
D-dimer <0.4 mcg/mL (<3 nmol/L)	15 mcg/mL (112.5 nmol/L)
Creatine kinase (CK) 20–200 U/L (20–215 U/L)	140 U/L (150.5 U/L)
C-reactive protein (CRP) <1 mg/dL (<10.0 mg/L)	10.2 mg/dL (102 mg/L)
Troponin I <0.03 ng/mL (<0.35 mcg/L)	0.01 ng/mL (0.17 mcg/L)
Blood culture: no growth	Pending
Urinalysis	
WBCs: 0–4 low-power field	0 (0)
Ketones: none	Positive
Urine culture: no growth	Pending
Arterial Blood Gases (ABGs)	
pH: 7.35–7.45	pH 7.30
PCO$_2$: 35–45 mm Hg	PCO$_2$ 27 mm Hg
HCO$_3$: 21–28 mEq/L	HCO$_3$ 14 mEq/L
PO$_2$: 80–100 mm Hg	PO$_2$ 85 mm Hg
SARS-CoV-2: PCR negative	Positive

Practice Question 10.13 — Unfolding Case Study 3—cont'd

History and Physical	Nurses' Notes	Laboratory Results	Diagnostic Results
			Chest x-ray: Bilateral pulmonary infiltrates compatible with COVID-19 pneumonitis ECG: NSR

Select the **4** laboratory findings that require **immediate** follow-up.

- ☐ A1c
- ☐ BUN
- ☐ Sodium
- ☒ Glucose
- ☒ D-dimer
- ☒ Potassium
- ☐ C-reactive protein
- ☒ Arterial blood gases

Rationale: Diabetic ketoacidosis (DKA) is a complication of diabetes mellitus (DM) and is characterized by uncontrolled hyperglycemia, metabolic acidosis, and increased production of ketones. This condition results from the combination of insulin deficiency and an increase in hormone release that leads to increased liver and kidney glucose production. The most common precipitating factor for DKA is infection. Other precipitating factors include an inadequate insulin dose. COVID-19 is a viral infection, and this client demonstrates manifestations of COVID-19 in addition to a positive test for the virus. This is one of the client's precipitating factors for DKA. The client also reports being unable to eat and discontinuing medications 3 days ago because of the nausea and abdominal pain and the inability to tolerate food or fluids. The lack of insulin is also a precipitating factor for DKA. DKA is a life-threatening complication of DM. The nurse must recognize manifestations of this event early so interventions can be performed immediately. Classic symptoms of DKA include hyperglycemia, polyuria, polydipsia, polyphagia, a rotting citrus-fruity breath odor, nausea and/or vomiting, abdominal pain, dehydration, weakness, and confusion. Shock and coma can result. From the laboratory tests listed in the options, the nurse would be most concerned with the glucose, D-dimer, potassium, and arterial blood gases. The glucose level is extremely elevated at 440 mg/dL (24.4 mmol/L), which is significant, indicating hyperglycemia. This result along with the serum and urinary ketone results is an additional indication of DKA. Arterial blood gas results also indicate metabolic acidosis, another indication of DKA. The pH is low, and the HCO_3 is low, which are other indicators of DKA. The potassium level is elevated, and although this will return to normal once treatment begins, it is of immediate concern because of the risk associated with life-threatening dysrhythmias when the potassium level is outside of the normal range. Coagulopathy and thromboembolism are complications of COVID-19. The D-dimer test helps confirm coagulopathy; because this level is elevated, it is of immediate concern because of the risk for thromboembolism. The A1c is 7%; although a value of <7% indicates good diabetic control, this test is a long-term index of the client's average glucose level and is not of immediate concern. The sodium level is elevated, and although this is an abnormal value, it is not of immediate concern. This increase is expected because of the dehydration that occurs with illness. Once treatment begins and hydration is provided, the sodium level will likely return to normal. The slightly elevated BUN is expected because of the dehydration and is not an indication of renal involvement, especially as the creatinine is normal, and there are no other manifestations of kidney injury. The C-reactive protein is elevated; this finding is noted in the client with COVID-19 as a result of the infection and inflammation that occur. Elevated levels also occur in the client with hypertension, metabolic syndrome, or DM.

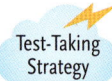

Test-Taking Strategy: First, note that this question is asking for the laboratory results that require *immediate* follow-up by the nurse. This indicates that there may be other results that are abnormal but not of immediate concern. Remember to first identify normal/usual or abnormal but expected results. These results would *not* require immediate follow-up by the nurse. Next, identify abnormal/not expected results to determine which results require immediate follow-up by the nurse. The laboratory results in the medical record can be categorized as shown in the table to help *Recognize Cues*.

Laboratory Results	Normal/Usual or Abnormal/Expected Not Requiring Immediate Follow-up	Abnormal/Not Expected Requiring Immediate Follow-up	Acute or Chronic Safety Implication if Not Addressed Immediately/Requires Immediate Follow-up? Yes or No
A1c 7%	☒	☐	Chronic No
Blood urea nitrogen (BUN) 22 mg/dL (9.0 mmol/L)	☒	☐	Acute No
Sodium 150 mEq/L (150 mmol/L)	☒	☐	Acute No
Glucose 440 mg/dL (24.4 mmol/L)	☐	☒	Acute Yes
D-dimer 15 mcg/mL (112.5 nmol/L)	☐	☒	Acute Yes
Potassium 5.9 mEq/L (5.9 mmol/L)	☐	☒	Acute Yes
C-reactive protein 10.2 mg/dL (102 mg/L)	☒	☐	Acute No
Arterial blood gases pH: 7.30 PCO_2: 27 mm Hg HCO_3: 14 mEq/L PO_2: 85 mm Hg	☐	☒	Acute Yes

Note that the question asks you to select the four options requiring immediate follow-up. Of all the options, the four options that are most concerning are the glucose, D-dimer, potassium, and arterial blood gas levels. These results could have immediate safety implications and acute findings and therefore need to be addressed immediately. The other results, although they could be relevant in some way to the acute condition or be abnormal, do not require immediate follow-up and could be safely addressed at a later time. They may also be related to a chronic condition and therefore would not require immediate follow-up.

CJ Cognitive Skill: Recognize Cues

Practice Question 10.14 — Unfolding Case Study 3

A 64-year-old client presents to the ED and reports a 2-week history of fever and chills, nausea and abdominal pain, sore throat, cough, fatigue and lethargy, and muscle aches.

History and Physical

1000: History of type 1 diabetes mellitus, hypertension, hyperlipidemia, and hypothyroidism. Denies chest pain or shortness of breath. Nonproductive cough, coarse crackles heard in lower lobes bilaterally. Blood glucose levels have been well controlled, but this morning the client reports a level of 375 mg/dL (20.8 mmol/L), prompting the visit to the ED. States recent glycated hemoglobin (A1c) level performed 2 months ago was 7%. Unable to eat, and reports discontinuing medications 3 days ago because of nausea and abdominal pain. Reports increased urination despite inability to tolerate food or fluids. Reports weakness and muscle aches and being confined to the bed for the past 3 weeks. Fruity breath odor noted. POC glucose 400 mg/dL (22.2 mmol/L). VS: T 100.4°F (38°C); HR 96; RR 24; BP 142/90; SpO$_2$ 91% on RA. Weight 175 lb (79.37 kg), height 5 feet 9 inches (stated). Voided: 250 mL.

Medications:

Levothyroxine 125 mcg/day orally
Lisinopril 2.5 mg/day orally
Simvastatin 20 mg/day orally
Insulin glargine 28 units/day subcutaneously
Semaglutide 1 mg/week subcutaneously

Laboratory Results

1120: The nurse reviews the recent laboratory and diagnostic results.

Test and Reference Range	Results
Glucose 74–106 mg/dL (3.9–6.1 mmol/L)	440 mg/dL (24.4 mmol/L)
Ketones <0 mg/dL (0.0–0.27 mmol/L)	86.4 mg/dL (4.8 mmol/L)
White blood cells (WBCs) 5000–10,000/mm³ (5–10 × 10⁹/L)	9900/mm³ (9 × 10⁹/L)
Blood urea nitrogen (BUN) 10–20 mg/dL (2.9–8.2 mmol/L)	22 mg/dL (9.0 mmol/L)
Creatinine 0.6–1.2 mg/dL (53–106 µmol/L)	1.0 mg/dL (88.3 µmol/L)
Potassium 3.5–5.0 mEq/L (3.5–5.0 mmol/L)	5.9 mEq/L (5.9 mmol/L)
Sodium 136–145 mEq/L (136–145 mmol/L)	150 mEq/L (150 mmol/L)
Thyroid-stimulating hormone (TSH) 2–10 mIU/mL (0.4–4.8 mIU/L)	4.0 mIU/mL (4.0 mIU/L)
D-dimer <0.4 mcg/mL (<3 nmol/L)	15 mcg/mL (112.5 nmol/L)
Creatine kinase (CK) 20–200 U/L (20–215 U/L)	140 U/L (150.5 U/L)
C-reactive protein (CRP) <1 mg/dL (<10.0 mg/L)	10.2 mg/dL (102 mg/L)
Troponin I <0.03 ng/mL (<0.35 mcg/L)	0.01 ng/mL (0.17 mcg/L)
Blood culture: no growth	Pending
Urinalysis	
WBCs: 0–4 low-power field	0 (0)
Ketones: none	Positive
Urine culture: no growth	Pending
Arterial Blood Gases (ABGs)	
pH: 7.35–7.45	pH 7.30
PCO$_2$: 35–45 mm Hg	PCO$_2$ 27 mm Hg
HCO$_3$: 21–28 mEq/L	HCO$_3$ 14 mEq/L
PO$_2$: 80–100 mm Hg	PO$_2$ 85 mm Hg
SARS-CoV-2: PCR negative	Positive

Practice Question 10.14 — Unfolding Case Study 3—cont'd

History and Physical	Nurses' Notes	Laboratory Results	Diagnostic Results

Chest x-ray: Bilateral pulmonary infiltrates compatible with COVID-19 pneumonitis

ECG: NSR

For each client finding, specify if the finding is consistent with the disease process of DKA or COVID-19. Each finding may support more than one disease process.

Client Findings	DKA	COVID-19
Fever and chills	☐	☒
Nausea	☒	☒
Abdominal pain	☒	☒
Increased urination	☒	☐
Cough	☐	☒
Lung crackles	☐	☒
High C-reactive protein level	☒	☒
High glucose level	☒	☐
ABG results	☒	☐

Rationale: The signs and symptoms of COVID-19 that present at illness onset vary, but over the course of the disease, most individuals experience fever and chills, cough, shortness of breath or difficulty breathing, fatigue, muscle or body aches, headache, new loss of taste or smell, sore throat, congestion or a runny nose, nausea and/or vomiting, abdominal pain, and diarrhea. Fine or coarse crackles are heard in the lungs, and a chest x-ray reveals pulmonary infiltrates characteristic of COVID-19 pneumonitis. In addition to a positive SARS-CoV-2 PCR test, other findings include, depending on the severity of the disease, lymphopenia, neutropenia, elevated liver enzyme levels, high C-reactive protein levels, high ferritin levels, and elevated D-dimer levels. Respiratory failure is a concern in clients with COVID-19. If the client's condition deteriorates, arterial blood gas values would be indicative of respiratory acidosis. The arterial blood gas values for this client are not indicative of respiratory acidosis. Classic symptoms of DKA include hyperglycemia, polyuria, polydipsia, polyphagia, a fruity breath odor, nausea and/or vomiting, abdominal pain, dehydration, weakness, and confusion. An elevated C-reactive protein level is a normal finding in DM. Arterial blood gas results also indicate metabolic acidosis.

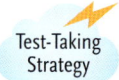

Test-Taking Strategy: Considering the two conditions, DKA and COVID-19, think about the pathophysiology that occurs with each of these conditions. The client findings in the medical record can be categorized, as shown in the table, to help *Analyze Cues*. Remember that with *Analyze Cues*, you are thinking about what could be happening to the client based on the information in the clinical scenario.

Client Finding and Disease Process	Pathophysiology
Fever and chills: COVID-19	COVID-19: Immune response related to infectious process
Nausea: Both	DKA: Metabolic decompensation COVID-19: Virus in GI tract
Abdominal pain: Both	DKA: Metabolic decompensation COVID-19: Virus in GI tract
Increased urination: DKA	DKA: Kidneys remove excess glucose, and water is excreted along with the glucose
Cough: COVID-19	COVID-19: Cough as a compensatory mechanism to respiratory injury and infection
Lung crackles: COVID-19	COVID-19: Fluid develops as part of the immune response and compensatory mechanism to respiratory injury and infection
C-reactive protein level: Both	DKA: Inflammation from metabolic imbalance COVID-19: Inflammation from infectious process
Glucose level: DKA	DKA: Insulin deficiency leading to hyperglycemia
ABG results: DKA	DKA: Buildup of ketone bodies when diabetes is uncontrolled

Think about DKA primarily as a metabolic process and COVID-19 primarily as a respiratory process. Remember that absolute insulin deficiency is the main cause of DKA. Recall that metabolic decompensation and acidosis occur, causing a number of signs and symptoms including nausea, abdominal pain, increased urination, inflammation, and elevated glucose levels. With COVID-19, remember that respiratory infection and subsequent injury is the main manifestation; however, other bodily processes are also affected. Fever and chills, nausea, abdominal pain, cough, lung crackles, and elevated C-reactive protein are all common findings associated with COVID-19. Thinking about the pathophysiology of each condition and considering all of the data available to you will help you *Analyze Cues* and direct you to the correct options.

CJ Cognitive Skill: Analyze Cues

Practice Question 10.15 — Unfolding Case Study 3

A 64-year-old client presents to the ED and reports a 2-week history of fever and chills, nausea and abdominal pain, sore throat, cough, fatigue and lethargy, and muscle aches.

History and Physical

1000: History of type 1 diabetes mellitus, hypertension, hyperlipidemia, and hypothyroidism. Denies chest pain or shortness of breath. Nonproductive cough, coarse crackles heard in lower lobes bilaterally. Blood glucose levels have been well controlled, but this morning the client reports a level of 375 mg/dL (20.8 mmol/L), prompting the visit to the ED. States recent glycated hemoglobin (A1c) level performed 2 months ago was 7%. Unable to eat, and reports discontinuing medications 3 days ago because of nausea and abdominal pain. Reports increased urination despite inability to tolerate food or fluids. Reports weakness and muscle aches and being confined to the bed for the past 3 weeks. Fruity breath odor noted. POC glucose 400 mg/dL (22.2 mmol/L). VS: T 100.4°F (38°C); HR 96; RR 24; BP 142/90; SpO$_2$ 91% on RA. Weight 175 lb (79.37 kg), height 5 feet 9 inches (stated). Voided: 250 mL.

Medications:
Levothyroxine 125 mcg/day orally
Lisinopril 2.5 mg/day orally
Simvastatin 20 mg/day orally
Insulin glargine 28 units/day subcutaneously
Semaglutide 1 mg/week subcutaneously

Laboratory Results

1120: The nurse reviews the recent laboratory and diagnostic results.

Test and Reference Range	Results
Glucose 74–106 mg/dL (3.9–6.1 mmol/L)	440 mg/dL (24.4 mmol/L)
Ketones <0 mg/dL (0.0–0.27 mmol/L)	86.4 mg/dL (4.8 mmol/L)
White blood cells (WBCs) 5000–10,000/mm^3 (5–10 × 10^9/L)	9900/mm^3 (9 × 10^9/L)
Blood urea nitrogen (BUN) 10–20 mg/dL (2.9–8.2 mmol/L)	22 mg/dL (9.0 mmol/L)
Creatinine 0.6–1.2 mg/dL (53–106 µmol/L)	1.0 mg/dL (88.3 µmol/L)
Potassium 3.5–5.0 mEq/L (3.5–5.0 mmol/L)	5.9 mEq/L (5.9 mmol/L)
Sodium 136–145 mEq/L (136–145 mmol/L)	150 mEq/L (150 mmol/L)
Thyroid-stimulating hormone (TSH) 2–10 mIU/mL (0.4–4.8 mIU/L)	4.0 mIU/mL (4.0 mIU/L)
D-dimer <0.4 mcg/mL (<3 nmol/L)	15 mcg/mL (112.5 nmol/L)
Creatine kinase (CK) 20–200 U/L (20–215 U/L)	140 U/L (150.5 U/L)
C-reactive protein (CRP) <1 mg/dL (<10.0 mg/L)	10.2 mg/dL (102 mg/L)
Troponin I <0.03 ng/mL (<0.35 mcg/L)	0.01 ng/mL (0.17 mcg/L)
Blood culture: no growth	Pending

Urinalysis

WBCs: 0–4 low-power field	0 (0)
Ketones: none	Positive
Urine culture: no growth	Pending

Arterial Blood Gases (ABGs)

pH: 7.35–7.45	pH 7.30
PCO$_2$: 35–45 mm Hg	PCO$_2$ 27 mm Hg
HCO$_3$: 21–28 mEq/L	HCO$_3$ 14 mEq/L
PO$_2$: 80–100 mm Hg	PO$_2$ 85 mm Hg
SARS-CoV-2: PCR negative	Positive

Practice Question 10.15 — Unfolding Case Study 3—cont'd

History and Physical	Nurses' Notes	Laboratory Results	Diagnostic Results

Chest x-ray: Bilateral pulmonary infiltrates compatible with COVID-19 pneumonitis

ECG: NSR

Complete the following sentence by selecting from the lists of options provided.

The client is at **highest** risk for developing **thromboembolism** as evidenced by **D-dimer level** and **immobility**.

Options for 1	Options for 2	Options for 3
Seizures	BUN	Chills
Acute kidney injury	Fever	Creatinine level
Myxedema coma	D-dimer level	Chest x-ray result
Respiratory failure	Lung crackles	TSH level
Thromboembolism	History of hypothyroidism	Immobility

Rationale: Thrombus formation has been associated with stasis of blood, endothelial injury, and/or hypercoagulability, known as the *Virchow triad.* Immobility is one condition that can promote thrombus formation. COVID-19 can cause severe inflammation, which can trigger alteration of the clotting mechanism. Older adults and those individuals who have underlying medical conditions such as heart or lung disease or diabetes seem to be at higher risk for developing more serious complications from COVID-19 illness. In severe cases of COVID-19, these individuals may develop abnormal blood clots—from PE in the lungs and DVT in the legs to clots that lead to strokes or heart attacks. This client is at highest risk for developing thromboembolism because of the report of immobility for the past 3 weeks and the elevated D-dimer level. The client is experiencing chills and has a temperature of 100.4°F (38°C). However, it is unlikely for the client to experience seizures related to this temperature reading; seizures are most likely to occur with a sustained high fever. There is no evidence of kidney injury. Although the BUN level is elevated, this elevation is most likely due to the dehydration that occurs in DKA. In addition, the creatinine is normal. Myxedema coma, sometimes called *hypothyroid crisis,* is a serious complication of untreated or poorly treated hypothyroidism. This client has a history of hypothyroidism, but the thyroid-stimulating hormone level is within the normal reference range, indicating that the condition is controlled. There is no evidence of respiratory failure. Although the client has lung crackles bilaterally and the chest x-ray shows pneumonitis, the client is not experiencing difficulty breathing or shortness of breath. The arterial blood gases show evidence of metabolic acidosis and not a respiratory condition.

Test-Taking Strategy: Note the strategic word *highest* in this question. The ability to use judgment and prioritize potential complications and associated evidence is needed in order to *Prioritize Hypotheses.* Considering the possible complications in the context of the clinical scenario and deciding which definitive evidence would support and apply to each complication listed can direct you to the correct options. Using a thinking process as illustrated in the table may help you *Prioritize Hypotheses.*

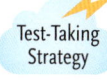

Potential Complication	Definitive Evidence/Supportive or Not Supportive of Complication?
Seizures	Fever, chills; not supportive
Acute kidney injury	BUN, Creatinine, normal; not supportive
Myxedema coma	History of hypothyroidism, TSH level normal; not supportive
Respiratory failure	Lung crackles, chest x-ray result; not supportive
Thromboembolism	D-dimer level, immobility; supportive: D-dimer level is highly suggestive of this risk, and immobility is a major risk factor

Remember that in order to *Prioritize Hypotheses,* you need to decide on the potential complication that is of *highest* priority first and then decide on the definitive evidence that is supportive of the complication. For each condition, there are risk factors present, but the only option that has definitive evidence of risk is thromboembolism, with an elevated D-dimer level and immobility as a major risk factor for this complication.

CJ Cognitive Skill: Prioritize Hypotheses

Practice Question 10.16 — Unfolding Case Study 3

A 64-year-old client presents to the ED and reports a 2-week history of fever and chills, nausea and abdominal pain, sore throat, cough, fatigue and lethargy, and muscle aches.

History and Physical

1000: History of type 1 diabetes mellitus, hypertension, hyperlipidemia, and hypothyroidism. Denies chest pain or shortness of breath. Nonproductive cough, coarse crackles heard in lower lobes bilaterally. Blood glucose levels have been well controlled, but this morning the client reports a level of 375 mg/dL (20.8 mmol/L), prompting the visit to the ED. States recent glycated hemoglobin (A1c) level performed 2 months ago was 7%. Unable to eat, and reports discontinuing medications 3 days ago because of nausea and abdominal pain. Reports increased urination despite inability to tolerate food or fluids. Reports weakness and muscle aches and being confined to the bed for the past 3 weeks. Fruity breath odor noted. POC glucose 400 mg/dL (22.2 mmol/L). VS: T 100.4°F (38°C); HR 96; RR 24; BP 142/90; SpO$_2$ 91% on RA. Weight 175 lb (79.37 kg), height 5 feet 9 inches (stated). Voided: 250 mL.

Medications:
Levothyroxine 125 mcg/day orally
Lisinopril 2.5 mg/day orally
Simvastatin 20 mg/day orally
Insulin glargine 28 units/day subcutaneously
Semaglutide 1 mg/week subcutaneously

1120: The nurse reviews the recent laboratory and diagnostic results.

Laboratory Results

Test and Reference Range	Results
Glucose 74–106 mg/dL (3.9–6.1 mmol/L)	440 mg/dL (24.4 mmol/L)
Ketones <0 mg/dL (0.0–0.27 mmol/L)	86.4 mg/dL (4.8 mmol/L)
White blood cells (WBCs) 5000–10,000/mm³ (5–10 × 10⁹/L)	9900/mm³ (9 × 10⁹/L)
Blood urea nitrogen (BUN) 10–20 mg/dL (2.9–8.2 mmol/L)	22 mg/dL (9.0 mmol/L)
Creatinine 0.6–1.2 mg/dL (53–106 μmol/L)	1.0 mg/dL (88.3 μmol/L)
Potassium 3.5–5.0 mEq/L (3.5–5.0 mmol/L)	5.9 mEq/L (5.9 mmol/L)
Sodium 136–145 mEq/L (136–145 mmol/L)	150 mEq/L (150 mmol/L)
Thyroid-stimulating hormone (TSH) 2–10 mIU/mL (0.4–4.8 mIU/L)	4.0 mIU/mL (4.0 mIU/L)
D-dimer <0.4 mcg/mL (<3 nmol/L)	15 mcg/mL (112.5 nmol/L)
Creatine kinase (CK) 20–200 U/L (20–215 U/L)	140 U/L (150.5 U/L)
C-reactive protein (CRP) <1 mg/dL (<10.0 mg/L)	10.2 mg/dL (102 mg/L)
Troponin I <0.03 ng/mL (<0.35 mcg/L)	0.01 ng/mL (0.17 mcg/L)
Blood culture: no growth	Pending
Urinalysis	
WBCs: 0–4 low-power field	0 (0)
Ketones: none	Positive
Urine culture: no growth	Pending
Arterial Blood Gases (ABGs)	
pH: 7.35–7.45	pH 7.30
PCO$_2$: 35–45 mm Hg	PCO$_2$ 27 mm Hg
HCO$_3$: 21–28 mEq/L	HCO$_3$ 14 mEq/L
PO$_2$: 80–100 mm Hg	PO$_2$ 85 mm Hg
SARS-CoV-2: PCR negative	Positive

Practice Question 10.16 — Unfolding Case Study 3—cont'd

History and Physical	Nurses' Notes	Laboratory Results	Diagnostic Results

Chest x-ray: Bilateral pulmonary infiltrates compatible with COVID-19 pneumonitis.
ECG: NSR

1145: Hospital admission is planned and the nurse reassesses the client.

History and Physical	Nurses' Notes	Laboratory Results	Diagnostic Results

1145: VS: T 100.4°F (38°C); HR 98; RR 24; BP 146/92; SpO₂ 89% on RA. POC glucose reading is 500 mg/dL (27.7 mmol/L). The client is alert but lethargic yet arousable. Voiding 200 mL/h. Dry cough. No shortness of breath. Coarse crackles heard in lower lobes bilaterally.

Specify whether the following potential nursing actions are indicated or not indicated for the client at this time.

Potential Nursing Actions	Indicated	Not Indicated
O₂ via NC	X	
0.45% NS infusion	X	
Insulin glargine bolus		X
Continuous infusion of regular insulin diluted in NS	X	
IV potassium		X
Continuous cardiac monitoring	X	
Enoxaparin subcutaneously daily	X	
Ceftriaxone		X

Rationale: DKA is a complication of DM and is characterized by hyperglycemia, metabolic acidosis, and increased production of ketones. The hyperglycemia leads to osmotic diuresis and electrolyte loss. Fluid therapy and the administration of regular insulin are needed to treat this condition. The first outcome of fluid therapy is to restore blood volume and maintain perfusion to vital organs. Dehydration is treated with IV infusions of 0.9% or 0.45% normal saline as prescribed. Hyperglycemia is treated with regular insulin as prescribed. An IV bolus dose of regular insulin is prescribed, followed by a continuous infusion of regular insulin mixed in 0.9% or 0.45% normal saline. Insulin glargine is a long-acting insulin that works slowly over 24 hours. Thus it is not helpful in treating DKA when blood glucose levels are critically high and need to be lowered. When treating DKA, the electrolyte levels are monitored closely. This client's potassium level is 5.9 mEq/L (5.9 mmol/L), which is elevated, so administering potassium would be contraindicated at this time. In addition, continuous cardiac monitoring is necessary because of the risk of dysrhythmias associated with an elevated potassium level. This client also tests positive for COVID-19 and exhibits signs of the viral infection. Although the client has no shortness of breath or difficulty breathing, the SpO₂ reading is 89% on RA, which warrants the need for oxygen. COVID-19 is a viral infection; therefore there is no need for ceftriaxone, an antibiotic that treats bacterial infections. An antibiotic would not be helpful and could actually be harmful in treating a viral infection because of its effect on the immune system and could lead to a superinfection. Although the blood culture is pending, there is no evidence of bacterial infection warranting the use of an antibiotic. Older adults and those individuals who have underlying medical conditions such as diabetes seem to be at higher risk for developing more serious complications from COVID-19 illness. In severe cases of COVID-19, these individuals may develop abnormal blood clots. This client is at high risk for developing VTE because of the report of immobility for the past 3 weeks and the elevated D-dimer level. Therefore prophylaxis with enoxaparin, a low-molecular-weight anticoagulant, is warranted. This client has an elevated C-reactive protein level, indicating the presence of inflammation, and an SpO₂ of 89% on RA.

Test-Taking Strategy: Note that the question is asking for potential interventions that are either indicated or not indicated for the client with DKA complicated by COVID-19 infection. Think about the clinical scenario and what each of the listed interventions

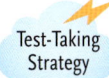

would do for this client. Look at each option provided, and think about the potential effect of that information and how it relates to promoting safe client care. Organize your thought process as illustrated in the table.

Intervention	Potential Effect	Promotes or Inhibits Safety
O$_2$ via NC	Treats hypoxemia related to respiratory infection	Promotes
0.45% NS infusion	Hypotonic, does not add to the glucose load; administered with regular IV insulin	Promotes
Insulin glargine bolus	Long-acting insulin, not useful in treating acutely elevated blood glucose levels	Inhibits
Continuous infusion of regular insulin diluted in NS	Treats elevated blood glucose levels associated with DKA	Promotes
IV potassium	Currently hyperkalemic	Inhibits
Continuous cardiac monitoring	Helps detect complications of condition and need for treatment	Promotes
Enoxaparin subcutaneously daily	Helps prevent VTE	Promotes
Ceftriaxone	Antibiotic: not necessary because infection is viral; may contribute to superinfection risk	Inhibits

Consider the rationale behind each action in the context of whether it would promote or inhibit safety. Each intervention categorized as promoting safety would be chosen as an indicated action, whereas each intervention categorized as inhibiting safety would be chosen as not indicated. Remember that in order to *Generate Solutions,* you need to think about expected outcomes and use your hypotheses to define a set of interventions that will enable the client to achieve the expected outcomes.

CJ Cognitive Skill: Generate Solutions

Practice Question 10.17 — Unfolding Case Study 3

1345: The ED physician orders are initiated, and the client with DKA and COVID-19 is transferred to the acute care medical unit for hospital admission. The admitting physician prescribes laboratory studies, and the nurse contacts the laboratory for the test results.

History and Physical	**Nurses' Notes**	Laboratory Results	Diagnostic Results

1345: Client is alert and oriented on admission. VS: T 99.4°F (37.4°C); HR 88; RR 20; BP 138/90; SpO₂ 90% on RA. Lab contacted for testing.

Based on the client assessment and laboratory findings, select the **3 priority** actions.

- ☒ Administer IV potassium.
- ☐ Offer a sports drink for sipping.
- ☒ Check hourly output measurements.
- ☐ Teach the client about ways to prevent dehydration.
- ☒ Administer 5% dextrose in 0.45% NS.

1415: The laboratory results are reported, and the nurse reviews the results and subsequent orders.

History and Physical	Nurses' Notes	**Laboratory Results**	Diagnostic Results

Test and Reference Range	Results
Glucose 74–106 mg/dL (3.9–6.1 mmol/L)	240 mg/dL (12.6 mmol/L)
Blood urea nitrogen (BUN) 10–20 mg/dL (2.9–8.2 mmol/L)	18 mg/dL (5.22 mmol/L)
Creatinine 0.6–1.2 mg/dL (53–106 µmol/L)	1.2 mg/dL (106 µmol/L)
Potassium 3.5–5.0 mEq/L (3.5–5.0 mmol/L)	4.0 mEq/L (4.0 mmol/L)
Sodium 136–145 mEq/L (136–145 mmol/L)	150 mEq/L (150 mmol/L)

Rationale: During treatment for DKA, it is critical for the nurse to monitor the client's fluid and electrolyte status along with glucose levels. When treating dehydration, 0.9% or 0.45% normal saline solution is infused. A continuous infusion of regular insulin is administered to lower the blood glucose level. During the first hour of treatment, the potassium level will decrease rapidly as the dehydration and acidosis are treated. To prevent hypokalemia, potassium replacement is initiated after the potassium level decreases below 5.0 mEq/L (5.0 mmol/L). This client's potassium level has decreased from 5.9 mEq/L (5.9 mmol/L) to 4.0 mEq/L (4.0 mmol/L), warranting the need for potassium. Therefore this would be a priority action by the nurse. Because potassium is excreted through the kidneys, the nurse would ensure adequate renal function before potassium is administered; therefore another priority action would be to check hourly urine output to ensure that the client is urinating a minimum of 30 mL/h. This is another important action because potassium accumulation could occur if renal function is altered, leading to life-threatening dysrhythmias. The blood glucose level is monitored closely. When the blood glucose level reaches 250 mg/dL (13.8 mmol/L), 5% dextrose in 0.45% normal saline is administered to help prevent hypoglycemia and cerebral edema, which can occur when serum osmolarity declines too rapidly. If the blood glucose level decreases too low or too quickly before the brain has time to equilibrate, water is pulled from the blood to the cerebrospinal fluid and the brain, causing cerebral edema and increased intracranial pressure. Teaching the client about self-care is important, but this would not be a priority action and can wait until the emergent situation is stabilized. The nurse would teach the client about ways to prevent dehydration because dehydration can precipitate DKA. The nurse would teach the client that liquids containing both glucose and electrolytes, such as sports drinks, should be consumed when nausea is present. The nurse would also teach the client not to discontinue medications for diabetes when ill.

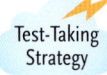

Test-Taking Strategy: Note that this question is asking you about the priority actions the nurse would take based on updated assessment findings and laboratory results. Create a table as illustrated below, and list the actions, if it is related to a new finding, and if it is a correct priority action.

Action	Related to New Finding	Correct Priority Action?
Administer IV potassium.	Yes—decreased K level	Yes
Offer a sports drink for sipping.	Yes—decreased K level	No
Check hourly urine output amounts.	Yes—assess renal function, which can be affected by condition and treatment	Yes
Teach the client about ways to prevent dehydration.	No—being managed with IV fluids	No
Administer 5% dextrose in 0.45% NS.	Yes—decreased blood glucose level, IV insulin	Yes

Once you determine which interventions are specifically related to a new finding (which could be related to the condition itself or to the treatment for the condition), then you need to think about whether it would be a correct *priority* action. Administering IV potassium is needed because of the decreased potassium level and would be a correct priority action to prevent hypokalemia from IV insulin therapy. Hourly urine output measurements are important to ensure adequate renal function as both the conditions and treatments can cause renal impairment leading to additional complications. A sports drink may be helpful for treating dehydration, but the question asks for the three priority actions; considering the options provided, this would not be a priority but could be performed once the others have been implemented. Teaching about ways to prevent dehydration may be important at some time, but not as a priority action. The client's condition is being treated with IV fluids, and ultimately this measure could wait until a later time once the acute issues have been resolved. Administering 5% dextrose in 0.45% normal saline is important to prevent hypoglycemia from the treatment. Because the blood glucose level has decreased, this is an important action to prevent complications of the insulin therapy. Remember that in order to *Take Actions,* you need to think about the solutions that address the highest priorities and relevant problems. In this scenario, the actions are focused on managing the acute condition and preventing complications related to treatment.

CJ Cognitive Skill: Take Actions

Practice Question 10.18 — Unfolding Case Study 3

0700: The hand-off report from the night nurse to the day nurse has been completed. The night nurse reports that the prescriptions to treat the client's DKA were implemented on the previous evening shift. The night nurse also reports that the client had a comfortable night and that laboratory results and vital signs were checked every 4 hours during the night and remained stable.

0730: The day nurse assesses the client and reviews the most current laboratory results, which were drawn at 0600.

History and Physical	Nurses' Notes	Laboratory Results	Diagnostic Results

Test and Reference Range	Results
Glucose 74–106 mg/dL (3.9–6.1 mmol/L)	240 mg/dL (12.6 mmol/L)
Blood urea nitrogen (BUN) 10–20 mg/dL (2.9–8.2 mmol/L)	18 mg/dL (5.22 mmol/L)
Creatinine 0.6–1.2 mg/dL (53–106 µmol/L)	1.2 mg/dL (106 µmol/L)
Potassium 3.5–5.0 mEq/L (3.5–5.0 mmol/L)	4.0 mEq/L (4.0 mmol/L)
Sodium 136–145 mEq/L (136–145 mmol/L)	150 mEq/L (150 mmol/L)

For each client finding, select whether the finding indicates that the treatment plan is effective or ineffective.

Previous Client Finding	Current Client Finding	Effective	Ineffective
Glucose 240 mg/dL (12.6 mmol/L)	Glucose 190 mg/dL (10.64 mmol/L)	☒	☐
Potassium 4.0 mEq/L (4.0 mmol/L)	Potassium 4.0 mEq/L (4.0 mmol/L)	☒	☐
Urine output 200 mL/h	Urine output 45 mL/h	☒	☐
Sodium 150 mEq/L (150 mmol/L)	Sodium 150 mEq/L (150 mmol/L)	☐	☒

Rationale: In DKA, the priority is treating the dehydration with fluids, managing the electrolyte imbalances, and treating the hyperglycemia. DKA is considered resolved when the blood glucose level is less than 200 mg/dL (11.2 mmol/L); therefore a blood glucose level of 190 mg/dL (10.64 mmol/L) indicates resolution and effectiveness of the treatment. The client's initial potassium level was 5.9 mEq/L (5.9 mmol/L), and it decreased to 4.0 mEq/L (4.0 mmol/L), which indicates a normal level. Although the nurse would continue to monitor the potassium level closely and for signs of an imbalance, the normal level indicates effectiveness of treatment. A manifestation of DKA is polyuria, which was an initial report by this client, and urine output has been 200 mL/h. Once the dehydration and acidosis are treated, the urine output will return to normal. An output of 45 mL/h is within the range, indicating effectiveness of treatment. The sodium level of 150 mEq/L (150 mmol/L) could indicate that further resolution of the dehydration status is necessary. The nurse would report this finding to the physician to further investigate the reason it remains elevated and to determine further necessary treatment measures.

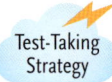

Test-Taking Strategy: This question is asking you to evaluate treatment effectiveness for DKA. Remember that treatments for this condition may result in a number of other effects that need to be monitored for and addressed if they occur. Think about each assessment finding, and determine how it has changed. Then decide whether this is in line with improvement or worsening of the condition or if the condition remains unchanged. If the result is evidence of improvement, then it would be considered effective; however, if it is evidence of worsening or is unchanged, then it would be considered ineffective. Use a thinking process as illustrated in the table.

Assessment Finding	Improvement, Worsening, or Unchanged
Glucose 190 mg/dL (10.64 mmol/L)	Improvement—indicates resolving DKA
Potassium 4.0 mEq/L (4.0 mmol/L)	Improvement—indicates resolution of hyperkalemia and avoidance of hypokalemia as a result of insulin therapy
Urine output 45 mL/h	Improvement—indicates stable renal function despite acute condition and treatment measures
Sodium 150 mEq/L (150 mmol/L)	Unchanged—indicates hypernatremia and possible continued dehydration; could lead to neurologic problems and must be reported

Remember that in order to *Evaluate Outcomes,* you need compare observed outcomes against expected outcomes and then look for evidence that the interventions were effective. In this case, you need to determine whether the assessment findings demonstrate improvement, worsening, or no change with regard to DKA treatment.

CJ Cognitive Skill: Evaluate Outcomes

Unfolding Case Study 4

Content Area: Medical-Surgical Nursing
Priority Concept: Gas Exchange; Perfusion
Reference(s): Ignatavicius et al., 2024, pp. 677–679; 783–807

Practice Question 10.19 — Unfolding Case Study 4

A 70-year-old client presents to the ED.

*Highlight the findings that require **immediate** follow-up.*

History and Physical	Nurses' Notes	Vital Signs	Laboratory and Diagnostic Results

1200: 70-year-old client admitted to ED reporting ==chest heaviness and difficulty breathing for 2 days==. Symptoms increase with activity and subside with rest after a few minutes. Past medical history of type 2 DM, hypertension, hyperlipidemia, hypothyroidism, and osteoarthritis. Currently smokes 1 pack of cigarettes per day × 20 years. Medications include sliding-scale insulin aspart prior to meals and at bedtime, insulin glargine at bedtime, lisinopril, atorvastatin, levothyroxine, and naproxen.

History and Physical	Nurses' Notes	Vital Signs	Laboratory and Diagnostic Results

1200: Appears nontoxic, well nourished, and well hydrated. Skin warm, dry, and intact. Lungs clear to auscultation bilaterally, no adventitious sounds. No use of accessory muscles. ==HR irregularly irregular==. S1 and S2 noted, no S3 or S4; no murmurs, rubs, or gallops. No peripheral edema. Abdomen soft, nontender, and nondistended. Bowel sounds present × 4. Cranial nerves II to XII grossly intact.

History and Physical	Nurses' Notes	Vital Signs	Laboratory and Diagnostic Results

1200: VS: T 97.5°F (36.4°C) oral; ==HR 130 and irregular==; RR 20; BP 108/59; SpO$_2$ 95% on RA. Height: 165 cm (5 feet 5 inches) Weight: 180 lb (81.6 kg) BMI: 30.
1200: I: 120 mL water (oral)
1230: O: 140 mL clear, yellow urine

History and Physical	Nurses' Notes	Vital Signs	Laboratory and Diagnostic Results

ECG:
==Atrial fibrillation with rapid ventricular response, rate 130==
==Acute anterior and lateral MI==
==Intraventricular conduction delay==
No ST elevation

Test and Reference Range	Results
Sodium 136–145 mEq/L (136–145 mmol/L)	136 mEq/L (136 mmol/L)
Potassium 3.5–5.0 mEq/L (3.5–5.0 mmol/L)	3.8 mEq/L (3.8 mmol/L)
Calcium 9–10.5 mg/dL (2.25–2.62 mmol/L)	9.2 mg/dL (2.4 mmol/L)
Chloride 98–106 mEq/L (98–106 mmol/L)	98 mEq/L (98 mmol/L)
Glucose 74–106 mg/dL (3.9–6.1 mmol/L)	212 mg/dL (11.8 mmol/L)
Blood urea nitrogen (BUN) 10–20 mg/dL (2.9–8.2 mmol/L)	22 mg/dL (7.8 mmol/L)
Creatinine 0.6–1.2 mg/dL (53–106 μmol/L)	1.0 mg/dL (88.3 μmol/L)
Glomerular filtration rate >60 mL/min/1.73 m²	70 mL/min/ 1.73 m²
White blood cells (WBC) 5000–10,000/mm³ (5.0–10 × 10⁹/L)	6000/mm³ (6.0 × 10⁹/L)
Red blood cells (RBCs) 4.2–6.1 × 10¹²/L (4.2–6.2 × 10¹²/L)	4.6 × 10¹²/L (4.6 × 10¹²/L)
Hemoglobin (Hgb) 12–18 g/dL (120–180 g/L)	13 g/dL (130 g/L)
Hematocrit (Hct) 37%–52% (0.37–0.54 volume fraction)	38% (0.38 volume fraction)
Cardiac Markers	
Troponin T <0.1 ng/mL (0.1 mcg/L)	==0.8 ng/mL (0.8 mcg/L)==

Rationale: Client findings that are of immediate concern to the nurse include reports of chest heaviness, difficulty breathing for the past 2 days, irregularly irregular heart rate at 130, atrial fibrillation with rapid ventricular response, acute anterior and lateral myocardial infarction (MI), intraventricular conduction delay on ECG, and a troponin T level of 0.8 ng/mL (0.8 mcg/L). These findings support an acute problem with the cardiovascular system and confirm that the client had an MI. In order to promote optimal outcomes, the nurse would follow up on these findings immediately. Other items in the health history, such as the past medical history, social history, and medications, are important and may relate to the acute condition, but they are not of *immediate* concern to the nurse. The findings in the Nurses' Notes that are of immediate concern would be the cardiovascular and respiratory findings. An irregularly irregular, elevated heart rate is consistent with atrial fibrillation with rapid ventricular response, which is a potentially life-threatening dysrhythmia. The assessment findings in all other body systems are normal or stable. The troponin T level is elevated, with a normal level being <0.1 ng/mL (<0.1 mcg/L), which indicates cardiac muscle damage and is consistent with myocardial ischemia and MI. All other laboratory results are normal or only slightly out of range.

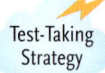

Test-Taking Strategy: First, note that this question is asking which findings are of *immediate* concern to the nurse. This indicates that there may be findings that are abnormal but not needing immediate follow-up. Remember to first identify normal/usual or abnormal/expected client findings. These findings would *not* be of immediate concern to the nurse. Next, identify abnormal/not expected findings to determine which findings need immediate follow-up. The client findings in the medical record can be categorized as shown in the table in order to help *Recognize Cues*.

Client Finding	Normal/Usual or Abnormal/Expected Not Requiring Immediate Follow-up	Abnormal/Not Expected and Requiring Immediate Follow-up
Chest heaviness	☐	✗
Difficulty breathing	☐	✗
Past medical history	✗	☐
Current smoker	✗	☐
Current medications	✗	☐
General assessment findings	✗	☐
Integumentary assessment findings	✗	☐
Respiratory assessment findings	☐	✗
Cardiovascular assessment findings	☐	✗
Gastrointestinal assessment findings	✗	☐
Neurologic assessment findings	✗	☐
T 97.5°F (36.4°C)°	✗	☐
HR 130 and irregular	☐	✗
RR 20	✗	☐
BP 108/59	✗	☐

Client Finding	Normal/Usual or Abnormal/Expected Not Requiring Immediate Follow-up	Abnormal/Not Expected and Requiring Immediate Follow-up
SpO₂ 95% on RA	☒	☐
I&O	☒	☐
Atrial fibrillation with rapid ventricular response, rate 130	☐	☒
Acute anterior and lateral MI	☐	☒
Intraventricular conduction delay	☐	☒
No ST elevation	☒	☐
Sodium: 136 mEq/L (136 mmol/L)	☒	☐
Potassium: 3.8 mEq/L (3.8 mmol/L)	☒	☐
Calcium: 9.2 mg/dL (2.4 mmol/L)	☒	☐
Chloride: 98 mEq/L (98 mmol/L)	☒	☐
Glucose: 212 mg/dL (11.8 mmol/L)	☒	☐
Blood urea nitrogen (BUN): 22 mg/dL (7.8 mmol/L)	☒	☐
Creatinine: 1.0 mg/dL (88.3 µmol/L)	☒	☐
Glomerular filtration rate: 70 mL/min (2 m²)	☒	☐
White blood cells (WBCs): 6000/mm³ (6.0 × 10⁹/L)	☒	☐
Red blood cells (RBCs): 4.6 × 10¹²/L (4.6 × 10¹²/L)	☒	☐
Hemoglobin (Hgb): 13 g/dL (130 g/L)	☒	☐
Hematocrit (Hct): 38% (0.38 volume fraction)	☒	☐
Troponin T: 0.8 ng/mL (0.8 mcg/L)	☐	☒

Chest heaviness; difficulty breathing; cardiovascular assessment findings (specifically heart rate and rhythm); ECG findings indicating dysrhythmia, MI, and conduction delay; and the troponin T level are all findings that are of immediate concern to the nurse because they specifically relate to a life-threatening condition and require immediate follow-up to promote optimal outcomes. Although the other options could be abnormal or may be relevant in some way to the acute condition, they do not require immediate follow-up and could be safely addressed at a later time.

CJ Cognitive Skill: Recognize Cues

Practice Question 10.20 — Unfolding Case Study 4

A 70-year-old client presents to the ED.

History and Physical

1200: 70-year-old client admitted to ED reporting chest heaviness and difficulty breathing for 2 days. Symptoms increase with activity and subside with rest after a few minutes. Past medical history of type 2 DM, hypertension, hyperlipidemia, hypothyroidism, and osteoarthritis. Currently smokes 1 pack cigarettes per day × 20 years. Medications include sliding-scale insulin aspart prior to meals and at bedtime, insulin glargine at bedtime, lisinopril, atorvastatin, levothyroxine, and naproxen.

Nurses' Notes

1200: Appears nontoxic, well nourished, and well hydrated. Skin warm, dry, and intact. Lungs clear to auscultation bilaterally, no adventitious sounds. No use of accessory muscles. HR irregularly irregular. S1 and S2 noted; no S3 or S4; no murmurs, rubs, or gallops. No peripheral edema. Abdomen soft, nontender, and nondistended. Bowel sounds present × 4. Cranial nerves II to XII grossly intact.

Vital Signs

1200: VS: T 97.5°F (36.4°C) oral; HR 130 and irregular; RR 20; BP 108/59; SpO$_2$ 95% on RA. Height: 165 cm (5 feet 5 inches) Weight: 81.6 kg (180 lb) BMI: 30.
1200: I: 120 mL water (oral)
1230: O: 140 mL clear, yellow urine

Laboratory and Diagnostic Results

1200:
ECG:
Atrial fibrillation with rapid ventricular response, rate 130
Acute anterior and lateral MI
Intraventricular conduction delay
No ST elevation

Test and Reference Range	Results
Sodium 136–145 mEq/L (136–145 mmol/L)	136 mEq/L (136 mmol/L)
Potassium 3.5–5.0 mEq/L (3.5–5.0 mmol/L)	3.8 mEq/L (3.8 mmol/L)
Calcium 9–10.5 mg/dL (2.25–2.62 mmol/L)	9.2 mg/dL (2.4 mmol/L)
Chloride 98–106 mEq/L (98–106 mmol/L)	98 mEq/L (98 mmol/L)
Glucose 74–106 mg/dL (3.9–6.1 mmol/L)	212 mg/dL (11.8 mmol/L)
Blood urea nitrogen (BUN) 10–20 mg/dL (2.9–8.2 mmol/L)	22 mg/dL (7.8 mmol/L)
Creatinine 0.6–1.2 mg/dL (53–106 μmol/L)	1.0 mg/dL (88.3 μmol/L)
Glomerular filtration rate >60 mL/min/1.73 m^2	70 mL/min/ 1.73 m^2
Complete Blood Count (CBC)	
White blood cells (WBCs) 5000–10,000/mm^3 (5.0–10 × 10^9/L)	6000/mm^3 (6.0 × 10^9/L)
Red blood cells (RBCs) 4.2–6.1 × 10^{12}/L (4.2–6.2 × 10^{12}/L)	4.6 × 10^{12}/L (4.6 × 10^{12}/L)
Hemoglobin (Hgb) 12–18 g/dL (120–180 g/L)	13 g/dL (130 g/L)
Hematocrit (Hct) 37%–52% (0.37–0.54 volume fraction)	38% (0.38 volume fraction)
Cardiac Markers	
Troponin T <0.1 ng/mL (0.1 mcg/L)	0.8 ng/mL (0.8 mcg/L)

The nurse monitors for complications based on the data collection findings. Complete the following sentence by selecting from the lists of options provided.

The client is at **highest** risk for developing **diminished cardiac output** as evidenced by **cardiovascular assessment**.

Options for 1	Options for 2
Fluid volume overload	I&O
Diminished cardiac output	Respiratory assessment
Decreased renal perfusion	Neurologic assessment
Venous thromboembolism	Cardiovascular assessment

Rationale: Atrial fibrillation is a cardiac dysrhythmia in which the atria quiver as a result of chaotic electrical signals. This dysrhythmia is often accompanied by a rapid ventricular response, causing a rapid heart rate. As a result of the ineffectiveness of this rhythm, there is a risk for diminished cardiac output. In addition, the ECG results indicate MI, which is tissue necrosis of the heart muscle. This can also contribute to diminished cardiac output. The cardiovascular assessment findings are characteristic of diminished cardiac output. Fluid volume overload, decreased renal perfusion, and VTE could also occur as potential complications for the client experiencing atrial fibrillation and MI; however, the highest-risk complication would be diminished cardiac output. Diminished cardiac output would be a predisposing factor to these other complications and can affect all body organ systems.

Test-Taking Strategy: Looking at each complication listed in the first set of options, determine the supportive data from the clinical scenario for each condition. The client findings in the medical record can be categorized as shown in the table to help *Analyze Cues*. Remember that with *Analyze Cues,* you are thinking about what could be happening to the client based on the information in the clinical scenario.

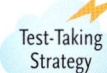
Test-Taking Strategy

Complication	Supportive Data
Fluid volume overload	Chest heaviness Difficulty breathing Past medical history Cardiovascular assessment (although there is no peripheral edema, which is usually noted) Vital signs (heart rate specifically)
Diminished cardiac output	Chest heaviness Difficulty breathing Past medical history Cardiovascular assessment Vital signs (heart rate and blood pressure) ECG results
Decreased renal perfusion	Past medical history BUN level (although creatinine is not elevated and glomerular filtration rate is not low)
VTE	Chest heaviness Difficulty breathing Past medical history ECG results

The complication with the most supportive data would be the one that is the highest risk. Chest heaviness and difficulty breathing could both be present with fluid volume overload, diminished cardiac output, and VTE. The client's past medical history could also predispose the client to any of these complications. The vital signs and cardiovascular assessment, which shows a rapid irregular heart rate and atrial fibrillation, could potentially lead to fluid overload and diminished cardiac output. In fluid overload, however, it is very common to see peripheral edema, and this is not present, making this complication less likely in comparison with diminished cardiac output. The laboratory results show an elevated BUN, but the creatinine and glomerular filtration rate are both normal; therefore decreased renal perfusion would be less likely compared with diminished cardiac output. Although the ECG shows evidence of atrial fibrillation, there are no findings on the physical assessment that increase the suspicion of VTE, such as redness, swelling, and pain in an extremity, therefore this is less likely than diminished cardiac output. Thinking about the pathophysiology of each of the listed complications and considering all of the data available to you will assist in *Analyzing Cues* and will direct you to the correct options. Remember that in the Drop-Down Rationale item type, you need to select the correct potential complication first in order to select the correct evidence to support that complication.

CJ Cognitive Skill: Analyze Cues

Practice Question 10.21 — Unfolding Case Study 4

A 70-year-old client presents to the ED.

History and Physical

1200: 70-year-old client admitted to the ED reporting chest heaviness and difficulty breathing for 2 days. Symptoms increase with activity and subside with rest after a few minutes. Past medical history of type 2 DM, hypertension, hyperlipidemia, hypothyroidism, and osteoarthritis. Currently smokes 1 pack cigarettes per day × 20 years. Medications include sliding-scale insulin aspart prior to meals and at bedtime, insulin glargine at bedtime, lisinopril, atorvastatin, levothyroxine, and naproxen.

Nurses' Notes

1200: Appears nontoxic, well nourished, and well hydrated. Skin warm, dry, and intact. Lungs clear to auscultation bilaterally, no adventitious sounds. No use of accessory muscles. HR irregularly irregular. S1 and S2 noted, no S3 or S4; no murmurs, rubs, or gallops. No peripheral edema. Abdomen soft, nontender, nondistended. Bowel sounds present × 4. Cranial nerves II to XII grossly intact.

Vital Signs

1200: VS: T 97.5°F (36.4°C) oral; HR 130 and irregular; RR 20; BP 108/59; SpO$_2$ 95% on RA. Height: 165 cm (5 feet 5 inches) Weight: 81.6 kg (180 lb) BMI: 30.
1200: I: 120 mL water (oral)
1230: O: 140 mL clear, yellow urine

Laboratory and Diagnostic Results

1215:
ECG:
Atrial fibrillation with rapid ventricular response, rate 130
Acute anterior and lateral MI
Intraventricular conduction delay
No ST elevation

Test and Reference Range	Results
Sodium 136–145 mEq/L (136–145 mmol/L)	136 mEq/L (136 mmol/L)
Potassium 3.5–5.0 mEq/L (3.5–5.0 mmol/L)	3.8 mEq/L (3.8 mmol/L)
Calcium 9–10.5 mg/dL (2.25–2.62 mmol/L)	9.2 mg/dL (2.4 mmol/L)
Chloride 98–106 mEq/L (98–106 mmol/L)	98 mEq/L (98 mmol/L)
Glucose 74–106 mg/dL (3.9–6.1 mmol/L)	212 mg/dL (11.8 mmol/L)
Blood urea nitrogen (BUN) 10–20 mg/dL (2.9–8.2 mmol/L)	22 mg/dL (7.8 mmol/L)
Creatinine 0.6–1.2 mg/dL (53–106 µmol/L)	1.0 mg/dL (88.3 µmol/L)
Glomerular filtration rate >60 mL/min/1.73 m^2	70 mL/min/1.73 m^2

Complete Blood Count (CBC)

White blood cells (WBCs) 5000–10,000/mm^3 (5.0–10 × 10^9/L)	6000/mm^3 (6.0 × 10^9/L)
Red blood cells (RBCs) 4.2–6.1 × 10^{12}/L (4.2–6.2 × 10^{12}/L)	4.6 × 10^{12}/L (4.6 × 10^{12}/L)
Hemoglobin (Hgb) 12–18 g/dL (120–180 g/L)	13 g/dL (130 g/L)
Hematocrit (Hct) 37%–52% (0.37–0.54 volume fraction)	38% (0.38 volume fraction)

Cardiac Markers

Troponin T <0.1 ng/mL (0.1 mcg/L)	0.8 ng/mL (0.8 mcg/L)

The nurse has completed the admission assessment and is initiating the client's plan of care. The nurse notes that the cardiologist has been consulted and has ordered further diagnostic testing.

Based on this clinical scenario, complete the following sentence by selecting from the lists of options provided.

The **priority** and **most specific** diagnostic test would be **cardiac catheterization** to assess for **blockages and narrowed vessels**.

Options for 1	Options for 2
D-dimer level	Blood clots
Chest x-ray	Cardiomegaly
Cardiac catheterization	Hyperthyroidism
Trended electrolyte levels	Hypokalemia or hyperkalemia
Thyroid-stimulating hormone	Blockages and narrowed vessels

Rationale: For acute coronary syndrome, which includes acute MI, a number of diagnostic tests could be ordered to assess for various causes contributing to this health problem. The priority diagnostic test would be cardiac catheterization as this is the most definitive test in diagnosing heart disease. Indications for cardiac catheterization include confirmation of suspected heart problems such as congenital abnormalities, coronary artery disease, myocardial disease, valvular disease, and valvular dysfunction. It is also performed to determine the location and extent of the problem; determine the best therapeutic option, such as angioplasty, stenting, bypass graft, or valve replacement; and evaluate the effects of medical or invasive treatment for cardiac problems. Because the ECG indicates MI, the client needs to undergo cardiac catheterization for further diagnostic determination of the extent of the problem as well as for treatment of the problem. The D-dimer level is helpful in evaluating for the presence of blood clots; however, this is a nonspecific test, and the result can be elevated by several conditions, such as pregnancy, liver disease, inflammation, malignancy, and hypercoagulable states. Given the client's symptoms, a D-dimer test would be helpful but would not be the priority diagnostic test. A chest-x-ray may be performed to assess for cardiomegaly or other complications of ischemia such as pulmonary edema, but it will not determine further treatment measures for this client. This would not be the priority diagnostic test because it would not provide information needed to treat the causative factors. Trending electrolyte levels are important because electrolyte imbalances, particularly potassium, can result in cardiac dysrhythmias that may lead to myocardial ischemia or MI and diminished cardiac output. This client's electrolyte levels were all within normal range 1 hour ago, and so this would not be the priority diagnostic test at this time. Because the client is already experiencing MI, this laboratory test is of lesser priority in comparison with cardiac catheterization at this time. A thyroid-stimulating hormone level may provide information on other, less common causes of MI, such as hyperthyroidism. This diagnostic test may be performed, especially if there are no blockages or narrowed vessels causing the ischemia or infarction. As with the other tests, this test is of a lesser priority in comparison with cardiac catheterization at this time.

Test-Taking Strategy: Note the strategic word *priority* in this question. The ability to use judgment and prioritize client needs is necessary to *Prioritize Hypotheses*. Considering the client's needs in the context of the current health problem the client is experiencing can help you decide on priorities of care and the most important diagnostic test to further direct client care. Think about whether the test would be the *initial* step in determining further treatment. Using a thinking process as illustrated in the table may be helpful to *Prioritize Hypotheses*.

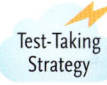
Test-Taking Strategy

Diagnostic Test	Initial Step in Determining Further Treatment	Helpful but Not an Initial Step in Determining Further Treatment
D-dimer level	☐	☒
Chest x-ray	☐	☒
Cardiac catheterization	☒	☐
Trended electrolyte levels	☐	☒
Thyroid-stimulating hormone	☐	☒

Another way to look at this is whether the diagnostic test would address the *highest priority* problem for the client based on the clinical scenario, which would be narrowed or blocked cardiac blood vessels. Use this thinking process as illustrated in the table.

Diagnostic Test	Addresses Narrowed or Blocked Vessels
D-dimer level	No
Chest x-ray	No
Cardiac catheterization	Yes
Trended electrolyte levels	No
Thyroid-stimulating hormone	No

Once you determine that cardiac catheterization is the *priority* diagnostic test because it is the *most important* in promoting optimal outcomes, you then need to choose the correct indication. Use your nursing knowledge of the indications for cardiac catheterization to assist in choosing the correct option of assessing for blockages or narrowed cardiac vessels as the second answer. Remember that in order to *Prioritize Hypotheses,* you need to decide on the diagnostic test that is of *highest priority* first and then decide on the correct indication.

CJ Cognitive Skill: Prioritize Hypotheses

Practice Question 10.22 — Unfolding Case Study 4

Progress Notes

1400: The consulting cardiologist ordered cardiac catheterization for a 70-year-old client with a suspected MI. Stents were placed, and blood flow was re-established to the affected areas of the heart. The procedure has been completed, and the nurse is monitoring the client on the intermediate care unit. The left femoral vein was used as the insertion site for the procedure.

Which of the following actions would the nurse plan for this client following cardiac catheterization? **Select all that apply.**

- ☒ Assess for shortness of breath.
- ☐ Keep both extremities straight.
- ☐ Encourage activity as tolerated.
- ☒ Apply a soft knee brace to the left leg.
- ☒ Position the client in the supine position.
- ☒ Monitor the client for changes in mental status.
- ☒ Monitor vital signs every 15 minutes initially.
- ☒ Assess the insertion site for bloody drainage or hematoma.
- ☐ Apply sequential compression devices to both lower extremities.
- ☒ Assess circulation, sensation, and motion of the affected extremity.

Rationale: For a cardiac catheterization procedure, the client is taken to the catheterization laboratory ("cath lab") and securely positioned on the table. The cardiologist or technician injects a local anesthetic into the insertion site. A catheter is then inserted into the access site, usually through the femoral vein to the inferior vena cava or through the basilic vein to the superior vena cava. The catheter is advanced into the right atrium, through the right ventricle, and through the pulmonary artery if needed. Intracardiac pressures are measured, and blood samples are obtained. The contrast medium is injected to detect cardiac shunts or regurgitation from the valves or to detect narrowed or blocked cardiac vessels. If the left side of the heart needs to be examined, then the catheter is advanced up the aorta, across the aortic valve, and into the left ventricle. Abnormalities are visualized, and blood samples are obtained as indicated. Follow-up care after this procedure is important to prevent complications of cardiac catheterization. The nurse would closely monitor the client after the procedure. The nurse would assess for shortness of breath and monitor the client's mental status because pulmonary edema, dysrhythmias, PE, MI, cardiac tamponade, and bleeding are all complications of this procedure. Vital signs are monitored every 15 minutes initially, and then every 30 minutes for 2 hours or until they are stable, as per agency policy. The affected extremity (not both extremities) must be kept straight for 2 to 6 hours after the procedure to prevent bleeding; therefore activity as tolerated would be avoided. A soft knee brace on the affected extremity can help remind the client to keep the leg straight. Typically, the client is placed in the supine position, and the head of the bed would not be elevated above 30 degrees as prescribed by the cardiologist. The nurse would assess the insertion site every 15 to 30 minutes to monitor for bloody drainage or hematoma. Sequential compression devices are used to improve blood flow to the lower extremities but are not indicated following cardiac catheterization and could potentially increase the risk for bleeding at the insertion site.

Test-Taking Strategy: Note that the question is asking about planning care for the client following cardiac catheterization. Think about the clinical scenario, what is involved with the procedure, and the potential complications of the procedure. Look at each option provided, and think about the potential effect of the intervention and how it relates to promoting safe client care. Organize your thought process as illustrated in the table.

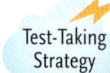

Intervention	Potential Effect After Cardiac Catheterization	Promotes/Inhibits Safety or Neither
Assess for shortness of breath.	Helps detect complications associated with the procedure.	Promotes
Keep both extremities straight.	Keeping affected extremity straight is necessary, but it is not necessary to keep both extremities straight.	Promotes for the affected extremity, neither for the other extremity
Encourage activity as tolerated.	Bed rest must be maintained to prevent bleeding and promote hemodynamic stability.	Inhibits
Apply a soft knee brace to the left leg.	May help remind the client to keep the affected extremity straight.	Promotes
Position the client in the supine position.	Helps maintain hemodynamic stability, minimizes pain, prevents bleeding at the insertion site.	Promotes
Monitor the client for changes in mental status.	Helps detect complications associated with the procedure.	Promotes
Monitor vital signs every 15 minutes initially.	Helps detect complications associated with the procedure.	Promotes
Assess the insertion site for bloody drainage or hematoma.	Assesses for postprocedural bleeding.	Promotes
Apply sequential compression devices to both lower extremities.	May increase the risk for bleeding.	Inhibits
Assess circulation, sensation, and motion of the affected extremity.	Helps detect complications associated with the procedure.	Promotes

Consider the rationale behind each intervention in the context of whether it would promote or inhibit safety or if it would not make a difference either way. Assessing for shortness of breath; monitoring the client's mental status; monitoring vital signs frequently initially; and assessing circulation, sensation, and motion of the affected extremity all help detect complications of the procedure and therefore promote safety and are correct. Regarding the option that states to keep both extremities straight, note that although it would promote safety to keep the affected extremity straight, it would not make a difference for the unaffected extremity, therefore this option is incorrect. Remember that for an option to be a correct answer, all aspects or parts of the option need to be correct. Encouraging activity as tolerated may increase the risk for bleeding and hemodynamic instability and therefore inhibits safety and is incorrect. Applying a soft knee brace may help remind the client to keep the extremity straight and therefore would help prevent bleeding at the insertion site; this promotes safety and is correct.

Positioning the client in the supine position helps promote hemodynamic stability, minimizes pain, and helps prevent bleeding at the insertion site and therefore promotes safety and is correct. Assessing the insertion site for bloody drainage or hematoma also promotes safety and is correct. Applying sequential compression devices to both lower extremities, although it promotes circulation, may increase the risk for bleeding following this procedure and therefore inhibits safety and is incorrect. All options that promote safety should be selected as correct answers, and all options that inhibit safety or neither promote nor inhibit safety would be incorrect and should not be selected. Remember that in order to *Generate Solutions*, you need think about expected outcomes and use your hypotheses to define a set of interventions that will enable the client to achieve the expected outcomes.

CJ Cognitive Skill: Generate Solutions

Practice Question 10.23 — Unfolding Case Study 4

A 70-year-old client was diagnosed with acute MI and postmyocardial heart failure with an ejection fraction of 30%. The nurse is initiating discharge teaching related to medication therapy.

*The nurse is teaching the client about discharge medications. Choose the **most likely** options for the missing information in the table by selecting from the lists of options.*

Medication	Dose, Route, Frequency	Drug Class	Indication
Aspirin	81 mg/day orally	Antiplatelet	MI prevention
Carvedilol	6.25 mg twice a day orally	Beta blocker	**Heart failure with reduced ejection fraction**
Atorvastatin	20 mg/day orally	**HMG-CoA reductase inhibitor**	Atherosclerotic cardiovascular disease
Lisinopril	5 mg/day orally	Angiotensin converting enzyme inhibitor	**Heart failure with reduced ejection fraction**
Nitroglycerin	**0.4 mg sublingually every 5 minutes as needed up to 3 times**	Vasodilator	Acute angina

Options for 1	Options for 2	Options for 3	Options for 4	Options for 5
Aspirin	0.6 mg sublingually every 15 minutes as needed up to 5 times	Fibrate	Acute angina	Hypertension
Ibuprofen	0.4 mg sublingually every 5 minutes as needed up to 3 times	Bile acid sequestrant	Hypertension	Hyperlipidemia
Diclofenac	0.6 mg sublingually × 1 before strenuous activity	HMG-CoA reductase inhibitor	Heart failure with reduced ejection fraction	Heart failure with reduced ejection fraction

Rationale: Aspirin, an antiplatelet medication, in the dose of 81 mg/day orally, is used for MI prevention and is prescribed at discharge following acute MI. Ibuprofen and diclofenac are similar in that they are also nonsteroidal antiinflammatory drugs, but these medications are not used for MI prevention. Nitroglycerin is a vasodilator and, when prescribed at a dose of 0.3 to 0.6 mg sublingually every 5 minutes as needed up to three times, is indicated for acute angina (not every 15 minutes or up to 5 times). For acute angina, clients are also taught that if there is no relief after the first dose, they need to call EMS and then take a second and third dose if still no relief occurs while waiting for help to arrive. Nitroglycerin may also be prescribed sublingually × 1 before strenuous activity for acute angina prevention, but it can be used up to three times for treating an acute angina episode. Atorvastatin is classified as an HMG-CoA reductase inhibitor. One use is to treat atherosclerotic cardiovascular disease and lower cholesterol. Fibrates can be used to lower cholesterol, and fenofibrate and gemfibrozil are examples of fibrates. Bile acid sequestrants are also used to lower cholesterol and include medications such as cholestyramine and colestipol. Carvedilol is a beta blocker used for post-MI heart failure with reduced ejection fraction, and it works by preventing cardiac remodeling and thereby improving contractility of the heart. It can also be used for hypertension, but hypertension is not usually the reason in post-MI management. Carvedilol is not used to manage acute angina. Lisinopril is an angiotensin-converting enzyme inhibitor and also helps with post-MI heart failure with reduced ejection fraction by the same mechanism as carvedilol. Like carvedilol, lisinopril can also be used for hypertension, but this is not usually the reason in post-MI management. It is not used for hyperlipidemia.

Test-Taking Strategy: Note that this question is asking you about the information you will provide the client during discharge teaching following acute MI with subsequent heart failure. You will need to draw on your knowledge of pharmacology in order to answer this question correctly. Use strategies for answering pharmacology questions, including recognizing common letters such as the prefix or suffix, to place the medication into a classification, as illustrated in the table. Once you have placed the medication into a classification, then you can think about the indications for use. This strategy will help you with four of the five medications in this question.

Medication	Prefix/Suffix	Medication Classification
Carvedilol	-lol	Beta blocker (e.g., carvedilol, metoprolol, atenolol)
Lisinopril	-pril	Angiotensin-converting enzyme inhibitor (e.g., lisinopril, enalapril, captopril)
Atorvastatin	-statin	HMG-CoA reductase inhibitor (e.g., atorvastatin, simvastatin, rosuvastatin)
Nitroglycerin	Nitro-	Vasodilator

Once you are able to determine the classifications and indications for four medications, think about the last medication, *aspirin,* and recall that it is an antiplatelet agent. In the baby aspirin dose (81 mg), it is used for MI prevention. You will need to rely on your pharmacology knowledge to determine the correct dose for the nitroglycerin. Remember that in order to *Take Actions,* you need to think about the solution that addresses the highest priorities. In this scenario, the teaching is focused on the discharge medications, and the actions are focused on which information is included.

CJ Cognitive Skill: Take Actions

Practice Question 10.24 — Unfolding Case Study 4

The nurse is caring for a 70-year-old client who had a cardiac catheterization yesterday to confirm an MI and has completed discharge teaching using the teach-back method. This morning the nurse is reinforcing teaching with the client.

Select whether the following client statements indicate understanding or no understanding of the discharge teaching provided.

Client Statements	Understanding	No Understanding
"I should walk 1 mile at least once a day in the beginning."	☐	☒
"I will be sure to carry my nitroglycerin with me."	☒	☐
"I will check my pulse before, during, and after I do my exercises."	☒	☐
"I won't exercise if I notice that my pulse is more than 5 BPM higher than what it usually is."	☐	☒
"I will exercise indoors as much as possible."	☐	☒
"I will make sure to walk at least 3 times per week."	☒	☐
"I need to avoid straining, so I won't do push-ups or pull-ups."	☒	☐

Rationale: Cardiac rehabilitation is an important part of the recovery process following acute MI. Usually a cardiac rehabilitation specialist will provide direction on an activity and exercise schedule, depending on the specific cardiac condition and the cardiac procedures performed. The client should remain near home during the first week after discharge and should engage in a walking program, light housework, or any activity performed while standing that does not cause angina. Then, during the second week, the client can increase social activities and may even be able to return to work part-time depending on the severity of the cardiac event and treatment procedures. By the third week, the client can begin lifting objects and engaging in progressively more intense activity. The client with coronary artery disease and stent placement, as in this scenario, should begin by walking approximately 400 feet three times each day. Walking 1 mile is an eventual goal, but not immediately following discharge. Clients should carry their nitroglycerin with them in the event they experience angina. They should check their pulse before, during, and after exercise. If their pulse increases more than 20 BPM above what it usually is, they should not continue with the activity. They should also discontinue the activity if they experience shortness of breath, angina, or dizziness. They should exercise outdoors when the weather is good and do not necessarily have to exercise indoors all the time. The client should progressively increase activity, with a goal of walking at least three times a week and increasing the distance every other week, until the total distance is 1 mile during exercise sessions. The client needs to avoid straining, such as with lifting, push-ups, pull-ups, and straining during bowel movements because of the stress these activities place on the heart.

Test-Taking Strategy: This question is asking you to evaluate understanding of discharge teaching for the client following acute MI. Remember that cardiac rehabilitation is a mainstay in long-term treatment, and activity or exercise is integral to health promotion. Think about each of the client statements in the context of safety in the immediate discharge period. If the client statement describes a safe action during this period, then you should categorize it as understanding. If it is potentially unsafe during this time, then you should categorize it as no understanding. Use a thinking process as illustrated in the table.

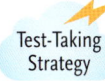
Test-Taking Strategy

Client Statement	Safe/Not Safe/Incorrect in the Immediate Discharge Period
"I should walk 1 mile at least once a day in the beginning."	Not safe
"I will be sure to carry my nitroglycerin with me."	Safe
I will check my pulse before, during, and after I do my exercises."	Safe
"If I notice my pulse is more than 5 BPM higher than what it usually is, I won't exercise."	Incorrect
"I will exercise indoors as much as possible."	Incorrect
"I will make sure to walk at least 3 times per week."	Safe
"I need to avoid straining, so I won't do push-ups or pull-ups."	Safe

Carrying nitroglycerin; checking the pulse before, during, and after exercise; walking at least 3 times per week; and avoiding straining are all safe actions during the immediate discharge period. Walking at least 1 mile per day in the immediate discharge period is potentially unsafe, and activity needs to be gradually increased. It is safe to exercise unless the pulse rate is greater than 20 BPM higher than what it usually is, and exercising outdoors is also acceptable. Remember that in order to *Evaluate Outcomes,* you need to compare observed outcomes with expected outcomes and then look for evidence that the interventions were effective. In this case, you need to determine whether the client statements demonstrate understanding or no understanding with regard to post-MI discharge teaching related to self-care and activity and exercise.

CJ Cognitive Skill: Evaluate Outcomes

Stand-Alone Item 1: Trend

Content Area: Medical-Surgical Nursing
Priority Concept: Elimination; Perfusion
Reference(s): Ignatavicius, et al., 2024, pp. 690–693, 675–676, 1455–1456; Pagana, et al., 2023, pp. 150–151, 179–181, 296–297, 451–453, 476–478, 479–480, 707–708, 803–804

Practice Question 10.25 — Stand-Alone Item 1: Trend

The nurse is caring for a 56-year-old client admitted 2 days ago from the ED for recurring atrial fibrillation.

History and Physical

History of atrial fibrillation, heart failure, and hypertension. Cardiac status has been well controlled with medications. Reports feeling skipped heartbeats and heart fluttering over the past 24 hours and swelling in the feet.

Vital Signs

	1100: Day 1	0800: Day 2	0800: Day 3
T	98°F (36.6°C)	97.6°F (36.4°C)	98.2°F (36.7°C)
HR	84 and irregular	86 and regular	88 and regular
RR	20	20	22
BP	148/90	154/92	168/99
SpO$_2$	96% on 2 L/min O$_2$ via NC	96% on 2 L/min O$_2$ via NC	96% on 2 L/min O$_2$ via NC
Weight	164 lb (74.38 kg)	165 lb (74.84 kg)	168 lb (76.2 kg)
	2400: 24-hour urine output 750 mL	2400: 24-hour urine output 535 mL	

Nurses' Notes

1100 Day 1: Reports feeling skipped heartbeats and heart fluttering over the past 24 hours. Reports dyspnea on exertion. Lung sounds clear bilaterally. Oxygen administered. ECG shows atrial fibrillation. Labs drawn. IV catheter inserted. Treated with IV diltiazem, converted to NSR. 1+ ankle edema.
0800 Day 2: Denies feeling skipped heartbeats or heart fluttering. Reports feeling better, but still experiencing dyspnea on exertion. Slight crackles heard in right lung base. Normal sinus rhythm on heart monitor. 1+ ankle edema.
0800 Day 3: Labs drawn. Denies feeling skipped heartbeats or heart fluttering. Reports ankles feel swollen, and is worried about another episode of heart failure; still experiencing dyspnea on exertion. Bilateral rhonchi heard in lung bases. Normal sinus rhythm on heart monitor. 3+ ankle edema.

Laboratory Results

Test and Reference Range	Results Day 1	Results Day 3
Sodium 136–145 mEq/L (136–145 mmol/L)	141 mEq/L (141 mmol/L)	138 mEq/L (138 mmol/L)
Potassium 3.5–5.0 mEq/L (3.5–5.0 mmol/L)	5.0 mEq/L (5.0 mmol/L)	5.5 mEq/L (5.5 mmol/L)
Glucose 70–110 mg/dL (3.9–6.1 mmol/L)	106 mg/dL (6.0 mmol/L)	100 mg/dL (5.5 mmol/L)
Calcium 9.0–10.5 mEq/L (9.0–10.5 mmol/L)	9.0 mEq/L (9.0 mmol/L)	8.6 mEq/L (8.6 mmol/L)
Blood urea nitrogen (BUN) 8.0–23.0 mg/dL (2.9–8.2 mmol/L)	28 mg/dL (10.0 mmol/dL)	38 mg/dL (13.6 mmol/L)
Creatinine 0.6–1.2 mg/dL (53–106 μmol/L)	1.8 mg/dL (157.2 μmol/L)	3.1 mg/dL (274.1 μmol/L)
Hemoglobin (Hgb) 14.0–18.0 g/dL (140–180 g/L)	14.2 g/dL (142 g/L)	14.0 g/dL (140 g/L)
Hematocrit (Hct) 42%–54% (0.42–0.54 volume fraction)	46% (0.46 volume fraction)	44% (0.44 volume fraction)

*Based on the client assessment findings, select the **5** orders the nurse would anticipate.*

- ✗ Prepare the client for kidney imaging studies.
- ✗ Prepare the client for an echocardiogram.
- ☐ Administer a fluid challenge.
- ✗ Begin diuretic therapy.
- ✗ Maintain strict I&O, and record output hourly.
- ✗ Insert an indwelling urinary catheter.
- ☐ Prepare the client for hemodialysis.

Rationale: The client has a history of heart failure, atrial fibrillation, and hypertension. The clinical scenario indicates that the client is retaining fluid as evidenced by worsening ankle edema, increase in weight, dyspnea on exertion, and adventitious lung sounds. The client also has a decreased 24-hour urinary output on day 2 that totaled 535 mL, which is only about 22 mL/h. The minimum normal urinary output is 30 mL/h, which the client produced on the first hospital day. Due to the history of heart failure and recent episode of atrial fibrillation, an echocardiogram would be performed to determine the function of the heart chambers and the ejection fraction. The decreased urinary output may be the result of impaired kidney function. There is also a consistent increase in blood pressure. On day 3, the client's laboratory results revealed hyperkalemia and hypocalcemia. Although there are a number of causes for these electrolyte imbalances, the rapid increase in serum creatinine indicates possible acute kidney injury (AKI). Creatinine is a protein waste product that is normally excreted via the kidneys to keep the serum level of this toxin as low as possible in the body. An increase of 1 to 2 mg/dL of serum creatinine per day accompanied by decreasing urinary output is consistent with AKI. An acute impairment of kidney function results in increased potassium and phosphate levels. Phosphate and calcium have an inverse relationship in the body; an increased phosphate level causes a decrease in serum calcium, thus the low calcium level. The client's BUN is increased, which could be due to dehydration or AKI; urea is also a protein waste product that is eliminated by the kidneys. Although both BUN and creatinine are associated with kidney function, creatinine is the most reliable and kidney-specific test that when elevated indicates kidney impairment.

Given that the client is likely beginning to have manifestations of AKI, the nurse would anticipate the need for collaborative interventions. Computed tomography, ultrasonography, and/or other kidney imaging studies would likely be ordered to help determine the cause of the impaired kidney function. Diuretic therapy is used to rid the body of excess fluid, which the client is experiencing. The client's fluid status is best monitored by taking accurate daily weights using the same scale before breakfast. Strict I&O with hourly urinary output measurements helps monitor the effectiveness of diuretic therapy and kidney function. Hourly urine output can be measured accurately if the client has an indwelling urinary catheter. A fluid challenge would not be performed in this case because the client has fluid retention with a history of heart failure. It is too soon to determine if the client will need kidney replacement therapy such as hemodialysis.

Test-Taking Strategy: To answer this test item correctly, you will need to approach it in a stepwise manner because it measures several cognitive skills. First, review the clinical scenario and the client's assessment findings and laboratory results to identify findings that are currently abnormal, as noted on hospital day 3. Next, create a table like the one shown here to help determine which of those abnormal client findings are relevant and require immediate attention by the nurse. This step enables you to *Recognize Cues* that you will then need to analyze.

Abnormal Client Finding	Abnormal Client Finding That Is Relevant and of Immediate Concern	Abnormal Client Finding That Can Be Addressed at a Later Time or Is Not of Immediate Concern
History of atrial fibrillation, heart failure, and hypertension	☐	☒
RR 22	☐	☒
Increase in pitting ankle edema	☒	☐
Decrease in 24-hour urinary output	☒	☐
Increase in blood pressure	☒	☐
Increase in weight	☒	☐
Dyspnea on exertion	☒	☐
Rhonchi in lung bases	☒	☐
Increase in potassium	☒	☐
Decrease in calcium	☒	☐
Increase in BUN	☒	☐
Increase in creatinine	☒	☐

As you can see from the table, most of the abnormal client findings are relevant in this clinical scenario and are of immediate concern to the nurse. *Analyze Cues* to determine what these data mean. The client's increasing ankle edema, increased blood pressure, increased weight, dyspnea on exertion, and rhonchi in the lung bases indicate that the client likely has fluid retention (hypervolemia). However, the client's kidneys are not working adequately to rid the body of the excess fluid. Instead the 24-hour urinary output demonstrates that the client is eliminating less than the minimum normal output of at least 30 mL/h. Given that the client has impaired urinary elimination, you then need to review the laboratory results and compare the previous results with the day 3 results. Four of the eight laboratory tests show significant changes between day 1 and day 3. All of these changes in potassium (increased), calcium (decreased), BUN (increased), and creatinine (increased) are associated with the client's *priority* condition of AKI *(Prioritize Hypotheses).*

Once you have determined the client's condition supported by abnormal physical and laboratory findings, you need to answer the test item by thinking about the interventions that are needed for clients with heart failure and early-stage AKI. Use this table to help you answer the test item to measure *Generate Solutions.*

Potential Physician Order	Indicated for Heart Failure or Early Acute Kidney Injury	Not Indicated for Heart Failure or Early Acute Kidney Injury, or Contraindicated for This Client
Prepare the client for kidney imaging studies.	☒	☐
Prepare the client for an echocardiogram.	☒	☐
Administer a fluid challenge.	☐	☒
Begin diuretic therapy.	☒	☐
Maintain strict I&O, and record output hourly.	☒	☐
Insert an indwelling urinary catheter.	☒	☐
Prepare the client for hemodialysis.	☐	☒

Note that the client has a history of heart failure and a recent episode of atrial fibrillation and early-stage AKI. Apply your knowledge of pathophysiology to determine the potential interventions for these conditions. Also consider the client's coexisting problems and how the interventions may affect those conditions. Use the options checked in the "Indicated" column as the correct responses for this Stand-Alone item.

CJ Cognitive Skills: Recognize Cues, Analyze Cues, Prioritize Hypotheses, Generate Solutions

Stand-Alone Item 2: Trend

Content Area: Medical-Surgical Nursing
Priority Concept: Gas Exchange; Perfusion
Reference(s): Ignatavicius, et al., 2024, pp. 565–568

Practice Question 10.26 — Stand-Alone Item 2: Trend

The nurse in the surgical unit is caring for a 51-year-old who had a thoracotomy for non–small-cell lung cancer.

Nurses' Notes

1300: Arrived from the PACU. Alert and oriented × 4. Resting comfortably in bed, no restlessness. Closed chest tube drainage system intact. Upper tube is near the right front lung apex; occlusive dressing dry and intact. Lower tube is on the right side near the base of the lung; occlusive dressing dry and intact. Drainage chamber 70 mL red fluid. Water seal chamber fluctuation of fluid, no bubbling. Suction control chamber gently bubbling. No subcutaneous emphysema. No shortness of breath or difficulty breathing. Lung sounds clear bilaterally. HOB elevated. Trachea midline. O_2 2 L/min via NC. Having difficulty with coughing and deep-breathing exercises and using an incentive spirometer. Pain rated 4/10.

1400: Alert and oriented × 4. Reports nausea. Restless, reports pain rated 8/10. Closed chest tube drainage system intact. Occlusive dressings dry and intact. Drainage chamber 170 mL red fluid. Water seal chamber fluctuation of fluid with intermittent bubbling. Suction control chamber gently bubbling. No subcutaneous emphysema. States difficulty breathing due to pain. Lung sounds clear bilaterally. HOB elevated. Trachea midline. O_2 2 L/min via NC. Refusing to cough and deep breathe or use incentive spirometer due to pain. Able to tolerate respiratory treatment with assistance of respiratory therapist. Nausea and pain medication administered as prescribed.

1500: Sleepy but arousable. Restless; reports nausea subsided and pain rated 7/10. Closed chest tube drainage system intact. Occlusive dressings dry and intact. Drainage chamber 170 mL red fluid. Water seal chamber continuously bubbling. Suction control chamber gently bubbling. Small amount subcutaneous emphysema around upper tube near the right front lung apex. States difficulty breathing. Lung sounds crackles in lower lobes bilaterally. Trachea slight deviation to the left. O_2 2 L/min via NC. Refusing to cough and deep breathe.

Vital Signs

	1300	1400	1500
T	99.6°F (37.5°C)	100.4°F (38°C)	101.6°F (38.6°C)
HR	88	96	110
RR	18	22	26
BP	100/62	128/88	140/90
SpO₂	94% on 2 L/min O₂ via NC	92% on 2 L/min O₂ via NC	90% on 2 L/min O₂ via NC

Select whether the following potential nursing actions are indicated or not indicated for the client at this time.

Nursing Action	Indicated	Not Indicated
Contact the surgeon.	☒	☐
Clamp the chest tube.	☐	☒
Request an order for a stat chest x-ray.	☒	☐
Request an order for additional pain medication.	☐	☒
Flush the chest drainage tube.	☐	☒
Increase the amount of suction in the suction control chamber.	☐	☒

Rationale: Postoperative care of a client who underwent thoracotomy requires closed-chest drainage to drain air and blood that collect in the pleural space. Chest tube drainage systems, such as the Pleur-evac system, use a water-seal mechanism that acts as a one-way valve to prevent air or liquid from moving back into the chest cavity. The first chamber in the system is the drainage collection chamber, located where the chest tube(s) from the client connects to the system. Drainage from the tube(s) collects in this chamber, which has a series of calibrated columns for measurement of the drainage. The second chamber in the system is the water seal to prevent air from moving back up the tubing system and into the chest. Water oscillates (fluctuates) in this chamber (moves up as the client inhales and moves down as the client exhales). The third chamber is the suction control chamber, which provides suction when attached to a suction device, such as wall suction. The nursing care priorities for a client with a chest tube are to monitor the client closely for changes in cardiopulmonary status, ensure the integrity of the system, promote comfort, ensure chest tube patency, and prevent complications. Common complications of chest tube placement are malpositioning and empyema. Malpositioning can lead to pneumothorax or tension pneumothorax. A pneumothorax is air in the pleural space that causes a loss in negative pressure in the chest cavity, an increase in chest pressure, and a reduction in vital capacity, which can lead to lung collapse. A tension pneumothorax is a life-threatening complication of pneumothorax in which air continues to enter the pleural space during inspiration and does not exit during expiration. If not promptly detected and treated, tension pneumothorax can quickly be fatal. Empyema is the collection of purulent material in the pleural space, which can develop following lung surgery. The nurse would closely monitor for complications associated with chest tubes and report any unexpected findings to the surgeon immediately. The amount of drainage from the chest tubes should be no greater than 70 to 100 mL/h. The nurse would notify the surgeon immediately if drainage amounts are greater, if drainage becomes bright red, or if drainage in the tube stops in the first 24 hours postoperatively. According to the Nurses' Notes, the client had no drainage between 1400 and 1500. Continuous bubbling in the water seal drainage is unexpected and could indicate an air leak in the system; the nurse would notify the surgeon if continuous bubbling is noted. The nurse would ensure that there is continuous, gentle bubbling in the suction control chamber. There are assessment findings that indicate deterioration in the client's condition. The client has become restless because the reported pain level decreased from 8/10 to only 7/10 after administration of pain medication. There is continuous bubbling in the water seal chamber, and some subcutaneous emphysema is noted around the upper tube near the right front lung apex. The client also reports difficulty breathing. Crackles are heard on auscultation of the lungs bilaterally, and there is slight deviation of the trachea to the left. In addition, the temperature, heart rate, respiratory rate, and blood pressure have increased, and the SpO_2 has decreased. Contacting the surgeon is the immediate nursing action, along with requesting a stat chest x-ray. The chest x-ray will assist in determining the cause of the deterioration in the client's condition. Clamping the chest tube is not indicated and is contraindicated, and it may increase pressure and tension in the lungs. Requesting an order for additional pain medication is not indicated and is *not* a safe action. The client received pain medication 1 hour prior, and administering additional pain medication may make the client sleepier and mask signs of worsening deterioration. Flushing the chest tube is not indicated and is contraindicated. Disconnecting a chest drainage system can cause a pneumothorax. Increasing the amount of suction in the suction control chamber will not increase the drainage outflow and would not be helpful. In fact, increasing the amount of suction could be harmful to lung tissue because too much suction can cause mechanical injury.

Test-Taking Strategy: Note that this question is asking you to determine nursing actions based on assessment findings for a client with a chest tube following thoracotomy. Use your nursing knowledge to interpret each finding. Looking at each action listed in the options, determine whether it will help or not help the client, and also think about the rationale as to why it would help, not help, or not be needed or potentially worsen the client's condition.

Action	Helps or Does Not Help/Potentially Worsens/Not Needed	Why?
Contact the surgeon.	Helps	Assessment findings suggestive of tension pneumothorax; contacting surgeon for further orders for necessary interventions
Clamp the chest tube.	Does not help/potentially worsens	Increases pressure and tension in lungs
Request an order for a stat chest x-ray.	Helps	Allows visualization of lungs and chest tube placement to determine the possible cause of the deteriorating condition
Request an order for additional pain medication.	Does not help/potentially worsens/not needed	May mask signs of further deterioration; does not address cause of pain
Flush the chest drainage tube.	Does not help/potentially worsens	Can cause further respiratory compromise; can cause or worsen pneumothorax
Increase the amount of suction in the suction control chamber.	Does not help/potentially worsens	Does not address the problem, and could potentially worsen pneumothorax and harm lung tissue

You need to identify relevant data *(Recognize Cues)* and analyze these data and interpret their meaning in the clinical scenario *(Analyze Cues)*. Then you need to determine the priority concerns *(Prioritize Hypotheses)* and think about solutions that address these concerns. Finally, determine the interventions that would promote safe care of the client with a chest tube *(Generate Solutions* and *Take Actions)*.

CJ Cognitive Skills: Recognize Cues, Analyze Cues, Prioritize Hypotheses, Generate Solutions, Take Actions

Stand-Alone Item 3: Trend

Content Area: Pediatric Nursing
Priority Concept: Gas Exchange; Perfusion
Reference(s): Hockenberry, et al., 2024, pp. 891–892

Practice Question 10.27 — Stand-Alone Item 3: Trend

A 2-year-old child is seen in the ED, where the ED physician diagnoses moderate acute laryngotracheobronchitis.

Nurses' Notes / Vital Signs

1000: Client is alert and responsive. Resting comfortably in bed, no restlessness. Responsive to verbal and tactile stimuli. Chest symmetrical. Suprasternal retractions with nasal flaring. RR 34. Barking cough, labored breathing, use of accessory muscles. Inspiratory wheezes bilaterally. S1 and S2 noted, pulse 110. No murmurs, rubs, or gallops. No cyanosis, edema, clubbing, or pulsations. Radial pulses 2+ bilaterally. Pedal pulses 2+ bilaterally.

Based on the assessment findings, which interventions would the nurse anticipate the ED physician will order? **Select all that apply.**

- ☒ Oral dexamethasone
- ☒ Supplemental oxygen
- ☒ Cool mist via facemask
- ☐ Intubation with ventilation
- ☐ Strict NPO status
- ☒ Nebulized epinephrine every 20 to 30 minutes prn
- ☐ Limited interaction between the parents and child

Vital Signs

	1000	1015	1030
T	99.6°F (37.5°C)	99.4°F (37.4°C)	99.6°F (37.5°C)
Apical pulse	110	112	112
RR	34	36	34
BP	100/62	98/60	98/60
SpO₂	94% on RA	92% on RA	90% on RA

Rationale: Acute laryngotracheobronchitis (LTB) is a type of croup usually experienced by children 6 to 36 months of age. Parainfluenza virus types 1, 2, and 3; adenoviruses; respiratory syncytial virus; and *Mycoplasma pneumoniae* are common causes. The illness is preceded by an upper respiratory infection, which descends to the lower airway structures. Clinical manifestations include low-grade fever and a barky, brassy cough after awakening, sometimes with inspiratory stridor. Agitation and crying exacerbate the symptoms and are often worse at night. A major concern with acute LTB is inflammation of the larynx and trachea, causing a narrowing of the airway. Inhaling air past the inflammation into the lungs can be difficult. This is the cause of the classic sign, inspiratory stridor. Other common manifestations include hoarseness, nasal flaring, intercostal retractions, tachypnea, and continuous stridor. Hypoxia and decreased oxygen saturation can occur when the obstruction is severe enough, which can lead to respiratory acidosis and respiratory failure. Maintaining airway patency and providing adequate respiratory support are the mainstays of treatment for acute LTB. Oral dexamethasone is given to decrease subglottic edema. Intravenous or intramuscular dexamethasone may be given if the child is unable to tolerate oral administration. Supplemental oxygen, sometimes with mist, may be needed if hypoxemia is present. Cool mist may be provided via facemask or as blow-by to help constrict edematous blood vessels in the airway, thereby reducing narrowing. This child's SpO₂ is decreasing, therefore use of supplemental oxygen and cool mist is anticipated. Intubation and ventilation may be required if the airway obstruction is severe. Signs of impending airway obstruction include increased pulse rate and respiratory rate; substernal, suprasternal, and intercostal retractions; nasal flaring; and increased restlessness. The child is not exhibiting signs of severe airway obstruction. It is important to allow the child to drink beverages of choice if able to tolerate fluids. IV fluids may be needed if airway obstruction is severe or if the child is intubated. Nebulized epinephrine is administered every 20 to 30 minutes prn for moderate to severe cases and causes mucosal vasoconstriction and subsequent decreased subglottic edema. Children need the security of a parent's presence to minimize crying as this can worsen the airway obstruction. Parents should be encouraged to use comfort measures such as rocking, holding, singing, and reading books with their child.

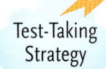

Test-Taking Strategy: Note that this question is asking you to anticipate physician orders based on assessment data in the question for the child with moderate acute LTB. Use your nursing knowledge to recall the pathophysiology associated with this condition. Recall that moderate acute LTB can cause severe airway obstruction and hypoxemia. Looking at each intervention listed in the options, determine whether it will help or not help this child. Also think about the rationale as to why it would help, not help or potentially worsen the child's condition, or not be needed.

Intervention	Helps or Does Not Help/Potentially Worsens/Not Needed	Why?
Oral dexamethasone	Helps	Reduces epiglottic edema
Supplemental oxygen	Helps	Treats hypoxemia related to airway narrowing
Cool mist via facemask	Helps	Reduces airway narrowing
Intubation with ventilation	Not needed	Condition not severe enough; pulse and respiratory rate are still normal; no restlessness
Strict NPO status	Does not help/potentially worsens	Because airway obstruction is not severe, oral fluids can still be taken in; without adequate hydration, condition could worsen
Nebulized epinephrine every 20 to 30 minutes prn	Helps	Reduces airway narrowing
Limited interaction between the parents and child	Does not help/potentially worsens	Can cause fear in the child and thus increase crying and worsen airway narrowing

You need to identify relevant data *(Recognize Cues)* and then analyze these data and interpret their meaning in the clinical scenario *(Analyze Cues).* Then you need to determine the priority concerns *(Prioritize Hypotheses),* think about solutions that will address these concerns, and decide which interventions would promote safe care of the child with moderate acute LTB *(Generate Solutions).* Oral dexamethasone will help reduce airway narrowing. Because the child's airway is still patent as noted in the Nurses' Notes and vital signs, this medication can safely be given orally; therefore this is a correct answer. Supplemental oxygen is indicated and will treat the hypoxemia as noted by the low SpO₂ level, and this option is correct. Cool mist via facemask may also help reduce airway narrowing and therefore is a correct option. Signs of impending airway obstruction are not present; therefore intubation and ventilation would not be anticipated at this time. Strict NPO status would be needed if airway obstruction were severe; because it is not severe, the child should be encouraged to continue oral fluids to prevent dehydration, therefore this is an incorrect option. Nebulized epinephrine every 20 to 30 minutes prn will help reduce airway narrowing and therefore is a correct option. Lastly, recall that interaction between the child and parents is important during stressful times and will reduce fear, distress, and crying, thereby helping with maintaining a patent airway, making this option incorrect.

CJ Cognitive Skills: Recognize Cues, Analyze Cues, Prioritize Hypotheses, Generate Solutions

Stand-Alone Item 4: Bow-tie

Content Area: Medical-Surgical Nursing
Priority Concepts: Cognition; Glucose Regulation
Reference(s): Ignatavicius et al., 2024, pp. 39–40; 1342–1343; 1352–1362; 1368

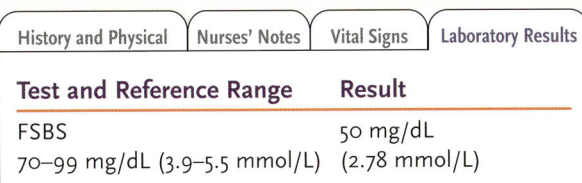

Stand-Alone Item 4: Bow-tie

0830: The nurse is assigned to care for a 70-year-old client in the ED for altered mental status.

History and Physical | Nurses' Notes | Vital Signs | Laboratory Results

0830: Client was brought to ED by a family member for altered mental status. Past medical history includes hypertension, overactive bladder, type 2 diabetes mellitus, and hyperlipidemia. According to the family member, the client has been feeling weak and confused since getting up this morning. Client's speech was slurred, and they appeared disoriented to time and place. Associated with decreased appetite and skipped meals. Client has been taking all medications as prescribed. Medications include lisinopril, oxybutynin, semaglutide, and atorvastatin.

History and Physical | **Nurses' Notes** | Vital Signs | Laboratory Results

0830: Client is restless, disoriented × 4, and agitated. Experiencing an altered level of consciousness, fluctuating between lucidity and confusion. Displays a disorganized thought process and speech pattern. Lungs clear to auscultation bilaterally. Regular cardiac rate and rhythm; no murmurs, rubs, or gallops. Visible skin clean, dry, and intact.

History and Physical | Nurses' Notes | **Vital Signs** | Laboratory Results

0830: T 98.6°F (37°C); HR 110; RR: 26; BP 152/88; SpO$_2$ 96% on RA

History and Physical | Nurses' Notes | Vital Signs | **Laboratory Results**

Test and Reference Range	Result
FSBS 70–99 mg/dL (3.9–5.5 mmol/L)	50 mg/dL (2.78 mmol/L)

Complete the diagram by selecting from the choices below to specify what potential condition the client is likely experiencing, 2 nursing actions that are appropriate to take, and 2 parameters the nurse would monitor to assess the client's progress.

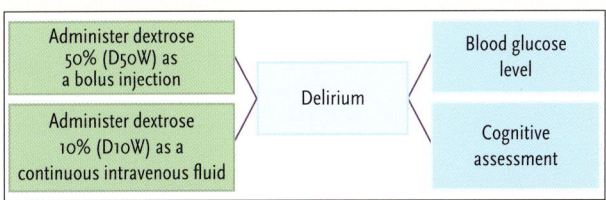

Actions to Take	Potential Condition	Parameters to Monitor
Coordinate neuropsychiatric testing	Anxiety	Suicidal ideation
Administer haloperidol intramuscularly	Delirium	Blood glucose level
Administer lorazepam intramuscularly	Dementia	Cognitive assessment
Administer dextrose 50% (D$_{50}$W) as a bolus injection	Psychosis	Quality-of-life assessment
Administer dextrose 10% (D$_{10}$W) as a continuous intravenous fluid		Extrapyramidal symptoms

Rationale: Altered mental status is a characterization of a clinical state rather than confirmation of the cause of the problem. The client has a history of metabolic issues (type 2 diabetes) and is taking medication that may affect mental status and cognition if the blood glucose decreases too low. The assessment findings documented in the Nurses' Notes support a problem with cognition and point to an underlying condition as the cause. The client takes semaglutide at home, has had a decreased appetite, and has a low blood glucose of 50 mg/dL (2.78 mmol/L). The client is most likely experiencing delirium related to hypoglycemia, which is a transient state of altered consciousness and cognitive function that arises from low blood glucose levels or hypoglycemia. Often, there will be acute and fluctuating disturbances in attention, awareness, perception, and cognition. With hypoglycemia, the brain is deprived of glucose, its main energy source, which leads to impairment in neuronal function and disruption of normal brain activity. The client is restless, disoriented, and agitated. The client is experiencing an altered level of consciousness, fluctuating between lucidity and confusion, and is having disorganized thought processes and speech patterns. Although these findings may also occur with dementia, psychosis, and even anxiety, delirium related to hypoglycemia is the most likely condition given the other physiologic findings. Dementia is a progressive and chronic condition characterized by a decrease in cognitive function that usually becomes severe enough to interfere with daily functioning. Psychosis is a mental condition that results in a loss of contact with reality, and it can manifest with a wide range of symptoms including disorganized thinking and altered mental status. Anxiety is an adaptive response to stress and perceived threats, and clients can also experience cognitive manifestations like intrusive thoughts and excessive worry. Anxiety does not usually cause altered mental status.

The main treatment for delirium associated with hypoglycemia is to increase the blood glucose level. The blood glucose level is 50 mg/dL (2.78 mmol/L), which necessitates immediate nursing action. Because the client's mental status is impaired, intravenous administration is the most appropriate and safe method to administer glucose. To increase the glucose level quickly, the nurse would administer $D_{50}W$ intravenously as a bolus injection and then provide continuous intravenous fluids to keep the blood glucose level steady and in range until the client's cognition improves and they are able to take in glucose on their own. Administering $D_{10}W$ would be another nursing action in this scenario. Neuropsychiatric testing would be premature and would be most appropriate if dementia was the most likely condition. Haloperidol may be administered if the client was experiencing psychosis, and lorazepam may be administered if the client was experiencing anxiety.

The nurse would monitor blood glucose levels to ensure that treatment is working and would perform ongoing cognitive assessments as the cognition should improve as the blood glucose increases. A quality-of-life assessment may be appropriate for a client with dementia confirmed with neuropsychiatric testing. Extrapyramidal symptoms and suicidal ideation are not priority assessments based on this scenario. Extrapyramidal symptoms are known adverse effects of haloperidol, and suicidal ideation has been known to occur when taking lorazepam.

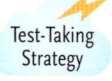

Test-Taking Strategy: To begin answering this question, organize your thought process into three parts. This question is asking you to decide on the potential condition by analyzing relevant data provided in the clinical scenario (*Recognize Cues* and *Analyze Cues*). List the potential conditions, and then think about each assessment finding to decide if it is associated with the condition listed.

Potential Condition	Relevant Assessment Findings
Anxiety	Restlessness, agitation HR 110 RR 26 BP 152/88
Delirium	Altered mental status Restlessness, disorientation, agitation Fluctuation between lucidity and confusion Disorganized thoughts and speech HR 110 RR 26 BP 152/88 Hypertension Type 2 diabetes mellitus Hyperlipidemia FSBS 50 mg/dL (2.78 mmol/L) Semaglutide Decreased appetite and skipped meals
Dementia	Altered mental status Restlessness, disorientation, agitation Fluctuation between lucidity and confusion Disorganized thoughts and speech Hypertension Type 2 diabetes Hyperlipidemia
Psychosis	Altered mental status Restlessness, disorientation, agitation Fluctuation between lucidity and confusion Disorganized thoughts and speech

Restlessness and agitation may occur with all four potential conditions. However, you would not note altered mental status and disorientation with anxiety. You would note altered mental status and disorientation with delirium, dementia, and psychosis. Anxiety is also different from the others in that you would not likely note fluctuation between lucidity and confusion with anxiety or disorganized thoughts and speech, but you could note this with delirium, dementia, and psychosis. Additionally, you would most likely note the acute vital sign changes with anxiety and delirium, and less likely with dementia and psychosis as longer-term conditions. When considering the past medical history, the metabolic conditions (hypertension, type 2 diabetes mellitus, hyperlipidemia) are relevant to delirium and dementia. To get to delirium as the correct answer, you need to consider the FSBS of 50 mg/dL (2.78 mmol/L) and the fact that the client is taking semaglutide and has skipped meals.

Now that you have identified the most likely potential condition that is the cause of the problem, the second part of your thought process will be to decide on client needs *(Prioritize Hypotheses)* and the most appropriate nursing actions for the care of the client with delirium *(Generate Solutions)*. To decide on the two actions the nurse would take *(Take Actions)*, think about what occurs with delirium. Next, determine whether there are data to support performing the listed actions, as illustrated in the table.

Action to Take	Supporting Data
Coordinate neuropsychiatric testing.	No *May be appropriate for dementia*
Administer haloperidol intramuscularly.	No *May be appropriate for psychosis*
Administer lorazepam intramuscularly.	No *May be appropriate for anxiety*
Administer dextrose 50% ($D_{50}W$) as a bolus injection.	Yes *Appropriate for delirium caused by hypoglycemia*
Administer dextrose 10% ($D_{10}W$) as a continuous intravenous fluid.	Yes *Appropriate for delirium caused by hypoglycemia*

The assessment findings supporting administration of $D_{50}W$ and $D_{10}W$ include the cognition findings, past medical history and medications, skipped meals, vital signs, and blood glucose level. Remember the importance of determining the cause of the cognitive changes, to be able to correct the cause with the appropriate actions.

The last part of the question asks you to determine parameters to monitor *(Evaluate Outcomes)*. List each parameter, and note if it is specifically related to the actions or potential condition.

Parameters to Monitor	Specifically Related to Actions/Potential Condition
Suicidal ideation	Not related to administering $D_{50}W$ or $D_{10}W$ Indirectly related to delirium
Blood glucose level	Related to administering $D_{50}W$ and $D_{10}W$ Related to delirium
Cognitive assessment	Related to administering $D_{50}W$ and $D_{10}W$ Related to delirium
Quality-of-life assessment	Not related to administering $D_{50}W$ or $D_{10}W$ Not directly related to delirium
Extrapyramidal symptoms	Not related to administering $D_{50}W$ or $D_{10}W$ Not directly related to delirium

You are considering the actions in the context of the potential condition and then linking them to the appropriate parameters to monitor. Suicidal ideation, quality-of-life assessment, and extrapyramidal symptoms are not related to administering $D_{50}W$ or $D_{10}W$. Suicidal ideation may be indirectly related to delirium, but it is not a clear connection in this case. Quality-of-life assessment and extrapyramidal symptoms, on the other hand, are not directly related to delirium. Blood glucose level and cognitive assessment as parameters to monitor are related to both the potential condition and the nursing actions.

CJ Cognitive Skills: Recognize Cues, Analyze Cues, Prioritize Hypotheses, Generate Solutions, Take Actions, Evaluate Outcomes

Stand-Alone Item 5: Bow-tie

Content Area: Medical-Surgical Nursing
Priority Concepts: Cognition; Mobility
Reference(s): Ignatavicius, et al., 2024, pp. 39–40; 256; 262; 648; 729; 895–899

Practice Question 10.29 — Stand-Alone Item 5: Bow-tie

The nurse working in a long-term care facility is caring for a 78-year-old client with Parkinson disease.

History and Physical | Nurses' Notes | Vital Signs

78-year-old client residing in long-term care has been experiencing difficulty with mobility and activities of daily living. Has been experiencing dizziness and weakness upon standing and increased confusion for the past week. Known history of Parkinson disease diagnosed 10 years ago. Symptoms have progressively worsened despite treatment adjustments. Symptoms include bradykinesia, rigidity, resting tremor, and postural instability. Lived alone prior to transitioning to long-term care, and is widowed. Occasional visits from adult children who live out of state.

History and Physical | Nurses' Notes | Vital Signs

1000: Skin warm, dry, and intact. Lungs clear to auscultation bilaterally, no adventitious sounds. No use of accessory muscles. S1 and S2 noted, no S3 or S4; no murmurs, rubs, or gallops. No peripheral edema. Abdomen soft, nontender, and nondistended. Bowel sounds present × 4. Urine output: 360 mL in the past 8 hours. Reduced facial expression, infrequent eye blinking.

History and Physical | Nurses' Notes | Vital Signs

Lying	Sitting	Standing
HR 86 and regular	HR 98 and regular	HR 110 and regular
BP 154/92	BP 120/80	BP 90/62

*Complete the diagram by selecting from the choices below to specify what potential condition the client is likely experiencing, **2** nursing actions that are appropriate to take, and **2** parameters the nurse would monitor to assess the client's progress.*

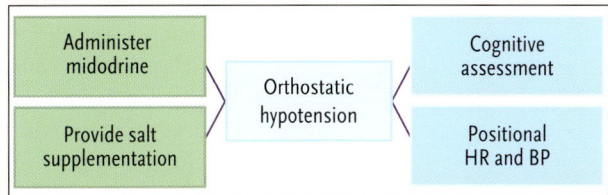

Actions to Take	Potential Condition	Parameters to Monitor
Assist with ambulation	Muscle atrophy	Urine output
Refer to physical therapy	Urinary retention	Gait assessment
Administer midodrine	Orthostatic hypotension	Muscle strength
Provide salt supplementation	Venous thromboembolism	Cognitive assessment
Perform straight catheterization		Positional HR and BP

Rationale: Parkinson disease is a progressive neurodegenerative disorder that mainly affects control of movement. A combination of motor symptoms is usually present, manifesting as tremors, bradykinesia, rigidity, and postural instability. Nonmotor symptoms also occur, including cognitive impairment, mood disturbances, and autonomic dysfunction. Complications of Parkinson disease include motor fluctuations, dyskinesia, gait freezing, cognitive decline, psychiatric symptoms, sleep disorders, autonomic dysfunction, speech and swallowing difficulties, fatigue, pain, falls, and medication-related complications. Orthostatic hypotension is characterized by a sudden decrease in blood pressure that occurs during position changes from lying to sitting to standing. *Orthostasis* is defined as a decrease in systolic blood pressure of 20 mm Hg or diastolic blood pressure of 10 mm Hg within 3 minutes of changing positions. The heart rate typically will increase to compensate for the decrease in blood pressure with orthostasis. Orthostatic hypotension can cause cognitive changes.

Nonpharmacologic interventions for orthostatic hypotension include salt supplementation to expand blood volume, hydration, compression garments, gradual position changes, and elevation of the head of the bed. Midodrine is an alpha$_1$-adrenergic agonist that works by constricting blood vessels to increase blood pressure. Other pharmacologic options include fludrocortisone, droxidopa, pyridostigmine, and octreotide. To determine the efficacy of the interventions for orthostatic hypotension, the nurse would monitor cognitive assessment findings using assessments like the Mini-Mental State Examination (MMSE) and would monitor for changes in heart rate and blood pressure during position changes.

Ambulation and physical therapy may be useful for muscle atrophy, urinary retention, and VTE, but it would not be recommended during an acute episode of orthostasis. Gait assessments and muscle strength testing may be performed to evaluate these interventions and therefore are not specifically related to evaluating treatments for orthostatic hypotension. Straight catheterization may be required for urinary retention, and urine output would be the measurement evaluated to determine efficacy of the intervention.

Test-Taking Strategy: Bow-tie items measure multiple clinical judgment cognitive skills. The question is asking you to decide on the most likely condition by recognizing and analyzing relevant data (*Recognize Cues* and *Analyze Cues*). Begin by listing the potential conditions, and think about each assessment finding to decide if it is consistent with the condition.

Potential Condition	Supportive Assessment Finding
Muscle atrophy	Difficulty with mobility and activities of daily living Bradykinesia, rigidity, resting tremor, postural instability
Urinary retention	Difficulty with mobility and activities of daily living Bradykinesia, rigidity, resting tremor, postural instability Urine output 360 mL in past 8 hours (adequate)
Orthostatic hypotension	Difficulty with mobility and activities of daily living Dizziness and weakness upon standing Increased confusion Bradykinesia, rigidity, resting tremor, postural instability Positional vital sign changes
Venous thromboembolism	Difficulty with mobility and activities of daily living Bradykinesia, rigidity, resting tremor, postural instability

Difficulty with mobility and activities of daily living may be seen with muscle atrophy and can also increase the risk for urinary retention, orthostatic hypotension, and VTE. Bradykinesia, rigidity, resting tremor, and postural instability may be seen with all four potential conditions as well. The increased confusion is specifically related to orthostatic hypotension because of the decreased perfusion to the brain that occurs. The vital sign changes are also specific to orthostatic hypotension. Also note that the urine output of 360 mL in the past 8 hours is adequate, equating to 45 mL/h.

Now that you have identified the condition most likely being experienced, the second part of your thought process will be to decide on client needs *(Prioritize Hypotheses)* and the most appropriate nursing actions for the care of the client with orthostatic hypotension *(Generate Solutions)*. To decide on the two actions to take *(Take Actions)*, think about what occurs with orthostatic hypotension. It is also helpful to think about whether there are data to support performing the listed intervention.

Action to Take	Supporting Data
Assist with ambulation.	No—Acutely hypotensive
Refer to physical therapy.	No—Acutely hypotensive
Administer midodrine.	Yes—Will help improve orthostasis
Provide salt supplementation.	Yes—Will help improve orthostasis
Perform straight catheterization.	No—Urine output is adequate

The last part of the question asks you to identify parameters to monitor *(Evaluate Outcomes)* based on the appropriate actions. Create a clear linkage between the parameter and the action.

Action	Associated Parameter
Assist with ambulation.	Gait assessment Muscle strength
Refer to physical therapy.	Gait assessment Muscle strength
Administer midodrine.	Cognitive assessment Positional heart rate and blood pressure
Provide salt supplementation.	Cognitive assessment Positional heart rate and blood pressure
Perform straight catheterization.	Urine output

Both parameters to monitor are associated with the appropriate nursing actions in this case and provide data specific to the efficacy of those interventions. Additionally, gait assessment and muscle strength are linked to two of the distracters: ambulation and physical therapy. Urine output is linked to another distracter: performing straight catheterization.

CJ Cognitive Skills: Recognize Cues, Analyze Cues, Prioritize Hypotheses, Generate Solutions, Take Actions, Evaluate Outcomes

Stand-Alone Item 6: Bow-tie

Content Area: Obstetric-Newborn Nursing
Priority Concepts: Gas Exchange; Perfusion
Reference(s): Lowdermilk, et al., 2024, pp. 204; 205–209; 272; 306–307; 872; 953

Practice Question 10.30 — Stand-Alone Item 6: Bow-tie

The nurse in the birthing suite performs an initial assessment on a newborn and documents the following data in the Nurses' Notes.

Nurses' Notes

0800: Newborn of 43 weeks' gestation born via vaginal delivery. Apgar score at 1 minute 3. Newborn limp, skin color bluish, RR 80, grunting during breathing with nasal flaring. Lacks cry with minimal response to gentle slap on soles. Nails and umbilical cord stained a yellow-green color. Blood glucose 40 mg/dL (2.2 mmol/L). Profuse scalp hair. Length 23 inches (58.42 cm), weight 5.5 lb (2500 g). SpO_2 90% on RA.

Complete the diagram by selecting from the choices below to specify what potential condition the client is likely experiencing, 2 nursing actions that are appropriate to take, and 2 parameters the nurse would monitor to assess the client's progress.

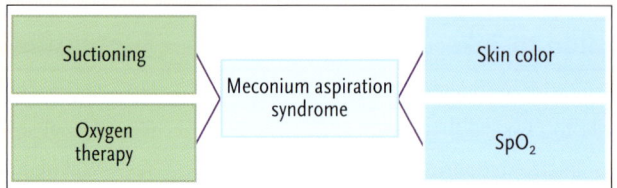

Actions to Take	Potential Condition	Parameters to Monitor
Suctioning	Acrocyanosis	Skin color
Oxygen therapy	Meconium aspiration syndrome	Umbilical cord color
Early feedings with dextrose	Large for gestational age	Blood glucose level
Phototherapy with a biliblanket	Transient tachypnea	Weight
Abdominal decompression with an NG tube		SpO_2

Rationale: Meconium aspiration syndrome is a condition that occurs when a newborn breathes a mixture of meconium and amniotic fluid into the lungs in utero around the time of delivery or during delivery. Meconium is a dark-green fecal material that is produced in the intestines of a fetus before birth. Normally the newborn will pass meconium stools after delivery for the first few days of life. If the fetus is stressed before or during birth, meconium stool may be passed while still in the uterus. The meconium stool then mixes with the amniotic fluid that surrounds the fetus. The fetus may then breathe the meconium and amniotic fluid mixture into the lungs shortly before, during, or immediately after birth. Fetal stress often results when the amount of oxygen available to the fetus is reduced. Common causes of fetal stress include a pregnancy that goes past the due date (more than 40 weeks), a difficult or long labor, maternal hypertension, diabetes, or infection. Respiratory distress is the most prominent sign, and the newborn may breathe rapidly or grunt during breathing. Therefore tachypnea, grunting, a bluish skin color (cyanosis), limpness, retractions, nasal flaring, and lung crackles may be present. The newborn's nails, skin, and umbilical cord may be stained a yellow-green color. Diagnosis is based on the newborn's clinical manifestations and the presence of meconium in the amniotic fluid. Blood gas analysis may be performed to evaluate oxygen and carbon dioxide levels, and a chest x-ray may be performed to determine if meconium has entered the newborn's lungs. If meconium aspiration occurs, the newborn needs immediate treatment via suctioning to remove the meconium from the airway. After emergency treatment is provided to remove the meconium, additional treatment may be needed to avoid complications. These interventions include oxygen therapy, use of a radiant warmer to help maintain body temperature, antibiotics to prevent or treat an infection from aspiration, possible use of a ventilator to help the newborn breathe, and extracorporeal membrane oxygenation (ECMO) if the newborn is not responding to other treatments or has pulmonary hypertension. Profuse scalp hair, dry and cracked skin without lanugo, and a long and thin body are characteristics of a postterm newborn. Although this newborn is postterm, this fact is not one of the options for a potential condition. Even though a newborn is postterm, it does not necessarily mean that the newborn is large for gestational age. Early feedings may be an intervention for a large-for-gestational-age newborn because of hypoglycemia. However, this would not be an intervention for meconium aspiration syndrome; feedings would not be initiated until the syndrome was treated and stabilized. Phototherapy may be prescribed for a newborn with hyperbilirubinemia. Abdominal decompression is not necessary in meconium aspiration syndrome but may be a necessary intervention in an acute inflammatory disease of the gastrointestinal tract such as necrotizing enterocolitis, which is most often seen in preterm newborns. Acrocyanosis is often seen in healthy newborns and refers to the peripheral cyanosis around the mouth and the hands and feet. It is normal in the first few hours after birth and may also be seen intermittently for 7 to 10 days after birth. A large-for-gestational-age newborn is one who is plotted at or above the 90th percentile on the intrauterine growth curve. Assessment findings would include respiratory distress, hypoglycemia, and signs of birth trauma or injury. Interventions include monitoring for and treating any respiratory distress that may occur, monitoring for hypoglycemia, and early feedings. Transient tachypnea of the newborn is a respiratory condition that results from the incomplete reabsorption of the fetal lung fluid in full-term newborns. This condition usually disappears within 24 to 48 hours. Assessment findings include tachypnea, retractions, nasal flaring, fluid breath sounds on auscultation, and cyanosis. Interventions include oxygen administration and supportive care. Following treatment for meconium aspiration syndrome, the newborn's skin color would improve as well as the SpO_2. Umbilical cord color, weight, and blood glucose level are unrelated to treatment for meconium aspiration syndrome,

Test-Taking Strategy: To begin answering this question, organize your thought process into two parts. This question is asking you to decide on the potential condition by analyzing relevant data provided in the clinical scenario (*Recognize Cues* and *Analyze Cues*). List the potential conditions, and then think about each assessment finding to decide if it is consistent with the condition listed, as illustrated in the table.

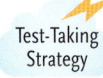

Supportive Assessment Finding[a]	Potential Condition
Bluish skin color	Meconium aspiration syndrome, transient tachypnea
Profuse scalp hair	Postterm (not an option)
Skin dry and cracked without lanugo	Postterm (not an option)
Length 23 inches (58.42 cm), weight 5.5 lb (2500 g)	N/A to any potential condition
Nails and umbilical cord stained a yellow-green color	Meconium aspiration syndrome

[a] No supportive assessment findings for acrocyanosis or large for gestational age.
N/A, Not applicable.

Bluish skin color and nails and an umbilical cord that is stained a yellow-green color are both specific to meconium aspiration syndrome. Profuse scalp hair and dry skin that is cracked without lanugo are both found in postterm newborns, but recall that this does not specifically mean that the infant is large for gestational age. The length and weight identified in the question are not supportive of any of the potential conditions listed, and there are no supportive assessment findings for acrocyanosis or large for gestational age in the clinical scenario. Now that you have identified the most likely potential condition that is the priority problem, the second part of your thought process will be to decide on the newborn's needs *(Prioritize Hypotheses)* and the most appropriate nursing actions for the care of the newborn with meconium aspiration syndrome *(Generate Solutions)*. To decide on the two interventions the nurse would take or *Take Actions,* think about what occurs in meconium aspiration syndrome. Next, determine whether there are data to support performing the listed intervention, as illustrated in the table.

Actions to Take	Supporting Data
Suctioning	Yes
Oxygen therapy	Yes
Early feedings	No
Phototherapy with a biliblanket	No
Abdominal decompression with a nasogastric tube	No

The Apgar score and the physical assessment findings, including muscle tone, skin color, respiratory rate and other respiratory findings, level of responsiveness, and umbilical cord findings, are all supportive for suctioning and oxygen therapy. Remember that with meconium aspiration syndrome, the first priority is to stabilize breathing and address potential or existing respiratory failure. There are no data to support early feedings, which would actually be contraindicated until the newborn is stabilized. There are also no data to support phototherapy with a biliblanket or abdominal decompression with a nasogastric tube.

Once you have determined the actions to take, think about the parameters that would measure effectiveness to *Evaluate Outcomes.*

Actions to Take	Would/Would Not Measure Effectiveness or Unrelated
Suctioning	Skin color—Would measure effectiveness Umbilical cord color—Would not measure effectiveness/unrelated Blood glucose level—Would not measure effectiveness/unrelated Weight—Would not measure effectiveness/unrelated SpO_2—Would measure effectiveness
Oxygen therapy	Skin color—Would measure effectiveness Umbilical cord color—Would not measure effectiveness/unrelated Blood glucose level—Would not measure effectiveness/unrelated Weight—Would not measure effectiveness/unrelated SpO_2—Would measure effectiveness

As noted in the table, you can see that skin color and SpO_2 would be the parameters to monitor to determine the effectiveness of treatment. Think about the pathophysiology of meconium aspiration syndrome and how it is treated to assist you in answering this question correctly.

CJ Cognitive Skills: Recognize Cues, Analyze Cues, Prioritize Hypotheses, Generate Solutions, Take Actions, Evaluate Outcomes

References and Bibliography

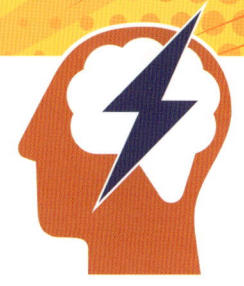

Benner, P., Sutphen, M., Leonard, V., Day, L., & Shulman, L. S. (2009). *Educating nurses: A call for radical transformation.* Stanford, CA: The Carnegie Foundation for the Advancement of Teaching; pp. 46, 118.

Halter, M. J. (2022). *Varcarolis' foundation of psychiatric-mental health nursing* (9th ed.). St. Louis: Elsevier.

Hockenberry, M. J., Duffy, E. A., & Gibbs, K. D. (2024). *Wong's nursing care of infants and children* (12th ed.). St. Louis: Elsevier.

Ignatavicius, D. D., Rebar, C. R., & Heimgartner, N. M. (2024). *Medical-surgical nursing: Concepts for clinical judgment and collaborative care* (11th ed.). St. Louis: Elsevier.

Lilley, L., Rainforth Collins, S., & Snyder J. (2023). *Pharmacology and the nursing process* (10th ed.). St. Louis: Elsevier.

Lowdermilk, D. L., Cashion, K., Alden, K. R., Olshansky, E. F., & Perry, S. (2024). *Maternity and women's health care* (13th ed.). St. Louis: Elsevier.

National Council of State Boards of Nursing (NCSBN). (2023). *Next-Generation NCLEX®. NCLEX-RN® Test Plan.* Chicago: NCSBN.

National Council of State Boards of Nursing (NCSBN). (2019). Clinical judgment measurement model and action model. *Next-Generation NCLEX®* News. Chicago: NCSBN.

National Council of State Boards of Nursing (NCSBN). (2018). Measuring the right things: NCSBN's Next Generation NCLEX® endeavors to go beyond the leading edge. *In Focus*; pp. 10–17.

Pagana, K. D., Pagana, T. J., & Pagana, T. N. (2022). *Mosby's manual of diagnostic and laboratory tests* (7th ed.). St. Louis: Elsevier.

Potter, P. A., Perry, A. G., Stockert, P., & Hall, A. M. (2023). *Fundamentals of nursing* (11th ed.). St. Louis: Elsevier.